Herbs by Body Systems

I've listed five popular single herbs under the body system that the herbs support. For instance, if you are having indigestion, try the herbs listed under the "Digestive System" heading. Be sure to read Part 1, "A Walk Through the Herbal Field," so that you can use these herbs safely and effectively. Happy herbal healing!

Digestive System (stomach, pancreas, esophagus, liver, gallbladder)
Papaya
Peppermint
Aloe vera
Ginger
Marshmallow

Intestinal System (small intestine, large intestine [colon])
Cascara sagrada
Slippery elm
Flax seed
Chlorophyll
Elecampane

Circulatory System (veins, arteries, blood capillaries, heart, blood)
Garlic
Capsicum
Hawthorn
Butcher's broom
Guggal lipid

Reproductive System (prostate/uterus, ovaries/testicles)
Male:
Ginseng
Yohimbe
Saw palmetto
Nettle
Sarsaparilla
Female:
Dong quai
Damiana
Wild yam
Red raspberry
Black cohosh

Glandular System (endocrine glands, thyroid, adrenals)
Kelp
Dulse
Licorice root
Blessed thistle
Evening primrose oil

alpha
books

Nervous System (brain, spinal cord, nerves)

Soothing:

Chamomile

Hops

Valerian

Kava kava

Feverfew

Boosting:

Ginkgo biloba

Gotu kola

St. John's wort

Spirulina

Bee pollen

Immune System (thymus, lymphatics, spleen)

Elderberry

Echinacea

Golden seal

Rose hips

Suma

Respiratory System (lungs, bronchials, sinuses)

Fenugreek

Thyme

Lobelia

Mullein

Horseradish

Structural System (bones, joints, ligaments, tendons, muscles, teeth, hair, skin, nails)

Horsetail

Alfalfa

Rosemary

Uña de gato

Devil's claw

Urinary System (bladder, kidneys, urinary tract)

Dandelion

Hydrangea

Juniper berries

Uva ursi

Parsley

Weight Management

Chickweed

Psyllium hulls

Garcinia cambogia

Kelp

Ephedra

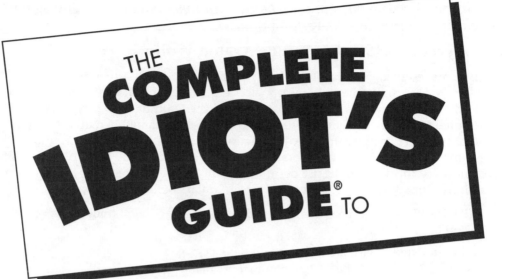

THE
COMPLETE
IDIOT'S
GUIDE® TO

Herbal
Remedies

by Frankie Avalon Wolfe

**alpha
books**

201 West 103rd Street
Indianapolis, IN 46290

A Pearson Education Company

This book is dedicated to all who wish to take more responsibility for health, healing, and prevention of disease.

Contents at a Glance

Contents

Foreword

After founding the Bio-Brain Center in Princeton, N.J., Dr. Karl Pfeiffer stated, "For every drug that benefits a patient, there is a natural substance that can achieve the same effect." Herb sales topped $339 million last year and, according to a new Gallup poll, herb usage among Americans increased by nearly 70 percent. Herbs like St. John's wort that enjoyed relative obscurity 20 years ago have now become common household medicines.

The surprising herbal frenzy we're seeing today is due to a variety of fascinating factors. The consequences of pollution, poor nutrition, and our unfortunate reliance on prescription and over-the-counter drugs have forced many of us to re-examine the value of natural, safe therapies. Moreover, within the last decade, scientific evidence continues to mount supporting the efficacy of herbs and the profound effect of diet and attitude on our health. The word is catching on.

I've been writing about and researching herbs and their medicinal value long before they came into the forefront of public review. After reading *The Complete Idiot's Guide to Herbal Remedies,* I feel confident in recommending it to anyone. The equivalent of a course in Herbology 101, this book offers a discussion on virtually every aspect of using medicinal plants. It not only equips the herbal novice with an essential herbal ready-reference, but offers seasoned practitioners invaluable information as well.

As a user-friendly herbal primer that covers virtually every aspect of herbal medicine including such timely topics as herbal activation, synergy, and elimination, Frankie Avalon Wolfe has selected the best of nature's power plants for everyone from children to pregnant mothers and the elderly to our beloved household pets. Because I strongly believe in the profound value of cleansing, I was delighted to see that she had aptly covered the subject and integrated it into an herbal regimen. Written with a step-by-step approach to successfully using herbal remedies, this book is like having your own personal herbal hotline to the latest herbal methods for not only treating a myriad of diseases and ailments but also for preventing them. Chock-full of practical information, it's an herbal source book that's fun to read. Ms. Avalon teaches us how to build an herbal first aid kit, how to decipher herbal lingo, how to grow our own medicinal plants, and how to go about finding a good herbalist. What I particularly like is her inclusion of herbal safety issues and possible drug interactions. I have to smile when I think about all the herbal skeptics I've encountered over the years and how the tide has turned.

Ironically, at the turn of the century, medical doctors still respected herbology and as late as 1930 took it as a course in medical schools. Even in 1960, some herbs were still listed in the *Physician's Desk Reference.* As scores of clinical studies continually emerge on the efficacy of herbs, even medical doctors are starting to pay attention to what we knew all along—Mother Nature offers us natural compounds capable of safely healing the human body. In addition, I wholeheartedly concur with what Frankie Avalon Wolfe stresses: None of us will truly enjoy good health until we discover the root causes of disease, which stem not only from physical factors but from emotional ones as well.

From the viewpoint of someone dedicated to educating the public about viable natural options for health, I not only recommend this delightfully written guide, I think it should be required reading for anyone interested in hobnobbing with the herbalists.

Louise Tenney, Master Herbalist (M.H.)

Louise Tenney is the author of the national best seller *Today's Herbal Health.* The author of nine books, her other publications include *Nutritional Guide, Health Handbook,* and *Today's Herbal Handbook for Women.* Ms. Tenney has been researching and writing about herbs for over 20 years and lectures throughout the United States and Canada on using herbal therapies.

Introduction

Here are some of the major reasons why I personally believe in herbs and their proper use. I have been working with clients with herbs as part of holistic nutritional counseling for years, and the following events are my greatest rewards. Besides my own "miraculous changes" over time using herbs, the following examples are what continues to deepen my "belief" in herbs as nutritional healing substances.

➤ Cysts that have melted and left the body unexplainably
➤ Eyesight that returned to 20/20 vision
➤ Asthma sufferers who no longer use an inhaler and who show no signs of asthma
➤ Chronic sinusitis sufferers who no longer have a need for a constant supply of tissues
➤ Diabetics who have gotten off their insulin or have been able to lower their dosage
➤ People who were exhausted because of an underactive thyroid, that now show no sign of hypothyroidism
➤ Smokers who quit smoking
➤ Surgeries that never had to take place
➤ Depressed individuals who have weaned themselves off of major psychotropic drugs
➤ Infertile couples now with healthy babies
➤ Women who say they "have a new lease on life"
➤ Suicidal tendencies turned toward a zest for life
➤ Healthy weight loss and maintenance of weight
➤ Acne that cleared up in days, never to return

Why, then, would I care about scientific evidence that supports the positive effects of herb use when I have hundreds of clients who are living testimonials to herbs? I don't, really, but the attention that scientists are showing herbs validates what herbologists have know for a long time—herbs work!

The studies emerging that prove the effectiveness of herbs are beginning to make the thought of using herbs much more mainstream here in the West. Many who have been closed-minded to using nature's plants as healers are now thinking that herbs just might be a viable choice for them! Most who use herbs are people who like to know why they are sick, they take responsibility for their health and their ailments, and they learn how to use herbs responsibly to gain and maintain wellness for themselves and their families. I am thrilled that you have taken a positive step toward understanding your ailments and reading about what herbs might help you with them, and I look forward to being your herb guide throughout this book.

Now that you're ready to learn, I need to make another important point about the information in this book. Any and all statements made in this book by the author, regarding any herbs, supplements, or any other therapies mentioned, have not been evaluated by the Food and Drug Administration. Information contained in the book is meant for *educational purposes only* and is not meant to diagnose, treat, cure, or prevent any disease.

Everyone's body is different and everyone will react to herbal preparations differently. All remedies described in this book are not for everyone. As I explain throughout the book, please work with a trained herbalist or practitioner who can help you choose the best herbs, combinations, supplements, and natural products for you. If you have doubts, consult your trusted medical physician first before taking any herb, and ESPECIALLY if you are on any medications. Always consult your physician for medical problems. Keep in mind that natural health and medical practice both have their respective place in your life, and utilize both accordingly.

How to Use This Book

Now let me tell you a little about how I wrote this book. You will notice that I have chosen a "best herb" to use for each particular ailment, then some combinations to try. Sometimes the single herb will be your miracle cure for what ails you! But, for most of us, it is the combination of herbs working synergistically that will prove most effective.

I purposely selected a new herb as the "best single" for each ailment to avoid discussing only a few popular herbs over and over. For instance, garlic, evening primrose oil, and echinacea are used for so many ailments and uses that I could have talked about these three in almost all the chapters. When you read about the herb, you will begin to see other uses for other ailments where it might come in handy.

I also believe that it is important to understand the nature and possible cause of your illness, and focus on eliminating, or at the very least, compensating, for the cause of your sickness in order for you to become truly healthy.

Although this book is meant as a quick, easy, and lighthearted text on herbs and remedies for common ailments, I hope that you will not view herbs as quick fixes and bypass holistic practices that can bring you overall total health and vibrancy.

First, read all of Part 1. This part gives you the background of herbs, gives you the dos and don'ts for safe and effective herb use, and explains the different applications of herbs and how to make them if you desire. This first section is meant to orient you on how to go about using herbs for ailments, and how to choose the right ones, and will also give you some tips on how to get the right dose for you.

Parts 2 through 4 are the meat of the book and contain the alphabetical layout of over 100 common (and sometimes not so common ailments) with charts at the end of each chapter to summarize your remedies for your specific ailment. For the quickest reference, see the end of each chapter under "The Least You Need to Know" section that summarizes the best herb for the ailment you are looking for. You can also consult the table at the end of each chapter for a summarized game plan to attack your ailment with natural remedies.

And finally, in Part 5, now that you have gotten over your ailments, you will want to read this section on how to stay well by maintaining with herbs. I'll give you some tips on finding and working with an herbalist and what to look for when working with one. Chapter 25 covers some interesting ways you can grow, harvest, and use herbs for more than just medicines. You'll even get a recipe for making your own herbal soap! The last chapter gives you an idea for an herbal first aid kit, what should be in it, and what the herbs can be used for during traveling, hiking, and camping or for any emergencies where medical care is unavailable.

I look forward to sharing these tried and true remedies with you so that you, too, may have life-changing events because of what herbs can do for you! And when you do, please don't forget to drop me a line and let me know, so we can continue learning about the miraculous changes that herbs can make.

How Does Your Herbal Garden Grow?

You will also see some very fun looking boxes throughout this book. These boxes do more than decorate the pages; let me explain what they are for:

Botanical Bit

Botanical Bit boxes are boxes for definitions and will give you an explanation of terms related to herbs or holistic health that may not be familiar to you.

Sage Advice

Sage Advice boxes will show up often as spaces for tips, hints, and enticing tidbits of information about overcoming an ailment with herbs, and other things you can do to get well. They also include such information as how to use an herb with better success.

Poison Ivy

Poison Ivy boxes are warnings about the use of specific herbs. If an herb is unsuitable for pregnancy or nursing mothers, for instance (many herbs are off-limits to pregnant moms), these boxes will let you know. These boxes will also tell you what to watch for when taking a certain herb.

Herb Lore

Herb Lore boxes give you pieces of interesting miscellaneous information related to holistic health.

Acknowledgments

I would like to thank, as always, my husband—without you I could not do all that I do, thank you for being my other half and one of my best guinea pigs over the years for herbal remedies! Thank you to some special women in my life who have taught me about the use of herbs, including Mary Frazee, Sherry Trenkle, Charlie Gruenwald, and Louise Tenney, whose books I treasure and whose foreword for this book is a great honor to me. And thanks to the men who certainly had a hand in shaping my philosophies in herbology such as Dr. Bernard Jensen, D.C., N.D., Ph.D.; Steven Horne, A.G.H., and Reverend George Dew—I'm much obliged. And my gratitude is extended to Reed and Nita Red Kettle (Brown) of the Rosebud Reservation, whose generous ways of teaching me about the Lakota ways, uses of plants, connection with the earth, philosophies, and powerful healing ceremonies will always be with me.

Thank you especially to the folks at Nature's Sunshine Products, Inc., whose dedication to integrity, quality, purity of product, and professionalism set the stage for the industry. Your efforts are unsurpassed. And again, thank you Jessica Faust at Macmillan Publishing, for your continued interest in my work, and to all the editors that pooled their talents to make this book a success.

Special Thanks to the Technical Reviewer

The Complete Idiot's Guide to Herbal Remedies was reviewed by an expert who double-checked the accuracy of what you'll learn here, to help us ensure that this book gives you everything you need to know about the many uses for herbs. Special thanks are extended to Elaine Nerland.

Elaine Nerland, B.S.N., M.N., has had over 20 years of experience in the medical field as a Health Educator and Director of Nursing. Through her private practice in Arlington, Washington, she assists clients to understand and correct the basis of their health problems. Elaine can be reached for consultation or mineral analysis at her office in Arlington.

Trademarks

All terms mentioned in this book that are known to be or suspected of being trademarks or service marks have been appropriately capitalized. Alpha Books and Macmillan USA, Inc. cannot attest to the accuracy of this information. Use of a term in this book should not be regarded as affecting the validity of any trademark or service mark.

Part 1
A Walk Through the Herbal Field

What are herbs? Why should I use them? Aren't witches, hippies, vegetarians, the uncivilized, and environmental radicals the only ones who take herbs for their food and medicine? This section will give you a more practical look at herbs—how herbs work on the body and why herbs are consumed by totally normal people like you and me!

Important: *If you bought this book to utilize herbal remedies, please read this section first to find out which herbs you should and shouldn't use when pregnant or on certain medications. If in doubt, don't take anything until consulting with a professional who can answer your questions.*

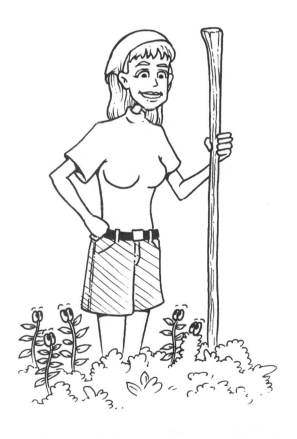

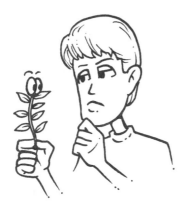

Chapter 1

What Are Herbs and Why Should I Use Them?

In This Chapter

➤ Find out exactly what herbs are

➤ Use herbs in a variety of forms

➤ Herbs and your diet

➤ How herbs differ from vitamin supplements

➤ How to get the most from herbs

"The spectacular advances made in therapeutics by industry during recent years tend to make us forget the medicinal value of plants. Their usefulness is far from negligible; their active principles are manifold and well-balanced." —Paul Fruictier, *Grandmother's Secrets*. Excerpted from Jean Palaiseul, *Compton's Reference Collection 1996*. Compton's NewMedia, Inc., 1995.

Welcome to the ever-popular subject of herbal remedies! This chapter will show you how useful and quite practical using herbs can be. You will see that herbs are a gift from nature and have been—and still are used—as foods, supplements, decorations, and medicines. I'll show you how herbs can be easily incorporated into any lifestyle, even somewhat hectic ones like yours, perhaps. So read on as we take a walk through the large field of herbs.

Herbs come in many different forms for internal and external use.

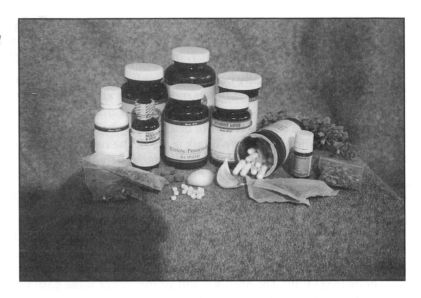

Different Applications of Herbs and How to Make Them

Form: Bulk herbs as teas, also called infusions.

Description: Usually the dried leaves, skins, and flowers of herbs in bulk form. Keep covered when in dried form, as bulk herbs can lose their essential oils rapidly if left open to the elements.

How to Make: Place bulk tea in a metal tea ball or press filter, which are both fairly inexpensive. Or, make sure to have some cheesecloth or coffee filters to strain tea when it is finished. Pour boiling water over herbs, and let sit for about five minutes or longer for a stronger taste. Teas only need a short exposure time to water to extract their oils and medicinal value.

How to Take: Drink right away, or refrigerate for later use. Teas work best on an empty stomach. Use approximately four tablespoons of herb per cup. If making tea from an encapsulated herb, use two to four capsules per cup. (Capsules are usually more concentrated than the bulk herb, so you will need to utilize more of the loose herb than the powder.)

Form: Decoctions.

Description: Usually stronger than teas. Decoctions are usually the twigs, stems, and dried roots of the herbs, which take a longer exposure time in hot water to extract their medicinal properties. Decoctions can be used for drinking or as enemas or douches.

How to Make: If your bulk herbs are not already cut into small pieces, slice all herb roots diagonally for maximum exposure to water. Place bulk herb into a pot of water, and bring water to a boil. Use approximately one ounce of herb for every one to two pints of water. Lower heat, and simmer covered for 20 to 30 minutes. Strain herbs before drinking.

How to Take: Treat the same as a tea and refrigerate if not taken right away. Again, this form of tea works best if your stomach is empty. It should also be drunk unsweetened.

Form: Compress or fomentation.

Description: For external use for injuries.

How to Make: Prepare decoction, or infusion (tea) as above.

How to Take: When decoction or infusion is ready, dip a clean rag into the mixture and place on injured area. As cloth cools, re-immerse into solution and re-apply to affected area. Repeat daily, if needed. This cloth may be wrapped with a bandage or even plastic wrap to keep it in place. A hot compress is also called a fomentation. This means that you apply extra heat on top of the soaked rag. You can place plastic over a soaked rag, then a dry towel, and then a heating pad or hot water bottle. Fomentations (or hot compresses) are best used for spastic or cold conditions such as muscle spasms or tension as they help relax and warm the body. Compresses can also be cold and are mostly used to decongest areas or inflamed conditions such as edema, constipation, poor urine flow, fevers, and sinus congestion. If you are really feeling energetic, you can also have your partner make you a hot and a cold compress and alternate them. This type of therapy stimulates circulation to the affected area and is helpful for injuries, sprains, bruising, lumps, bumps, and tumors.

Form: Poultice.

Description: A poultice is a paste made from herbs for an external application for injuries or infections, such as boils. The poultice's value is the rapid absorption of the herb through the skin. A poultice will generally stimulate circulation, reduce infection, pull out toxins through skin, reduce inflammation, and relieve irritations.

How to Make: Using herb powders is best for making poultices. Capsules can be opened and the powder dumped out, or you can make your own powder from bulk herbs by using a mortar and pestle to crush the herb into powder. If using a freshly cut herb grate, crush or chew it a bit first. Moisten dry powdered herb with a liquid herb, such as aloe vera (we'll talk about aloe later) until it has a pasty consistency. Other safe options to bind your herbs together with include egg whites, slippery elm, clay, or olive oil.

How to Take: Apply paste to injury, and cover with plastic, cheesecloth, wool, or muslin cloth and wrap with a bandage to hold in place. Change two to four times a day, or as necessary.

Form: Capsules or tablets.

Description: Probably the most convenient way to take herbs. Powdered herbs can come in a capsule form (usually made from gelatin or cellulose materials) or tablet form (usually a bit stronger than the capsules and made from a powdered herb that is compressed and coated to form a pill). Make sure that the company you get tablets from uses a natural coating, not plastic or synthetic coatings. All ingredients, including the binding or base materials used to form tablets, should be listed. If not, find out before you buy.

continues

Different Applications of Herbs and How to Make Them (continued)

How to Make: If you'd rather swallow your herbs in a capsule, but you bought or grew your own herbs in bulk form, you can purchase empty capsules at your local health food store and encapsulate your herbs yourself. (Nature's Way makes Vegicaps®, which are labeled kosher.) Crush your dried herbs into powder form with a mortar and pestle to make it easier to encapsulate. You will also get more herb in each capsule this way.

How to Take: Swallow with plenty of water.

Form: Liquid/tinctures.

Description: Liquid herbs, known as tinctures, are concentrated herbal extracts that can be preserved over longer periods of time. They are easier to administer to children, the elderly, and pets and are easily absorbed. Liquid herbs require a base, which is usually either glycerin or alcohol, to stabilize them. If an extract has an alcohol base that is disagreeable to taste, the herb can be placed in a small amount of very hot water before drinking. The hot water will evaporate the alcohol. Tinctures are not suited for those who lack tolerance to alcohol.

How to Make: To make your own liquid extracts use one pint of 60-proof or higher alcohol (brandy, gin, and vodka have all been used), glycerin, or apple cider vinegar to four ounces of herb powder. Combine in container with lid for two to six weeks. Vigorously shake the mixture two times per day. You will notice a slow change in the color. Strain tincture through cheesecloth and store in a dark-colored bottle (preferably with a dropper so that it can be easily administered).

How to Take: Take sublingually with a dropper, or by the teaspoon—usually a few drops will do. Or, place drops in water or juice, and drink. Tinctures may also be used externally.

Form: Chewable.

Description: Chewable herbs are another great way to get kids, the elderly, or anyone who hates to swallow pills to take herbs. Herbal manufactures make herbs in chewable forms that are usually sweetened with fruit juice.

How to Make: I have not found a palatable way to make my own, but here's an idea used by some if you have the gumption: Take a small amount of the powdered herb mixture, moisten with a small amount of marshmallow herb, add a tiny amount of water (just enough to mix but keep firm). Roll into pea-size balls and leave to dry. Then dip the balls in honey or peanut butter to cover the taste.

How to Take: Chew and swallow.

The Essence of It All

Herbs are also used in homeopathic and flower remedies and to make essential oils. Essential oils are the "essence" of a plant—the moisture you see when you tear a fresh plant leaf or the spray that you see when tearing a fresh tangerine peel in the sunshine. These oils give a plant their scent; they evaporate thoroughly when exposed to air.

The proper distillation process to extract these volatile oils is expensive and time-consuming, so you will more than likely have to purchase your oils. Try to find a Grade A type, 100 percent pure oil when you shop. Many in the market are adulterated with a chemical fragrance enhancer and/or another substance to stretch the company's bottom line. Unfortunately, manufactures who cheat by diluting their oils could do you more harm than good.

If you are in the wild and are positive that you have identified a plant correctly and want to use its essential oil, you can rub the leaves of the plant on you—the moisture from the plant is the plant's essence. However, it is important that you identify a plant correctly—the essence of poisonous plants, such as poison ivy and poison oak, can give you a terrible skin reaction if touched. Before you go rubbing yourself with nature, know exactly what you are getting yourself into, or rely on a purchased product.

Sage Advice

An old trick used by those who work with essential oils (known as aromatherapists) to test the purity of an oil is to dab a drop of oil on a piece of blotting paper and wait until it dries. If the spot leaves a mark or residue, it usually means that the oil has been cut with other chemicals; if it dries "clean," the oil is usually pure.

Quality: Being Picky

Some people find pleasure in learning about the plants that surround them. Harvesting your own herbs for some purposes is a good excuse to get in touch with nature while getting a nice tan. For instance, when I lived in a mountain cabin in Colorado, I had 10 herb-filled acres, which is where I first began to understand about herbs as helpful plants. I used to harvest my own rose hips from the wild rose plants growing out front, chamomile that grew in the driveway, and feverfew for my migraines from the valley. I felt very John Denver-ish as I walked around on my Rocky Mountain High property and learned about the plants firsthand.

Although this was a nice break from my busy routine, I realize now that this was a far cry from using herbs responsibly or very effectively. Let's take a quick look at why.

The Monotony of Botany

Picking my own herbs was nice and holistic, but the truth of the matter is that there's a lot more to herbalism than identifying a plant correctly and picking it.

The herb-picking party came to a screeching halt once I began to learn more about harvesting herbs. I learned that there are specific harvest times that need to be adhered to in order to capture a plant's medicinal value. I also learned that the drying process had to be done just so for the best effects—and then I saw under a microscope that I was getting a *whole* lot more than just my herb with my herb, including bug parts, animal feces, and other unidentifiable beasties. That's not to mention the dangerous possibility of incorrectly identifying a safe herb for a toxic or poisonous plant.

Poison Ivy

Picking your own herbs for occasional use is great but should be limited to external use. For internal use, you might want to rely on the experts to get you a cleaner and probably more potent plant. This will also eliminate the possibility of misidentifying a plant and picking and ingesting something that can make you sick!

A mistake like that could turn a Rocky Mountain High into a Rocky Mountain Spotted Fever!

Needless to say, I gave up on my little fantasy of picking all my own herbs very quickly! For my daily herb intake, I now rely on certain herbal manufacturers who not only send their specialists to the field to pick the herbs at the right time (important for capturing the best properties), but who also enforce strict quality-control standards that I am not capable of doing on my own. Besides, I wasn't too hip on getting my protein from microscopic bug parts left on my self-harvested herbs!

I haven't abandoned picking herbs completely, though. I still pick my own sagebrush once in a while and use it for incense, or I harvest some chamomile and add it to my shampoo to lighten my hair. For the herbs I use internally, however, I order in!

Of course, I don't want to discourage you from learning herbology from the ground up—this is a good way to get back to your roots. It's also very helpful for when and if we are alienated from commercial availability, as we will have to rely on our knowledge of plants and herbs for survival and emergency situations.

A lot of value comes from knowing the herbs around you. For the purposes of this book, though, you should probably stick to purchasing your herbs from a company whose reputation you can trust until you become an expert yourself.

So, every salesperson, distributor, manufacturer, and herbal advertisement tells you that their product is the best? Guaranteed? All natural? How do you *really* know what sets the quality products apart from the fly-by-nights? Here's a little checklist that you can use to find the best quality in your herbal products. Call the manufacturer of the product(s) you are considering and see if they match up to this strict test of quality and integrity:

❏ If the herb comes in a capsule are the capsules preservative-free? (Make sure they are not synthetic materials, petroleum by-products, or plastic.)

❏ Are herbs free of all synthetic ingredients including dyes, artificial sweeteners, and other chemical additives? (Don't we get enough chemicals in our daily lives without deliberately taking them with our daily herbs?)

❏ Does the bottle clearly state ALL ingredients and or additives? Does the label list the ingredients used as a base to bond the herbs into a tablet form? (Since the FDA does not require this disclosure on herb labels, those who volunteer this information on the label probably have nothing to hide.)

❑ If a preservative must be used to preserve freshness, is the source of the additive or preservative from a vegetable or fruit source? (You are again looking for hidden chemicals and synthetic materials with this question.)

❑ Does the manufacturer quarantine the bulk herbs for two to three days? (Any raw products left out to the elements can be spoiled or contaminated.)

❑ Are the herbs unsprayed? (It is customary in some countries to spray certain herbs and not so in others. Choose the manufacturer who knows this and gets the unsprayed herbs from the correct countries, or who tests all their herbs for any pesticides or chemical contamination.)

❑ Are the herbs you are considering more expensive than many others? (Unfortunately, cost is a factor in good herbs, just as cost is a factor in the quality of most products. Cutting costs at the cash register usually means cheating your body of the best herbal products.)

❑ Does the company use the most medicinal parts or the whole herb in their product? (Again, labels do not need to mention if the flower, stem, or root is used in a particular encapsulated herb, although there may be no value at all depending on which part is used. Another example is the age of a plant. Aloe vera, for instance, needs to be at least four years old to have any medicinal value. For greedy, impatient, or ignorant reasons, many manufactures will bottle and sell immature, and impotent plants because legally, they can.)

❑ Does the manufacturer test the "fingerprint" of each batch of herb they acquire to ensure it is what they ordered? (Many herbs look alike in bulk form. One large herb manufacturer told me that they once received cocoa bean from their supplier and was told it was pau d'arco. Visually the differences in the bulk herb were nil. The manufacturer's first quality-control check quickly uncovered the mistake and the shipment was sent back. Make sure the manufacturer has the quality equipment to undertake these types of tests.)

❑ Are the encapsulated herbs made without the use of high heat? (Heat damages enzymes, evaporates potent essential oils, and decreases an herb's value. Exception: concentrated tablets made from infusions or decoctions, liquid herbs, and extracts.)

❑ Are the herbs guaranteed pure? (There is a big difference between 100 percent refund guarantee and guaranteed 100 percent pure. It is more valuable to know that you are getting what you think you're getting than to get something that is questionable and have it not work or make you sick! Would you rather have a purity guarantee or would you rather just take your chances and have to get your money back on a terrible product?)

❑ Does the manufacturer run themselves to pharmaceutical standards? (Are outside doors sealed against dust, do workers wear masks, gloves, and sterile clothes, are herbs quarantined, are strict quality-control tests taken before, during, and after

Herbs or Vitamins: What's the Difference?

Vitamins are important in many cases—in fact, I have included a few helpful supplements for each ailment discussed in future chapters because many herbalists use other supplements in their practices along with the use of herbs. These supplements may be used in cases of great deficiency, or may even add an enhanced effect to your herbal program. Other natural supplements that will be mentioned in this book you might consider along with your use of herbs are:

➤ Bacteria (usually referred to as acidophilus or bifidophilus)

➤ Enzymes

➤ Essential oils

➤ Homeopathics

➤ Vitamins

➤ Minerals

Poison Ivy

Vitamins may be synthetically made because they are cheaper to manufacture than to obtain fresh, plant materials. Synthetics are not as highly usable by the body as natural materials are.

Botanical Bit

Vitamins are complex organic substances that occur naturally in plants (herbs) and animal tissue, and are essential for health and life. Vitamin pills differ from foods such as herbs and meat because they are usually a single, extracted vitamin from the plant (or animal) instead of the entire plant, which contains many phytochemicals, other vitamins, and minerals intact.

Because herbs are plants, they contain vitamins and minerals. Therefore, once you recover from your ailment, your need for the extra extracted vitamin supplements may decrease if you are using herbs as a part of your daily nutritional program.

Next let's check out the real difference between a vitamin supplement and an herb.

Foods from the earth are whole foods, which contain all the elements needed to sustain our body and maintain health. Herbs contain usable forms of vitamins and minerals from nature. For instance, natural forms of vitamin C can be found in many herbs, such as rose hips; rose hips provide many other substances such as vitamin A, vitamin E, rutin, B-complex sodium, calcium, selenium, magnesium, potassium, vitamin D, and zinc that herbalists believe enhance the positive effects of the vitamin C. Vitamins, on the other hand, are extracted from the whole plant and are used as an isolated substance.

Herbs provide the entire plant and all its constituents (minus the bug parts). In other words, you get Mother Nature's full meal and not an extracted piece of it.

So trust in your "Mother" to feed you correctly and provide you with everything you need to nourish your body. Mother Nature has lots of things to teach you, so honor thy mother if you know what's good for you!

You Are What You Graze Upon: The Right Diet *Helps*

Herbs are nutrients, and your body will use what it needs from them. However, herbs should not be thought of as a miracle drug that forces your body to do something or stop doing something that it wouldn't do naturally. Herbs are your assistants. They need your cooperation in order to get the best results, so think of herbs as your partners in health.

Not that downing your handful of herbal pills with your beer and pizza doesn't have any value at all, but your herbs will be better utilized if you take them with a proper diet. What do I mean by a "proper diet"? The simplest way to think about eating healthy is to think whole, raw, fresh, vine-ripened, organic fruits and vegetables; grains such as rice, millet, barley, and rye (don't eat wheat as your only grain—mix them up!); and organic, raw (if possible) dairy products in moderation. See the section, "Got Gas?" in Chapter 12, "G: Great Remedies," for more food-combining tips.

Don't Eat That!

I also believe in under-eating occasionally. Under-eating occurs when you may want more food, but you discontinue eating anyway. Most of us eat more than we really need, and it takes a lot of energy for your body to digest and assimilate food. Taking a load off your digestive organs once in a while by under-eating or fasting can—and will—help you feel better and will enhance your health.

When you fast (abstain from all food), your body has the opportunity to cleanse itself of toxins rapidly. If you begin to cleanse too rapidly, however, you may feel extremely ill. The toxins from your body may get stuck and form obstructions that can be fatal. So, although fasting is extremely beneficial when done correctly, you should know what you are doing or seek supervision before attempting a long fast. Under-eating by eating about three quarters to one half of your normal portions is a safer way to give your body a break occasionally and will help you maintain your ideal weight.

Poison Ivy

Don't fast without supervision unless you are a fairly healthy adult. If you have low blood sugar (hypoglycemia) or diabetes, fasting is not for you!

Sage Advice

Bee pollen is an excellent supplement to take while fasting because it won't require much digestive energy, but it will provide nourishment and can keep your energy up while you abstain from eating. If you are allergic to bee pollen, you can substitute barley green juice powder instead.

Sage Advice

Pure water is important, and you can purify your water in several ways. At the very least, a carbon filter for your tap will filter out chlorine, many viruses, and heavy metals such as lead. In my opinion, reverse-osmosis water is the best tasting and the cleanest drinking water available.

Herb Lore

After studying a civilization of centenarians, I learned about a strange commonality between the people: They all lost their teeth in their teens, and their foods had to be pulverized with a mortar and pestle before eating. My theory was that the pulverized "baby food" these people ate saved them an enormous amount of digestive energy, which the body then used to keep them healthy and alive for well over 100 years. Because of the long food preparation time, these people ate much less often than typical "civilized" peoples. So maybe less *is* more!

Some herbs can easily be taken on an empty stomach, just as you would eat a salad; others may make you nauseous. It depends on the herb. Teas seem to work best on an empty stomach. For best results, try eating lightly just before or after you take your herbs, especially if they are in a pill form. This will help you feel the subtle changes that the herbs will have upon your body, too.

Botanical Bit

Reverse osmosis (R.O.) is a process of filtering water using a pressure vessel made up of layers of extremely fine membranes. As water is pushed through, viruses, heavy metals, bacteria, and other pollutants are too large to pass through and are left behind. The end result is pure H_2O. These filters can be found through catalogs, home stores, health food stores, and independent distributors.

Water, How Dry I Am

Most of us suffer from chronic dehydration and are not even aware of the problem. Dr. F. Batmanghelidj's clinical research showed that many ailments—including adult-onset diabetes, stomach ulcers, headaches, depression, and general aches and pains—come from chronic dehydration alone. He discovered that he could cure most of his subjects of their chronic ailments using only water.

Here's a general formula for how much water you need daily: Divide your body weight by half; that number is how many ounces of water you need every day. Remember that a cup of water equals eight ounces. In addition, if you are drinking diuretics such as coffee or beer, you need four cups (or 24 ounces) to every one cup (eight ounces) of diuretic. This is on top of the daily water intake!

This formula is a rough estimate, but it is designed to keep a body hydrated. We loose up to three quarts of water every day just from our breath and our skin. We need to replace that water to remain healthy—most of us are all dried up!

One good thing that herbs will do if you take them in pill form is get you to drink more water! It is imperative that you do drink more water any time you are feeling ill. The extra water you drink will help your body to flush out the toxins, bacteria, and waste products and will help you heal more quickly. Water helps herbs do their job more efficiently, so drink up!

The Least You Need to Know

➤ Herbs are wild vegetables that have nutritional and medicinal value.

➤ Herbology is a vast field, and picking your own herbs can be dangerous. To start, use an herbalist and/or a manufacturer you can trust.

➤ Herbs can be used in place of vitamins because they contain vitamins and minerals and all the compounds necessary for nourishment.

➤ Herbs will work for you, but drinking enough water and eating wisely is essential to helping herbs work even better.

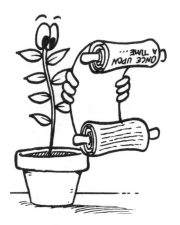

Chapter 2

A Little Herb Lore

In This Chapter

➤ Some herbs give clues to their use

➤ Learn some global history about medicine and herbs

➤ Herbs that can serve us medicinally

➤ Some medicines and herbs that don't mix

➤ Reasons why herbs are becoming mainstream again

➤ Learn some herbal alternatives to over the counter drugs

"Then God said, 'I give you every seed-bearing plant on the face of the whole earth and every tree that has fruit with seed in it. They will be yours for food. I give every green plant for food. And so it was." —Genesis 1:29–31

Could this quote be the earliest evidence of the use of herbs for health, life, nutrition, and medicine? We don't know for sure, but we do know that before the development of technology, our ancestors figured out many ways to use the plants as medicines. In this chapter, we'll take a look at the development of medicine from nature and then give you some up-to-date tips on drugs that don't mix with plant remedies.

Unmasking Nature's Secret Codes

Take a moment to look around your yard and outdoor surroundings. If you live in a rural, mountain, or agricultural environment, take a little walk around and see what plants you can identify. The herbs that grow will be herbs that are ideal for your particular area, climate, and soil type. This can teach you something about what you might need since you also live in the same environment. For instance, how many of you have dandelions growing in your pretty green lawn? Plenty I'm sure! But did you know that the dandelion can be used to cleanse the liver, support the urinary system, and work as a mild laxative?

Your liver is a major filter of the body. On a daily basis the liver has the job of filtering environmental toxins, pesticides in your food, chemicals in the water, air pollutants saturated fats in the diet, and excess hormones in the blood. Do you think Mother Nature could be trying to tell you something when she offers dandelions at every turn? Is this her way of subtly offering her help for your liver? Could be, after all, Mother knows what's best for us.

Of course, before we had advanced technology synthetics and a greater understanding of the body we had nature to look to for answers. Today we have research and science to back up and validate that herbs do in fact work through chemistry. In early days, we relied more on our observations, trial, and error. Technology is finally catching up to what many herbalists have believed and practiced for years and years. Let's take a look back and see how they came up with some of these uses.

The Doctrine of Signatures philosophy dates back as early as the 1600s and was popularized in the medical field by Paracelsus. This philosophy, now considered nonsense by the medical community, put forth the theory that an herb or plant had a certain characteristic or set of characteristics that would reveal its value to the thoughtful observer. The signature was recognized as several different characteristics of the plant, including its color, texture, shape, and/or the environment where the plant grew.

Sage Advice

Notice that the dandelions always seem to be the first ones out in the spring. Ever hear of spring cleaning? Our body can use a good dose of it, and dandelion is there to help. Its leaves can be picked and used in salads to offer a gentle cleansing to our system.

Herb Lore

The old Doctrine of Signatures theory held that plants with a yellow signature, such as dandelion or golden seal, could be used to treat conditions of the liver, such as jaundice (a yellowing of the skin). Furthermore, red signature plants were thought to be good for blood conditions (presumably because the color red matched the color of blood). The Doctrine of Signatures philosophy also stated that the walnut could be an effective brain food because of its close resemblance to our brain. Since then we've found that walnuts contain lecithin, an oil that protects our brain and nervous system.

It would be nice if this theory was completely valid—it would make learning herbology much simpler to the thoughtful observer. However, don't throw the entire theory away just yet. Coincidences or not, some things can validate this thinking and also help you remember the medicinal value of an herb or plant. For instance, hawthorn berries are bright red berries that are shaped like a heart, and hawthorn berries have been used by many to strengthen and build the heart and circulatory system.

We can take many factors into consideration when contemplating an herb and how we might find its value by looking at nature. Some native tribes believe that plants that are poisonous to man will crop up in areas where the soil needs to be replenished. These plants serve to protect the earth by repelling man. (Remember poison ivy and poison oak's nasty essential oils mentioned in Chapter 1, "What Are Herbs and Why Should I Use Them?") These herbs keep both man and woman away!

On the other hand, herbs that are extremely resistant to poisons and toxins—including the herb milk thistle, a tall, very prickly plant—grow plentifully in heavily polluted areas, such as near nuclear testing sites. Ironically, milk thistle is used medicinally to help rebuild the liver, which has the job of filtering out poisons and toxins from our body.

Some herbal teachers are very philosophical in nature, and others tend to make herbology more clinical. You can choose to see herbs in whatever way suits you. The important thing to remember is that foods can be your medicine, and herbs are foods.

> **Sage Advice**
>
> Ginseng root bears a strong resemblance to a human figure, and it is thought to be an all-over body tonic for this reason. Many of these theories based on the Doctrine of Signatures can now be confirmed by research.

The History of Herbs and Medicine Around the World

Herbs are used as medicines and nutrition all around the globe. Each culture seems to have its own philosophy and approach to herbal medicine, based on individual cultures and belief systems. And, of course, in different parts of the country, different plant species thrive, so each culture has its own selection of herbs considered sacred or common.

We are lucky to now have the use of transportation channels that provide us unique herbs from all parts of the globe, and we can study or utilize herbs from around the world when we visit our local health food store or herbalist. Some people seem to respond better to traditional Chinese herbs, whereas others do best on Ayurvedic remedies from India; still others respond most to traditional Western herbs. Let's take a look at a little history from a few places around the globe.

Herbs Around the Globe

Ancient Egyptians' favorite laxatives were figs, dates, and castor oil. More than 500 drug remedies were used in Mesopotamia, some of mineral origin. Hebrew medicine included dressing wounds with oil, wine, and balsam. Ancient Hindus discovered the calming effects of an Indian plant that was later made into one of the first tranquilizers in modern medicine.

Indeed, many modern medicines of today were originally made from herbs. Here are few:

➤ Quinine, derived from the bark of the cinchona tree, was used primarily to cure malaria before the production of synthetic drugs for this use. In 1944, the American chemists Robert Woodward and William Doering managed to synthesize quinine from coal tar.

➤ Digitalis is a heart-stimulating drug made from the foxglove plant.

➤ The bark of the white willow tree contains a compound known as salicin, from which a synthesized version has been made called acetylsalicylic acid, commonly known as aspirin.

➤ Local anesthetics, such as the numbing shot given to you by your dentist, originally was derived from the leaves of the coca plant.

Herb Lore

Some of the earliest-known medical practices included the use of purges, diuretics, emetics, laxatives, enemas, and plant extracts. At least 50 of these plants serve as the basis for our prescription medications of today. However, you can't patent a plant. Herbs are less profitable than patented prescription drugs. For instance, statistics show that for about every 24 million dollars of bulk herbs, three billion dollars of prescription drugs are made.

Maybe it was because of China's ancient religious beliefs against cutting open the human body that propelled them so far into healing with natural medicines. They excelled in acupuncture, herbs, and the understanding of "chi"—life force energy.

Today the Chinese still take natural healing very seriously. Chinese herbal medicine schools are equivalent to the West's medical schools, requiring years of intense study. Natural methods and more conventional methods of healing are utilized side by side.

So why didn't everyone's natural health philosophy evolve together and happily integrate with our medical procedures just like the Chinese? Well, the answer is too long to be contained in a fortune cookie, but let's take a look at how medicine and health care evolved over time.

Herb Lore

The Greek philosopher Empedocles conceptualized that disease was based on an imbalance of the four elements of air, fire, water, and earth, which is still used as a philosophy for many holistic approaches to life and health today. For instance, almost every holistic practitioner, especially those who follow Chinese healing philosophies, will take into consideration the "nature" of your ailments to find out which element(s) you are lacking or are overabundant in. Any natural practitioner, such as Reflexologists, herbalists, holistic nutritionists, and iridologists may incorporate the four-element model into their assessment of your health.

In the eighteenth century, there began a shift dividing the use of nature as a cure and the use of complicated medical procedures as two philosophies that arose from differing German physicians. One approach believed that the soul is the vital principle and that it controls organic development; the other considered the body a machine and life as a mechanical process. The mechanistic beliefs eventually overpowered German universities and put to rest the philosophy of the four elements and eliminated this idea from medical schools.

Let's take a look at some of the influential people who popularized herbal remedies in the West.

People of the Herb in the West

Everyone has a father, and to many Western herbalists, Samuel Thomson is known as the father of herbology. His gift was a deep understanding of nature and Indian folk medicine.

Thomson, born in the 1700s in New Hampshire, was instrumental in leading the public (at least two million followers have been accounted for) in the successful home use of herbal remedies. However, as no good deed goes unpunished, this had its consequences from physicians of the day. Those physicians who were using mercury, arsenic, and other known deadly poisons in their practice—and who were sometimes bleeding people to death—accused Thomson of poisoning people with herbs, many of which are still used safely today. Thomson served at least one jail sentence during his lifetime of helping others.

Thomson believed in nature and people's capacity to take responsibility for their own health. He had faith that people were intelligent enough to judge for themselves whether a remedy was helpful or hurtful to them—and the people (at least back then) agreed. Thomson cured many with his herbal remedies and was in such demand for his cures that he obtained a permit for his herbal formulas and methods and sold family rights to millions to teach them to use herbs correctly. Thomson's influence is the basis of much of today's Western use of herbology.

Another well-known herbalist who was certainly influenced by Thomsonian methods is Dr. John Raymond Christopher (1909–1983). As a baby, John Raymond Christopher had his work cut out for him. He was born with advanced rheumatoid arthritis and walked with a cane and was often confined to a wheelchair. He became interested in natural healing while witnessing his mother's sufferings with dropsy and diabetes. He once told his mother that he would find a way to heal people without the use of surgery.

Herb Lore

As a baby, John Christopher contracted a severe case of croup. In the middle of a cold winter night, as his parents fretted over his health, a strange, bearded man wearing no coat arrived at the door. The man gave little John's parents explicit directions on what natural remedies to use to help the child and told them that their son had an important mission to fulfill, and he would not die. When the parents went to fetch a coat for the stranger, the stranger disappeared, leaving no footprints in the deep snow.

With his life filled with unfortunate accidents and ailments, Christopher had plenty of opportunity to experiment with natural herbs and remedies. His faith in the power of herbs was certainly strengthened when he used only natural methods to cure himself of cancer. After years of study obtaining a Master Herbalist designation, naturopathic doctor degree, and an herbal pharmacist degree, he founded the School of Natural Healing in 1953. This school is currently directed by his son, David Christopher, and is responsible for making Master Herbalists out of thousands of motivated pupils.

Dr. Christopher's herbal formulas are sold by at least five of the largest herb manufactures in the United States, and his life still serves as an inspiration to many.

The Philosophy of Herbs and Medicines

These days, thousands of people are using herbs before, after, and during their regular medical treatments to not only enhance their recovery but also to help prevent disease in the first place. Just as we can eat the right foods to help us stay healthy, we can take herbs to produce the same effect. The only difference is that herbs can usually bring us quicker results, so they need to be used with discretion.

The difference in choosing herbs or synthetic drugs to heal the body is really in the philosophy of the user. Herbs are foods that help your body to do what the body is supposed to do naturally. Synthetically derived drugs many times have properties that force your body into a chemical reaction to change, stop, or suppress your normal bodily functions or symptoms.

Many people run to the doctor with every ache, pain, and sniffle, for which the doctor really doesn't have a cure or a medicine. This is where herbs come in as medicines. Most of our aches, pains, and sniffles can be effectively "cured" by utilizing some simple herbal remedies. Herbs can be a safer, healthier, and usually are a less-expensive solution to many ailments. However, because herbs are *not* medicines, they will not necessarily work like you expect a medicine to work. Therefore, you need to understand how herbs do work for you to fully take the time to benefit from them.

First, we need to have a little different view of our bodies. To use herbal remedies, you will need to trust in your body's innate intelligence.

Do not take for granted that your body takes over to do its best to digest, assimilate, and eliminate after you eat something. Just think if you had to consciously learn the exact chemistry, physiology, and anatomy that it would take to teach your body and all your cells how to do their jobs. And think of the time that it would take to oversee that process—I'll bet we would all eat much less if our digestion required a conscious process!

Sage Advice

Herbs are widely prescribed in Europe and are playing a larger role in America's health care. The World Health Organization estimates that 80 percent of the world's population rely on herbs for primary health care.

The point is that our body works hard for us every day doing things that we could not conceive of doing if we were suddenly handed the job. When we become more conscious of how hard our body tries to keep us healthy, then we might become a little kinder to it and learn about what we put into it and the effects it will have on us.

When used correctly, herbs are safe medicines because, just like our body, herbs are organic and are a product of nature. Every molecule in your body is made up of something inherent on earth—so are herbs. When something goes wrong in the body, it is usually because of a deficiency of some vital nutrient or a build-up of toxins. Because herbs can feed nutritional deficiencies and/or stimulate your body to release toxins, many ailments that are caused by these factors can be corrected with the use of the right quantity and quality of herbs. Herbs help keep our body healthy by performing the following actions:

1. Supplying the missing element(s) such as vitamins, minerals, enzymes, essential fatty acids, and other phytochemicals in a concentrated form.

2. Helping the body eliminate built-up toxins that could be causing our ailments. Herbs may aid the body in eliminating these toxins by stimulating the release of excess mucus, urine, compacted bowel material, flushing cholesterol from arteries, and increasing perspiration.

As products of nature, herbs will first go to the area of your body that needs it most. This means that your symptom (the reason you reached for an herb in the first place) may not be eliminated immediately. When using herbs, as with any nutrition, you will have to be patient and know that Mother Nature works on her own time schedule.

On the other hand, I have seen the right herb(s) taken at the right time bring almost instant relief. Either way, most herbs you purchase that are produced by a reputable manufacture are going to be safe to use and experiment with if you are a generally healthy adult. ("Experiment" means that if you are not seeing results, you can try taking more than what the bottle recommends. See the next chapter for more details on how much you might need.)

This book has been created to help you avoid the hit or miss game:

➤ To help you understand the possible cause of your ailment(s).

➤ To introduce you to a new herb for each ailment; you will be introduced to about 100 herbs by the time you are through.

➤ To help you choose the right combinations of herbs and supplements to ease you through many illnesses.

In the coming pages you will be introduced to many herbs using their most commonly used name, but all herbs have a Latin or scientific name, too. When you are first introduced to specific herbs beginning in Part 2, you will also be given its Latin name in parenthesis. This is so you can be sure the species that you are using matches the common herb being described. Most herbalists, however, will refer to an herb's common name.

You can also use this book as a reference for occasional illnesses after you find yourself a good herbalist to help you create a personalized, daily herbal program. This book is made to empower you so that you won't have to call your doctor or your herbalist for every little ache, pain, and sniffle!

Herb Lore

Here's a scenario to illustrate the difference between man's quick-fix philosophy and natural healing. If a house plant is turning brown, we feed it water and give it sunshine— both from nature. Soon, the plant is green again. But when we are impatient and believe that technology has a better way, we might resort to painting the plant green! The green paint will take care of the outward symptom, but which is better for the plant? The paint was a much quicker "fix," but it did not get to the core problem. Which solution will be best for the plant in the long run?

Of course, medications have their place in humankind and are responsible for saving lives. However, many medicines fix the symptoms but don't reach the true source of the problem. The way I see it, you need to cover your bases first before using medications. Assess your symptoms and see what you body is trying to tell you before you stop your body's natural processes with a chemical drug. If you have a runny nose, is there something in your environment irritating your sinus cavities? Or did you inhale an incoming bacterium that the nose is trying to rid itself of? Using herbs will help you and your body communicate and will help you become more empowered to take care of yourself.

Sage Advice

The more patience we have to heal with natural means, the less patients our doctors have.

You should engage yourself in understanding how herbs work with your body so that you can get the most out of your herbal remedies. Sometimes just understanding a little about how herbs versus medicines work might give you the patience you need to get back to health instead of just covering up your symptoms. Remember that herbs give your body the opportunity to heal itself.

The Difference Between Herbs and Medicines

Fundamentally, the body (via the brain) knows what to do and how to process a whole food, such as an herb, but a drug is a more aggressive substance that forces a chemical change in the body. This is why drugs need to be administered by doctors: They can be dangerous and are deadly substances if used incorrectly.

Herbs are much more forgiving. If you overdose on an herb, the worst you may experience is vomiting and a headache. In contrast, drugs need to be taken with much more caution and regulation, as they can cause death when taken in the wrong combination or dosage.

Be smart when taking herbs and medications. Although your herbs may make you feel like you do not need your medications anymore, it is very important to *never go off your medications* without working with your prescribing doctor.

Let me explain why this is so important. Let's say for example that you suffer from high blood pressure. First of all your body is raising your blood pressure in an attempt to improve your circulation that is being inhibited (many times due to fat clogging the arteries). Then the doctor gives you a blood pressure medicine that blocks the mechanisms that allow your blood pressure to raise. This is an artificial cure, because now your body *really* wants to raise your pressure in an attempt to get the nutrient, oxygen-rich blood to all areas of the body. In a sense, your body works harder and pressure builds as the medication works against your body's natural process. If you suddenly discontinue your medications, the cork can be blown out, so to speak, and your blood pressure can rise to dangerously high levels very fast. (I liken this example to pushing hard against a door to open it and suddenly someone opens the door.)

It is so much wiser and easier use herbs first, to get to the source of your problem, (in this case, cleaning the cholesterol) and have your blood pressure return to normal as your body was designed to do in the first place. This is the natural approach to health and is where many medical doctors and holistic practitioners differ.

Unlike using a synthetic medication designed to suppress a symptom immediately, nature tends to have her own time schedule. Depending on your genetic makeup, you will have to wait for the results, which vary from person to person. Sometimes you will use an herb that works overnight for you, and other times it will take a much longer time to notice changes.

Our bodies all work a little differently. For one person, an herb will work within 20 minutes; for you it might take two weeks. Remember, however, that your body is sick because it usually is missing one or many nutrients. How fast you will notice healing evidence depends on the extent of your deficiency and how long you have been deficient.

Poison Ivy

Do *not* go off medication in place of herbs—going cold turkey could cause serious problems or withdrawals. Always consult your medical physician when working with your prescription medications. If you decide to take herbs and medications, have your physician re-check your required dosage often.

Sage Advice

Take medications at a different time of day, at least one hour apart from your herbs. This allows each substance to help your body and not interfere with the other. In addition, you should not take some herbs if you are on a specific medication—check with your qualified health professional and your herbalist.

Remember that nature takes her time, so hang in there and continue feeding your body the nutrients it needs to heal itself!

Herbs with Medicine: Making It Complementary

Herbs work differently than medications. Sometimes herbs have a cleansing or a detoxifying effect (*detoxing* means to remove *toxins* from the body). Toxins can be construed as anything toxic, poisonous, or of no positive value to the body.

By strengthening you, herbs can make your body more effective at eliminating foreign substances from your system. Some medications have by-products that are unnatural to the body (synthetic materials), so the cleansing herbs may lessen the effect of your medications by pushing out these foreign substances.

Conversely, some herbal properties have the same effects as medications and can actually enhance the effects of each other. This can also be a cause for caution. Make sure your prescribing doctor monitors your prescription dosages if taking herbs and medications together. It is always wise to let both your prescribing doctor and your herbalist know any and all supplements and medications you are taking to avoid unpleasant interactions.

Following is a table with some common contraindications to be aware of when considering using herbs with medications.

Botanical Bit

Detoxing is a term used by herbalists for a process of internal cleansing. The body will eliminate waste materials, materials that it cannot use, or things that are harmful to the body when it is strong enough to do so.

Toxins are considered any substances that are harmful or poisonous, or that do not serve a positive function in the body.

Common Herbs and Medicine Contraindications

Herb	Not to Be Taken with...
Black cohosh	Medication for diabetes or high blood pressure
Echinacea	Immunosuppresant therapy (such as organ transplants)
Feverfew	Arthritis medication
Garlic, Irish moss, chlorophyll, white willow, ginkgo biloba	Anticoagulant drugs (blood thinners)
Hawthorn	Heart-failure medications, unless supervised
St. John's wort	MAO inhibitors (antidepressant drugs)
Licorice root	Diuretics (used to eliminate excess water retention from the body)

I have found that many of my clients who have been on medications when starting on an herbal program have been able to cut back or even eliminate their medication. This has happened with synthetic thyroid medications, insulin, and even antidepressants. However, do not attempt this yourself—supervision by a competent physician is important when working with herbs and medications together.

It's exciting to see how herbs can strengthen the body and lessen the need for drugs. The body is truly a sufficient manufacturing plant, which requires the correct raw materials to keep it running smoothly.

Herbs Are Popular Again—It's About Thyme!

Why we are turning back to home remedies? My guess is that, just like in the pioneer days of the West, people around the globe are realizing that there is not really any magic pill to cure all ills. They may be realizing (if even subconsciously) that we are products of nature, and that surgery and medicines do not change that fact.

Many people begin to look for answers elsewhere when their medical treatments don't prove effective or when physicians do not have all the answers. They seek a kinder, gentler approach to health. Herbs and nutritional information is widely available and is a healthy and safe solution for many.

Since herbs are a safer alternative to medications, many times you'll get well before you run out of patience and get a prescription for your ailment. Unlike synthetic materials, the body can eliminate herbs if they are not able to be utilized.

If you do experience "side effects" when using an herb, the effects are usually a result of your body rapidly eliminating wastes. Unless you have a known allergy to an herb, herbs are generally safe. Some common herbal cleansing side effects you could experience include:

➤ Sinus drainage: Herbs can loosen long-standing mucus deposits. Drainage is common especially if you have had a history of sinus or respiratory conditions. A client of mine went on an herbal program and began feeling mucus draining from her nose, inside her ears into her throat, and experienced many odd sensations in her head, despite the fact that she hadn't experienced allergies in a few years. After one week of copious drainage, her long-standing congestion was gone for good!

➤ Nausea: Cleansing of the digestive tract—predominately the liver—is taking place too rapidly. Cut back on the cleansing herbs slightly to slow your cleansing process.

➤ Vomiting: Cleansing is taking place to rapidly. Handle the situation the same as you would for nausea.

➤ Diarrhea: Too much of the bowel stimulant herbs can cause diarrhea. Loose stool is different than diarrhea, however, and is a positive cleansing sign. Diarrhea is characterized by griping pain in the intestines, and the stool is predominately liquid.

➤ Headaches: Circulation has been stimulated before the body has been cleansed. Work with your herbalist to go through a cleanse before you begin any herbs designed to increase your circulation. Blood carries waste materials to the head area.

➤ Rashes: Usually because the blood is eliminating wastes. Try going on a bowel-cleansing regimen first before working with herbs that cleanse the blood.

Many herbalists that I know got their start by first seeking answers to their own health issues and found herbs to be their solution. Their experience engaged them in a passionate study until folks began seeking them out for their knowledge and understanding of how herbs can also work for them, too. So, I guess it was about "thyme" for a resurgence of nature and a rediscovery of our responsibility to take care of our families and ourselves. This is one of the reasons why herbs are back in the spotlight once again.

Below are some of the most common, minor ailments that have been effectively remedied with the use of herbs. You might want to try the herbs for a few days before you resort to drug usage. More than likely you'll be surprised how fast you find relief!

Sage Advice

A survey taken in the United States in 1997 shows a marked increase in the prevalence of people seeking alternative medical therapies. Ninety-six percent of the respondents, who were chosen from a wide range of socioeconomic categories, saw an alternative practitioner within a year after visiting a medical doctor.

Ailment	Typical Drug Taken	Safer Alternative(s)
A cold	Cold/cough/fever medicine	Echinacea, golden seal, rose hips, slippery elm, ginger, licorice root
Allergies/hayfever	Antihistamines	Fenugreek, horseradish, and mullein
Sinus infection	Antibiotics	Golden seal, black walnut, parthenium, plantain, bugleweed, marshmallow
Bladder infection	Antibiotics	Cranberries, buchu root, golden seal
Influenza	Cold/cough medicines, ibuprofen or aspirin	Parthenium, golden seal, yarrow, capsicum
Constipation	Over the counter laxatives	Cascara sagrada
Diarrhea	Anti-diarrhea medicine	Slippery elm
Headaches	Ibuprofen or aspirin	White willow bark or feverfew

continues

continued

Ailment	Typical Drug Taken	Safer Alternative(s)
General aches and pains	Ibuprofen, pain killers	White willow bark and/or uña de gato
Stomach ache	Antacids or anti-nausea liquids	Peppermint tea
Heartburn	Antacids	Marshmallow, calcium, or chewable papaya tablets

Looking at this table you might think, "Why take all those herbs when I can take a drug in one pill?" There are two answers to that question.

First, most companies will offer you herbal products that combine several herbs geared toward a certain condition into one pill. Granted, you will need a few of these pills every few hours, versus one of the OTC (over-the-counter) drugs, but the effects herbs have on your body are positive. Synthetic drugs of any kind can have permanent negative effects on your body and can lead to a damaged liver, kidney failure, decreased immune, and even death.

Second, take a look at the long list of ingredients listed on the back of that package of drugs you wanted to take. You are not getting just one ingredient, but also several chemicals, dyes, and synthetic materials (mostly words you never knew existed) all combined into one pill or dosage. You will also see a list of warnings and cautions to take into consideration. Are you really taking that for your health or for convenience? Why not bear through what you can, while helping your body get well with the use of herbs? Consider using medications when you feel that you must stop your symptoms immediately. Then get home as soon as possible, get some rest, and take your herbs!

The Least You Need to Know

➤ Our first medicines came from the plants, and their value is still inherent today.

➤ Herbs should be taken at different times of the day (at least one hour apart) from any prescription medications.

➤ For minor problems, you might want to try herbs and rest first before resorting to an over-the-counter drug.

➤ Consult the known contraindication chart with your doctor before starting a complete herbal program if you are on any medication.

➤ Never go off your prescription medications without your qualified health professional's approval.

➤ The public's dissatisfaction with medical treatments, along with the resurgence of taking responsibility for our own lives and health, may be why herbs and nutrition are becoming so popular.

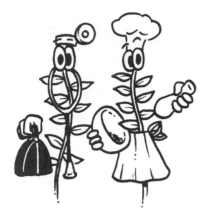

Chapter 3

What to Expect with Herbs

In This Chapter

➤ What to expect when first taking herbs

➤ Three ways herbs work in the body

➤ The importance of internal cleansing

➤ How herbs complement each other

➤ Assess the nature of your symptoms: a look at energetics

When I first became curious about herbs, I would browse the health food store aisles, pick up something that I had read about in a nutrition magazine, and give it a try. After several bottles of different herbs with no dramatic results or any noticeable changes, I came to my own conclusion: Herbs don't work! On the other side of the coin, however, I have met a few people who have abandoned the use of herbs completely because they had very strong reactions that they didn't expect and that caused them to come to the conclusion that all herbs are bad or poisonous.

Wait! Before you make any erroneous conclusions or actions, read this chapter. It will provide you some background on why some people believe both of these misinformed extremes. More important, it will help you use herbs safely and with good results.

How Herbs Work

Herbs work in three different ways: to activate, build, and cleanse the body. (You can remember this best by remembering your ABCs to using herbs.)

We'll talk about each of these separately so that you can assess the type of results you are looking for in using herbs.

Activating Properties

Herbs have activating qualities to them, also known as stimulation. This activation may be needed when an organ of the body is functioning sluggishly or under par. Some herbs have tonifying properties, meaning that they tone the glands or functioning of the body, much like exercise tones your muscles. Some herbs can actually stimulate and support your body to help it do its job better.

Activating herbs have a stimulating effect on the body organs and can give you a jump-start on health. This effect might be compared to the feeling of suddenly being pushed into an icy cold pool on a hot summer day. (Now *that's* activating!) These activating herbs are not necessarily used long-term, but they can be a catalyst to helping you recover.

An example of some stimulating herbs include:

Capsicum	Stimulates blood circulation
Horseradish	Stimulates respiratory passages
Peppermint	Stimulates alertness and digestion

Building: We're Going to Pump You Up!

The herbs you use to build the body can also be used in smaller doses to maintain your results. You can use the herbs as foods and nourishment to build and maintain your immune system so that you keep yourself from getting ill in the first place. When you're weak and need nourishment, you'll need more nutrients than when you are just maintaining your health. Be ready to take a lot of herbs until you reach that level.

Sage Advice

Well-known herbalist Dr. Jack Ritchason says that it takes five to seven times the normal amount of nutrition to build and repair than it does to maintain. And it takes a minimum of three months to produce change in the body with consistent good nutrition (herbs) and an additional one month for every year you have been sick.

Using herbs as nutrition will help build up and maintain your body and will help protect you from being vulnerable to disease. Most herbs considered building or nutritive herbs will be salty to the taste, which means they have a high mineral content. Minerals nourish your body and help build strong bones, hair, skin, and teeth.

A few examples of building herbs include:

Alfalfa	Rich in minerals; great for structural system
Horsetail	Rich in silica; feeds structural system, hair, and nails
Kelp	Rich in iodine and other minerals; nourishes and builds the thyroid

Usually you will build up with herbs after you go through a cleansing stage. Once the body has rid itself of the old toxins and irritants that were making you feel sick, you are in a much better position to be able to use herbs as foods to nourish your body and maintain your health and vibrancy. So let's talk about cleaning out those pipes!

Cleansing: The Process of Elimination

Herbs can have what herbalists call a *cleansing* effect on the body. Herbs that cleanse are herbs that help the body to eliminate built-up waste materials—some people refer to these waste products as toxins. When toxins build up in the body, they can be the cause of many irritating and depleting ailments. Many times, by just cleansing the body, the ailment you were suffering from disappears. Remember when we talked about detoxing the body in Chapter 2, "A Little Herb Lore"? This is basically what a cleanse is.

When we cleanse, the toxins will exit the body faster than normal. Therefore, you might expect some extra activity at your body's exits! These exits are the four elimination channels, which carry off waste products:

1. The bowel
2. The lungs
3. The kidneys
4. The skin

The skin eliminates uric acid waste products through the pores of the skin; the urinary tract carries off liquid waste products; the respiratory system (lungs and sinuses) carry off gaseous wastes and excess mucus; and the bowel eliminates solid waste matter.

This natural elimination process not only speeds up through an herbal cleansing, but it also speeds up naturally if the body is trying to rid itself of a foreign invader, such as a cold virus, bacteria, or a parasite.

The process of cleansing, eliminating, or detoxing may include a variety of symptoms, including a runny nose, a rash, or diarrhea. The mistake that many people make is to stop this natural process with a medication designed to stop or suppress these annoying symptoms. By medicating the symptoms,

Botanical Bit

A **cleanse** occurs when the body dumps excess toxins through one or more of the body's elimination channels; the skin, the bowel, the respiratory passages, or the urinary system.

Sage Advice

Think of your body as working for your protection when you experience minor cold symptoms. This is usually a result of the body detoxing itself, so think twice before medicating and stopping these symptoms. Think of herbs first to assist your body through the process.

however, you are actually plugging up the elimination channel and allowing the bug that caused your body the problem to stay inside your body. This can allow the toxins to settle back into your body tissues and cause another problem sometime later. I see this constantly with people who experience recurring sinus infections. When you help the body eliminate its invader, you will help put a stop to this vicious cycle.

Poison Ivy

The strong herbal bowel cleansers such as senna, turkey rhubarb, cascara sagrada, and others should be avoided if you suffer from IBS (irritable bowel syndrome) or colitis. You will need soothing herbs such as aloe vera and marshmallow instead to help heal your inflamed and irritated tissues.

Many times a cleanse offers a breath of fresh air to organs that have been suffocated with mucus build-up. The colon, for instance, can harbor wastes that can fester in the body for years—and sometimes even decades. Most people who are in general good health can benefit from an herbal cleansing before starting on a nutritional/herbal program. Cleansing the bowel and digestive tract periodically will help ensure that nutrients will be more efficiently absorbed and properly utilized by the body. Natural cleansing can consist of a three-day cleanse or several weeks, depending on the type of cleanse and how toxic your body tissues are.

The act of cleansing first and then building is like cleaning out your refrigerator before going shopping for more food. Ridding yourself of old, moldy cucumbers and cleaning the bins before you put new, fresh foods back in is a good idea for your body, too. See Chapter 4, "Herbs Are Not Just for Hippies Anymore," for the recipe for an effective herbal cleanse you can use.

Herb Lore

When a knowledgeable herbalist first put me on my herbal program, I was not truly ready for the results. After weeks of what seemed like non-stop trips to the bathroom, I thought I was becoming hollow! I stopped taking the herbs. What I did not understand was that the herbs were cleansing years of built-up toxins from my body (especially my colon). I went back several months later—after I read more on the subject—and began a process that has literally changed my entire health and well-being. Now I couldn't live (at least not as well) without my daily intake of herbs and supplements. I consider my herb program to be my best health insurance!

Many cleansing herbs will be bitter to the taste and are best taken in a pill form. Examples of some cleansing type herbs include:

Cascara sagrada	Helps clear the bowel
Burdock root	Helps cleanse the blood
Yellow dock	Helps cleanse the blood, liver, and bowel

An Energetic and Synergistic Look at Herbs

Sometimes you will hear about an herb's energetic effect on the body, or you will hear an herbalist say that a combination of herbs works synergistically together. What's all this about?

Energetics describes the personality, energy, and general characteristics of herbs. It's also used to categorize how an herb or a food reacts to our body when we taste, smell, and ingest it. *Synergy* is a term used to describe how herbs work together. We can have a synergistic relationship with our friends, but not our enemies! Working synergistically together is basically working in harmony to enhance the effects of each other.

Botanical Bit

Energetics describes an herb's personality, energy, and general characteristics. This term also can describe an herb's energetic effect on our body when we use it. **Synergy** is a term used to describe how herbs work together. Working synergistically together is basically working in harmony to enhance the effects of each other.

An Energetic Approach

Energetics is an interesting and complex approach to herbology, but once you get the hang of it, it can be fun and very effective in choosing the right herbal remedy for your body. Used in this context, energetics is considered the energy, the nature, or the personality of an herb and the effect it has on you when you take it. When you assess the nature of your illness, you can choose a herb with a more balancing or complementary energy.

For instance, if you don't take into account the energetics of a cough, then you might assume that a cherry bark cough syrup is what you need. After all, cherry bark has been used successfully by many to tame coughing. However, if you have a dry cough and you take cherry bark, your cough will worsen because cherry bark has a very drying effect on the tissues. It works great for those with a loose, phelgmy cough, but you are better off with a different remedy for a dry cough—you might try slippery elm or licorice root, which soothe dry, irritated tissues.

Energetics is a very deep subject that's just briefly introduced so that you can understand why not just one herb works for everyone's cough. Where appropriate throughout this book, I have provided suggestions for each ailment to help you choose the best remedy for your needs.

This quote, by Leonardo da Vinci, explains quite eloquently the holistic view of an energetic approach to healing:

> "You know that medicines when well used restore health to the sick: they will be well used when the doctor together with his understanding of their nature shall understand also what man is, what life is, and what constitution and health are. Know these well and you will know their opposites; and when this is the case you will know well how to devise a remedy."

Synergy

Why is it that one herb doesn't seem to help change how you feel, but three or four in combination can change your life? This is called *synergy*. Synergy is the effect you get when everything is working complementary with one another. You may require the benefits of the synergist effects of more than one herb to help your body get back into shape.

Many herbs work synergistically with each other just like a nice wine goes with a certain meal. On the contrary, some herbs can actually cancel each other out because they have opposite effects on each other. (Kind of like onions and ice cream!)

Sage Advice

You might have seen golden seal and echinacea together already. These two herbs are great for the immune system and, when taken together, seem to be very effective against colds. Golden seal is nature's antibiotic, and echinacea boosts the immune system and helps clear the respiratory tract.

Unfortunately, there is no such thing as the magic herb, although sometimes an herb added to a few other herbs can serve as a catalyst that helps boost the effects of the others. Some herbs just make good teams together; for instance, capsicum is an activating herb that works synergistically with many herbs to enhance the effect of the other. Herbal companies who know this will add a pinch of capsicum to their herbal formulas for this synergistic and enhancing effect.

Many herbalists and nutritionists believe that what can prevent a sickness also can cure it. If your disease was caused by a lack of nutrients in the first place, then it makes sense that feeding that nutrient back to your body will return you to your normal functions. Take scurvy, for example. It is caused by a lack of vitamin C. We not only use foods rich in vitamin C to prevent scurvy, but it is also the remedy for this disease.

Adjusting Herbal Remedies to Your Needs

If you aren't working with an herbalist, or someone educated in herbology, you will need to experiment somewhat on how much or how many herbs your body needs to get results. Larger people sometimes need larger doses, and smaller people need smaller doses. Children usually need very little amounts and respond quickly to herbal remedies (see Chapter 4 for guidelines for children).

If you are especially sensitive to medications or foods it is best to start out with smaller doses than what is recommended on a label. It's always best to get little or no results and work your way up than to bombard yourself with too much, which can bring on an uncomfortable cleansing.

Sometimes it takes a couple days to feel the effects of an herb. This is especially true with the cleansing-type herbs, so it's a good idea to take the recommended dosage for a few days and wait for any changes. If you are not seeing a change, in-crease what you are taking daily until you start seeing changes in your body.

Hot, Cold, Wet, or Dry: Which Do I Apply?

To get the right synergy and energetic combination, consider the nature of your symptoms. You can use four general descriptions—hot, cold, wet, and dry—to categorize your illness, and these can be matched to four general effects that herbs have on the body.

You can determine whether an herb is hot, cold, wet, or dry by its taste, smell, touch, and sometimes just by its appearance. For instance, slippery elm, when tasted, will have a slippery feel on your tongue. This means that the herb has a wet characteristic that can be used for dry conditions in the body. The slippery elm, being *mucilaginous*, is soothing to the body tissues; I use it if I get a dry, scratchy throat from talking too much!

An example of the hot category is the herb capsicum, which is the fruit of the cayenne pepper plant. Capsicum is a very hot herb indeed—and one taste on the tip of your tongue will prove it! Another clue that capsicum is hot is its red color. If you are cold and lacking circulation, capsicum would be a great herb to help you generate some heat.

Poison Ivy

If you have sensitivities to medications or other things, your system might need smaller amounts than what a label might recommend. Start out with smaller doses (such as one capsule or tablet daily) for a few days, and work your way up in dosage until you begin seeing results. Then maintain that dose as long as you are improving.

Botanical Bit

Mucilaginous is a quality of an herb that is soothing to irritated tissues. These herbs are usually slippery to the feel, are soluble fibers, and act as gentle laxatives. Other names for mucilaginous herbs include emollient, demulcent, or mucilants.

A dry herb in energetics is an herb that causes your tissues to dry up. Most of these herbs are referred to as astringents or sour herbs. A good example is white oak bark, which is used to tighten and dry up swollen tissues and blisters.

An example of a cooling (cold) effect from an herb is aloe vera, which is also a muci-laginous herb. This herb has both a cooling and a moistening effect on the body. If you were hot and dry, drinking a little aloe vera in your water would help you cool down and would moisten your tissues.

Try your own taste test with each of these herbs and see for yourself the effect it has on you. Open a capsule of capsicum and dab some on your tongue. It won't be long before you'll be reaching for that cooling sip of aloe vera! You will feel the white oak bark tighten your tongue, and you'll sense the sliminess of the slippery elm when you moisten it. This experiment will really get you in touch with energetics.

Choosing the Right Combinations

How do you know what combinations of herbs to choose? Don't worry—that's probably why you bought this book, and it will be spelled out for you. Combinations are excellent because you can take just one pill that contains several different herbs for a specific body system. For instance, instead of purchasing fenugreek and thyme separately to help you eliminate mucus and boost the immune (many take these herbs when suffering from bronchitis), you can obtain one combination pill that contains both these herbs. Hey, it saves space and allows you to take some other herbs without having a bottle of every single herb you need filling up your countertops! Taking combinations can save you money also since you only need to buy one bottle and not two or more to get the same synergistic effects one bottle of a combination provides.

Sage Advice

Besides being sure that you are taking a quality product, consider taking a single herb (especially if you have allergies or if you have a sensitive system) before taking a combination. This will get you familiar with how the herb makes you feel. You can then avoid combinations that contain the particular herb in the future if you're having difficulty with it. It's harder to tell which herb might not agree with you when using a combination.

When you see a combination of two or more herbs together in future tables, it's because the combinations are working synergistically and usually serve a few different purposes to help you with an ailment. If you cannot find a combination that I suggest in future tables (*hint*: I *know* they are out there) then don't hesitate to combine your own using singles or bulk herbs. Let's look at some other combinations that work synergistically.

Lobelia and St. John's wort is one combination that many smokers use to help them quit. The lobelia is calming and has an effect similar to nicotine in the body. St. John's wort has been used to fight mild depression sometimes associated with breaking an addictive physical habit.

Capsicum with garlic and parsley is another synergistic combination utilized for its positive effect on the circulatory system. The parsley serves as a deodorizer that helps mask the unpleasantness of garlic breath!

Combinations are excellent; nevertheless, each person is chemically a little bit different, so some will respond better to a few single herbs and others to combinations. You will find in this book that a couple options are listed for you.

The positive affirmation you made by purchasing and reading this book alone proves you are ready to continue learning and take more responsibility for your health and life. Although the road to total health through natural means is not necessarily a piece of tofu cake, the rewards you earn are vitality, clear thinking, emotional control, vibrancy, and energy—well worth working for, wouldn't you say? Once you begin using herbs, you instantly become more aware of your body and you will feel how herbs can enhance your life and health. If you are interested in studying herbology, start studying now because it's a vast and wonderful journey—oh, and don't forget to take your ginkgo biloba to boost your memory while you learn!

The Least You Need to Know

➤ Herbs have three major properties to activate, cleanse, and build the body.

➤ Herbs have their own "personalities," or effects on the body, which can be referred to as energetics.

➤ Cleansing is a good first step before trying to build or protect your body with herbs.

➤ Unfortunately, there is no one single magic herb that will cure all that ails you, but combinations of herbs can work synergistically to enhance the effects and get you the results you are seeking.

➤ Although you will usually need more than one type of herb at a time, for best results you should first try herbs as singles to get familiar with the effect they have on you.

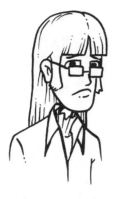
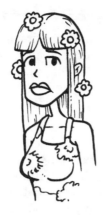

Chapter 4

Herbs Are Not Just for Hippies Anymore

In This Chapter

➤ How to use herbs safely before, during, and after pregnancy

➤ How to give herbs to children

➤ Using herbal remedies for your pets

➤ How to use herbs to counteract aging

➤ The best herbs for those well beyond retirement age

When I first began using herbs in my mid-20s, I was accused of being a hippie. I don't know whether the accuser made that conclusion because I was taking a handful of herbs, or whether it was the flowers in my hair, the paisley skirt, beaded necklace, and bubble-blowing that gave it away. But seriously, more than just hippies have used—and still use—herbs for health and to enhance their quality of life.

These days, athletes are discovering the benefits of using herbs and other natural supplements to boost their performance in sports—and because herbs are foods, taking them is perfectly legal! Movie stars are using herbs for energy and as beauty aids, and business people and students are using herbs to keep their mind sharp and their stress under control.

So relax, you won't have to get out your sandals and bell-bottoms to start using herbal remedies. In this chapter we will discuss herbs for kids, herbs for use before, during, and after pregnancy, and even herbs for pets! So put on some Bob Dylan music, and read on, 'cuz the times, they are a changin'!

Pregnancy and Herbs

Herbs can support an easier pregnancy by helping alleviate morning sickness, mood swings, leg cramps, hemorrhoids, constipation, and anemia. They can also be used for nourishing and strengthening the body to support a growing, healthy fetus.

Some herbs are best used to prepare your body before pregnancy. Then there are herbs you can use to support your body and the future health of your child during gestation; many of these herbs will help enrich your breast milk during the nursing period. Finally, thank goodness, other herbs can help your body get back into shape again. And some herbs, of course, should be completely avoided during pregnancy. This chapter will give you plenty of herbal information for use all along the way.

Before Planting the Seed

You can again remember your ABCs to herbs before, during, and after pregnancy. Before pregnancy you will be cleansing. During pregnancy you will be building and after pregnancy, and when nursing you will be activating your body to get it back into shape again.

The three steps to herbally plan for a smoother and healthy pregnancy are:

1. Cleansing with the use of herbs
2. Nourishing (building) the body with herbal nutrients
3. Activating and toning the body and reproductive organs

Sage Advice

The health and proper nourishment of the mother during pregnancy can reduce the risk of childhood health problems. Tell your doctor which herbs and supplements you are considering taking to boost your health during pregnancy.

Sage Advice

Potential dads can also prepare by using herbs and supplements before conception. Good herbs and supplements to build healthy sperm and to support male reproductive organs include: Siberian ginseng, sarsaparilla, parthenium, horsetail, saw palmetto, garlic, gotu kola, capsicum, damiana, and chickweed.

It is wise to begin preparing your body up to a year before conception. First, do some cleansing. An overloaded liver is usually the culprit that causes morning sickness, so a cleansing and building program for the liver and bowel can help prevent illness during those first few months of pregnancy.

You can use a wonderful general cleansing remedy designed by herbalist Ivy Bridge. This cleanse can be used and should only be used well before conception and then again after you deliver and have stopped nursing. Here's the recipe, generously donated by Ivy for your health:

Ivy Bridge's Colon Cleanse

$1/2$ glass of apple juice (organic and no sugar is best, but use your favorite brand otherwise)

2 tablespoons aloe vera juice (if using a whole-leaf aloe vera you'll only need 1 tablespoon)

2 tablespoons liquid chlorophyll

8 capsules psyllium hulls (or 1 teaspoon loose powder)

2 capsules cascara sagrada

Blend aloe vera juice and chlorophyll into apple juice. If you are using powdered psyllium instead of capsules, stir in the psyllium and drink down quickly; psyllium will expand in water. Swallow your cascara sagrada capsules with a full (at least 8 ounces) glass of pure water.

Use this formula mixture first thing in the morning every day for 60 days. Make sure to drink at least 8 to 10 glasses of water each day.

Ivy's formula has been used by many to cleanse the lower bowel of poisons, strengthen the digestive and intestinal track, lower cholesterol, build blood, soothe acid conditions, aid fat loss, and stimulate bile flow from the liver.

In addition to this cleanse, one to three capsules/tablets of milk thistle (or $1/2$ to 1 teaspoon of tincture) may be taken daily. Milk thistle helps the liver break down and excrete poisons, promotes bile flow, acts as a mild laxative, decongests blood circulation to the liver, and protects the liver cells from damage. (See Chapter 5 for more on this herb.)

As with any cleansing, you may experience new sensations you didn't know you could feel! Intestinal rumblings, stomach growls, initial intestinal gas, and many trips to the bathroom can all be part of the cleansing process. Use caution if you get diarrhea and cut back on your cascara capsules if you are too uncomfortable. The initial grumblings and mumblings of your intestines should settle down in a few days. Think of it as a power car wash blasting out years of built-up dirt. The cleaner you get, the less "mud splattering," until finally you are balanced and internally clean.

The more positive effects you may feel include a lighter feeling, clearer skin, weight loss, loss of cravings for junk food, clean breath, and less body odor. The psyllium hulls swell in water, which makes you feel satisfied and less hungry. This is one of the reasons why many lose excess weight on the program.

Poison Ivy

Herbal cleansing should be discontinued about three months before you decide to try to conceive. Do not cleanse at the same time you are trying to get pregnant, and never during gestation.

After cleansing, you will want to begin a nutritious herbal building program that can be continued from up to a year or any time before conception, through pregnancy, and all during nursing. Let's talk next about what herbs and nutrients are critical for a healthy pregnancy.

Herbs for Soon-to-Be Moms

So, now you've done your cleanse and broken those bad habits and are feeling clean, trim, and clear. Next you need to begin to build up your body with nutrients. Building your nutritional reserves with herbs rich in calcium, iron, and B vitamins will all work to ensure a healthy pregnancy for you and the little one. All these nutrients will be good not only prepare your body for pregnancy, but will carry you through your nine months and will even help nourish you and baby during nursing time.

If you are already pregnant and haven't had time to build up your reserves, don't fret! You can begin right now taking your nutrients. A non-synthetic pre-natal vitamin is excellent to cover your bases, and may be prescribed by your doctor. Your herbalist may have a quality source for you also. Compare your options and decide which is best for you. Make sure your prenatal vitamin contains extra folic acid and calcium.

Once a fetus begins to grow, the body will take what it needs from the mother. If you (as the mom) are not getting the right nutrients, your body can rob your body's reserves to support the growing fetus. This can lead to uncomfortable symptoms and ailments.

Anemia is a common problem during pregnancy. To avoid anemia, you will want to build a good red blood count. Herbs that can help are rich in iron and include dark green drinks, such as liquid chlorophyll or wheat grass juice. Others are not necessarily green but also are rich in organic iron; these include yellow dock, dandelion, and nettle leaves.

We all know that calcium helps build strong bones and teeth, and calcium is a mineral that helps in bone growth during fetal development. Many believe that we need to drink milk to receive calcium. If this is so, then how do you think the cows produce all that excess calcium-rich milk and maintain those strong bones and hoofs without drinking cow's milk throughout their life?

That's right—the grass! The green plants provide much usable calcium for the body. Calcium-rich herbs safe for pregnancy include alfalfa, liquid chlorophyll, fennel, parsley, horsetail, and oatstraw.

After you have constructed an nutritional herbal program to ensure you are getting enough vitamins and minerals to support a growing fetus, there are some extra herbs you can use to strengthen your body for the actual birthing process and to aid some symptoms that frequently accompany pregnancy. Let's take a look at some common symptoms and their herbal solutions.

Red raspberry is an herb that strengthens the uterus and reproductive organs and can even enhance fertility. Red raspberry tea can be sipped during pregnancy and has helped many moms to overcome nausea.

Sage Advice

Since calcium supplies can be stolen from the bones and teeth, your body should be properly nourished so that it has plenty of calcium before, during, and even after the baby comes. In days past, there was a saying that said, "You will lose one tooth for every child." That was before we knew about supplementing with calcium!

Herb Lore

"Got Milk?" is a great advertising campaign; however, it leads us to believe that cow's milk will give us strong bones and teeth and, of course, that flattering white moustache. Contrary to popular belief, cow's milk is not our best source of usable calcium for the body. The ratios of naturally occurring constituents in milk differ greatly from cow to human. In fact, there is 300 times more casein in cow's milk, which makes absorbing calcium difficult. Milk is difficult to digest because the enzymes renin and lactase needed to break it down are depleted by age three. Large fat globules and heavy protein content in milk are designed for the developing calf, not humans.

Some moms get constipated during pregnancy, because the same hormone that maintains the pregnancy also decreases the movement of the bowel. One of the safest herbs you can use for constipation during pregnancy is psyllium hulls, or psyllium husks (pronounced *silly-um*). Psyllium is a fiber that swells in water and that acts as a intestinal broom, picking up and sweeping away debris from the colon. The colon is a muscle that needs fiber foods that strengthen it by giving it something to resist against

Botanical Bit

Peristaltic action is the wavelike muscular contractions that move contained matter along the colon. Because the colon is a muscle, fiber will help strengthen the bowel by giving it something to resist against.

Sage Advice

Many pregnant women consider ginger root their miracle cure for morning sickness. Ginger can be taken in a tea or capsules, or purchased as a root and nibbled on raw. Ginger aids digestion and is safe for pregnant moms.

during *peristaltic action*. Peristaltic action is the wavelike movement the bowel makes to move things along. Most foods we eat offer no fibrous content, so our colon winds up getting flaccid and lazy, making constipation and hemorrhoids (because of pressure on the lower organs of the body) more common. Psyllium helps keep you going (so to speak) and is safe for the baby as well.

One of the best herbal remedies for nausea or morning sickness during pregnancy is ginger root. Used as a spice in many Indian dishes, ginger also can be taken in a tea or capsules, and some people even like the taste enough to purchase candied ginger for nibbling. Ginger is a restorative herb, which means that it activates the body to bring it into balance.

Push, Push—Herbs for a Smoother Delivery

The proper use of herbs will assist you through the entire birthing process, for before, during, and after pregnancy. A combination used by many moms in daily small doses, five weeks before the due date is a mixture of black cohosh, squawvine, dong quai, butcher's broom, and red raspberry. Moms who have tried it attest that the combination supported the uterus to carry to full term, prevented premature births, helped with the pain of childbirth, and decreased blood loss during and after delivery. Search out this combination or have an herbalist mix you up a batch. Every mom I know who has used it has reported excellent results. Consult your doctor or midwife before beginning to take this combination.

Congratulations! Now that you used herbs to cleanse, build, and prepare your body for conception, nourished your body and growing fetus for nine months, and used herbs to combat pregnancy discomforts and aid in your delivery, you can consider your baby an herbal baby! Don't be surprised if you earned the "Earth Mother" reputation with your OB/GYN, especially if you decide to name your baby Herb!

With all the efforts you put into your health up to this point, you will still need to continue this regimen during the nursing time for yourself and your child. Let's take a look at why breastfeeding is such a fantastic and natural part of life, and how to enhance the process with herbs.

Nursing for Health: Mutual Benefits

Breastfeeding your baby is one of the best ways to ensure a strong nutritional foundation for your child.

Babies' benefits from being nursed include these:

➤ Helps build a relationship with Mom

➤ Supports a strong nutritional foundation

➤ Builds the immune system

➤ Supplies the healthy intestinal flora in the intestinal tract

And for Mom:

➤ Tones the uterus

➤ Helps bond with the baby

➤ Burns excess calories

➤ Can serve as a relaxing experience

A mom can enhance her own breast milk using herbs that also give her baby good nourishment. Herbs taken during pregnancy should be continued during the nursing period to ensure proper nutrition for baby. Remember that all herbs, medications, and foods you take will be passed to your baby through your breast milk. So continue to eat well, and avoid taking any medications (unless prescribed by your physician), harsh herbs (see the following list of herbs to avoid), or very spicy foods because they can upset your baby's very small digestive system.

Herbs you can add to enrich breast milk include nettle leaves, spirulina (rich in chlorophyll, amino acids, and enzymes), and alfalfa.

And, as my friend who has borne seven (count them, seven) children of her own and breastfed every one wanted me to let you know that a mom also needs lots of extra water (beyond the normal daily intake) because the requirement for water goes up when breastfeeding.

Sage Advice

Varicose veins are another pregnancy-related condition and can be helped by using bilberry and rose hips, which will help to strengthen blood capillaries. These herbs will also aid if you are suffering from hemorrhoids.

Sage Advice

If you are ready to stop breast-feeding before your body is, keep in mind that sage and black walnut help dry up breast milk.

Shaping Up with Herbs

Although nursing your baby will help you burn up more calories and swing your body back in to shape more quickly, some moms still need a little quicker boost after baby is weaned.

Herbs to help get your body back into shape will include herbs that act as appetite suppressants and fat burners that increase thermogenesis. *Thermogenesis* is the process of raising body temperature to speed up the body metabolism, which in turn helps your body burn more calories.

If you haven't had the opportunity to cleanse before you were pregnant and nursing, after you are done nursing is a great time to go on a good cleansing. A weight-loss program following a good cleanse is a way to give your body a jump-start—and you might just lose the extra weight with only a cleanse! Try Ivy's Colon Cleanse drink recipe earlier in this chapter.

After cleansing, herbs can be combined and used for weight loss. Some single herbs used for weight loss include chickweed, psyllium hulls, lecithin, and ma huang. Chickweed acts as a mild appetite suppressant and is a natural source of lecithin; lecithin is a fat emulsifier; and psyllium grabs the fat from your foods before your body has a chance to absorb it. This is especially effective if taken 15 to 20 minutes before meals. For information on general weight loss, see Chapter 23, "V, W, X, Y, Z, and Other Technical Words."

Try these herbs to shape up with after nursing:

➤ Psyllium hulls

➤ Lecithin

➤ Chickweed

➤ Ma huang

➤ White willow bark

➤ Licorice root

Ma huang, a Chinese herb that's also known as Chinese ephedra, is an herb that is best combined with white willow bark, which helps balance its effect for weight loss. Ma huang promotes thermogenesis and should *never* be taken with caffeine—the intensified "upper" affect can push your body into overdrive. People with sensitive systems, heart problems, or hypertension can have serious trouble with this mixture. Responsible companies who have a deep understanding of herbology will not combine ma huang and caffeine-containing herbs in their products.

You've made it full circle! Congratulations again! You look better now than before you were pregnant, really! And please don't forget to check out the following list of herbs to avoid during pregnancy—just in case you plan to do this again. Happy parenting!

The following table summarizes all the herbs we've talked about and then some. Note which herbs are appropriate at what times during your family-building process.

Poison Ivy

Avoid taking herbs that combine ma huang with caffeine or caffeine-containing herbs. Herbs that are caffeine-rich include kola nut, colanitida, herba mate, bissy nuts, and guarana.

Herbs for Building a Family

Herbs	Before/During/Nursing	Uses
Cascara sagrada	Before	Bowel and liver cleansing; to prevent future morning sickness
Milk thistle	Before	Liver building; to help prevent morning sickness by strengthening the liver
Liquid chlorophyll	Before, during, and nursing	Rich in minerals; builds red blood count
Spirulina	Before, during, and nursing	Rich in nutrients and proteins; feeds baby and enriches breast milk
Psyllium hulls	During	Provides fiber to alleviate constipation
Red raspberry leaves	Before and during	Tones uterus and reproductive organs
Horsetail	Before, during, and nursing	Rich in calcium; helps build bone strength
Oatstraw	Before, during, and nursing	Rich in calcium; helps build bone strength
Ginger	During	Helps with morning sickness

Avoid these herbs during pregnancy or when nursing:

Caffeine-containing herbs such
as guarana, kola nuts, colanitida,
herba mate, and bissy nuts

Aloe vera

American ginseng

Angelica

Arnica

Barberry

Butcher's broom

Black cohosh

Blue cohosh

Bugleweed

Camphor

Castor bean

Cascara sagrada

Cayenne

Cedar berries

Chamomile, Roman

Clary sage

Clove bud

Dong quai

Elecampane

False unicorn

Fennel

Feverfew

Flax

Gentian

Golden seal

Hyssop

Juniper berries

Licorice root

Lobelia

Ma huang

Myrrh

Oregon grape

Pennyroyal

Peppermint

Rosemary

Safflower

St. John's wort

Sage

Sassafras

Senna

Squaw vine

Thyme

Wild ginger

Wild oregano

Wild yam

Wood betony

Wormwood (Artemisia)

Yarrow

Cautionary Note: Please be aware that this is just a partial list and includes herbs that are not recommended to be taken in large dosages as dietary supplements during pregnancy on a regular basis. Some of these herbs may stimulate the uterus into action, which can cause miscarriage. There are really only a handful of herbs that we know are completely safe all during pregnancy. So play it safe when going through this delicate time. Herbs used occasionally as a seasoning should not be a problem. When pregnant or nursing, use the guidelines in this book for safe herbals, or work with a qualified herbalist—if in doubt, don't take it!

A Childish Look at Herbs for Kids

Children generally respond very well and quickly to herbal remedies. This is because their bodies are small, and they haven't had years of polluting themselves to compensate for.

Children also usually respond better to single herbs versus herbal combinations; babies respond best to a single herb in a liquid form. The older they are, the better able children are to take a few different combinations. Herb manufacturers make chewable or liquid herbs that are easy to administer to children. Make sure that your child's chewable herbs or vitamins are not sweetened with artificial flavors and colored with dyes! The same quality that you find in your herbs apply to children's supplements as well. Artificial and synthetic materials are more likely to cause reactions in a child's body.

The same herbs that work gently for adults are also appropriate for kids. The following table includes several herbs that are ideal for children and that can be used safely in herbal remedies.

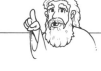

Sage Advice

Read the label of the formula you are using for a child, and begin with the recommend dosage for children or $1/2$ to $1/3$ the recommended adult dosage. Recommended dosages are usually smaller than what a person may need when ill, but starting slowly is the best caution. Also, the smaller the child, the less he or she will need.

Common Herbs Safe for Children's Use

Herb	Used For	Body System Support
Astragalus	Colds	Immune system
Catnip and fennel	Colic	Nervous and digestive systems
Catnip and garlic enema	Breaks fever	Immune and nervous systems
Chamomile	Calming, getting to sleep	Nervous system
Echinacea	Allergies, colds	Immune system
Elderberry	Mucus, runny nose, colds	Respiratory system
Garlic oil (externally)	Ear infections	Immune and respiratory systems
Licorice root	Energy, stress, coughs	Glandular system
Pau d'arco (externally)	Diaper rash	Immune system
Peppermint	Nausea, stimulant	Digestive system
Red Raspberry	Diarrhea	Intestinal system
Thyme	Stimulates thymus gland	Immune system (small doses)
White willow bark	Headaches	Nervous system

A good rule of thumb for discerning dosages for children is given here by Master Herbalist Humbart Santillio in his book *Natural Healing with Herbs* (Hohm Press, 1989):

Weight of child in pounds = fraction of adult dose to be used

Example: The average weight of an adult is 150 pounds. Divide the weight of the child by 150.

$$\frac{50 \text{ pound child}}{150 \text{ pound adult}} = \ ^{1}/_{3} \text{ of the adult recommended dosage}$$

When administering herbs to your children, it is best to start out with small doses and work your way up until results are achieved.

Here Kitty, Kitty: Herbs for Pets

Domestic pets need supplements because they are not part of the wild food chain in nature, which would supply them everything they need. Many domestic animals now suffer the same diseases that are suffered by humans, and pets can benefit from herbal supplements to help prevent these problems.

"Little Miss Outboard Kitty" relaxing after playing with her catnip stuffed sock. Herbs can be fed to our pets for their health, too.

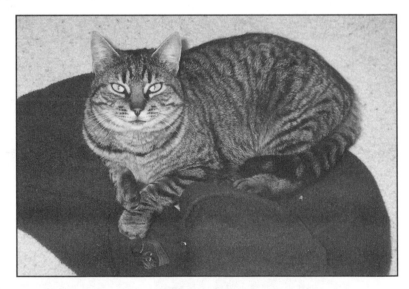

Usually when a pet has an upset stomach, it will try to find some grass to chew on. When your carnivorous pet chews on grass, it is because he is craving the chlorophyll from the green blades. Chlorophyll is rich in nutrients and minerals. You can put some liquid chlorophyll in your pet's water dish in the winter, when there might not be any grass available to munch on.

I tried an experiment with my own two dogs and chlorophyll: One had definite digestive troubles, and the other was lacking minerals, as recognized by his creaking joints. I set out three bowls of water, one with chlorophyll added, one with aloe vera added, and one just plain. After smelling each one, the dog that had arthritis drank up the chlorophyll. The one with digestive troubles chose the aloe vera. From then on, I added these to their water, with good results, including taking away my dogs' dog breath. The one with stiff joints seemed more limber, and the other was less gaseous—both made my home life much more pleasant.

Of course, liquid herbs are the easiest to administer to pets. You can also coat tablets or capsules in butter or some other food to get your dog to eat them. Most of the time they won't even know you have slipped them an herb! Cats are pickier eaters, so it may be wise to forget your carefully hidden pill placement and administer their herbs via a liquid or tincture.

The next table lists some common pet problems and some simple remedies you can use to help. Who knows, by feeding your dog herbs, you just might be able to teach an old dog new tricks!

Sage Advice

Another way to feed your pets herbs is to empty capsules into their dry food and mix this up with a little bit of olive oil. My dog loved the olive oil and never seemed to mind the herbs. The olive oil will also be beneficial to the animal, lubricating his joints and enhancing the shine on their fur coat.

Herbs for Pets

Problem: Dog Breath

Herbal Remedy: Liquid chlorophyll (Also it is a good idea to keep the kitty litter box inaccessible to dogs who take pleasure in dining on kitty 'treats.' This habit is definitely a breath destroyer!)

Administration: In water or straight; acts as a deodorizer in the body.

Problem: Fleas

Herbal Remedy: Garlic

Administration: Add to food. Externally, eucalyptus oil sprayed on fur is a natural repellent. You can also drip a few drops directly onto the skin and rub it in. The back of the neck is most effective, and makes it harder for your pet to lick off. Nutritional yeast flakes added to pet food have been helpful. Internally, high-potency garlic or garlic oil is best—this way you are getting a concentrated form over raw garlic, although raw garlic works well, too. Fleas and other pests hate the smell of garlic in the blood and will usually flee—this goes for some humans, too!

continues

Herbs for Pets (continued)

Problem: Foul gas

Herbal Remedy: Alfalfa pills or liquid chlorophyll

Administration: Crush and sprinkle on food, or add liquid chlorophyll to water. Has a deodorizing affect and will support digestion. (Hint: Make sure it is your pet and not your roommate that is the culprit. If so, offer some alfalfa or activated charcoal to your roommate!)

Problem: Structural problems

Herbal Remedy: Alfalfa, liquid chlorophyll, and olive oil

Administration: Crush alfalfa tablets, sprinkle on food, and mix with olive oil. Add liquid chlorophyll to drinking water.

Problem: Kidney/urinary tract problems

Herbal Remedy: Parsley

Administration: Chop fresh and add to food, or give in pill form if easier. Parsley helps clean the urinary tract, if stones are present, decreases pets' protein intake, and supplements them with hydrangea, an herb used as a stone solvent.

Age-Old Herbs to Help Old Age

What is "old age" anyway? I define old age as feeling old. If I can't get up in the morning, step out on my balcony and stretch my arms into the air, and stand on my toes while I breathe in some fresh mountain air without coughing and ripping a tendon—then that is old age. If I can't ride a bike, take a hike, lift my (someday) grandchildren, swim, laugh hard, stretch, or bend without pain and joy, then … that's what I believe is being old.

Sage Advice

Studies show that our health is improved and we may live longer when we have a pet to care for. Here's a hint: Adopt a pet, name it Joy, and you will always have Joy in your life.

If you are going to live a long life, why not feel good living it? No one wants to be a mentally active adult person trapped in an invalid body when it could be prevented with proper care! It is not the way life was meant to be lived! And who wants to look forward to burdening friends or relatives with having to take care of us, when we could have taken better care of ourselves and prevented debilitation in the first place?

The good news is that we now know that herbs can help you keep your mental and physical functions maintained. You can start now to prevent these diseases from creeping up. In addition to the right nutrients, stay active, keep running or at least walking briskly, and old age won't catch up with you as fast!

Take a look at the active "older" people around and see what there is to learn from them. Many 50+ adults can run circles around inactive folks half their age and younger! An inspirational example is astronaut and political leader John Glenn. He passed strenuous physical fitness tests in his 70s and went into space again! We can all do it, too. All the body needs to slow the aging process down to a more reasonable pace is to be provided the right materials.

Some preventative herbs you can begin taking now include herbs rich in antioxidants. Antioxidants are substances in foods and herbs that fight against the damaging effects of free radical activity in our body. The older you get, the more stress you have, the more toxins you ingest, the more free radical damage takes place. Free radical damage is one of the biggest factors in aging.

Herbs rich in antioxidants include peppermint, sage, spearmint, rosemary, oregano, red clover, savory, and thyme. Green tea is a great antioxidant drink. Consider having a cup or two of herb tea daily that includes any or all of the antioxidant herbs.

Other popular herbs to hold back the hands of time include ginkgo biloba, gotu kola, American ginseng, evening primrose oil, garlic, and milk thistle (preserves the liver).

Herb Lore

Did you know that your body is actually designed to live up to 120 years? Why then are so many checking out in our 70s? Most of you have a long life in front of you—why not make it a healthier one? Exercise the body and the mind and incorporate herbs and supplements along with a reasonable diet to help slow the aging process and deter age-related ailments.

Now, some of you might just want to help your elderly grandma or great grandparent with some herbs that will aid in some of their general discomforts and may be past the point of prevention, so let's take a look at how we can help these dear folks.

Fortunately, herbs come in so many different forms that there is an easy way for everyone to take them. Many times the elderly folks don't like to swallow pills and prefer a chewable or liquid form.

As we age, especially after age 50, digestion is usually less than optimum (unless, of course, you have been maintaining your health with herbs!). Folks into their 70s and 80s usually have very weakened digestion, and the liquid and chewable tablets will help them get better absorption than taking capsules or tablets.

The next table lists some of the top herbs that can be taken daily by elderly people for a healthier life. No matter what your age, it's not too late to begin taking these supplements to prevent premature aging.

Best Herbs for Elderly Folks

Herb	Description	How to Take
Liquid chlorophyll	Supports digestion, easily assimilated, aids tissue repair, purifies the liver, works as a body deodorizer, and provides easily assimilated minerals.	Add a tablespoon to a glass of water three times daily.
Chewable papaya and peppermint tablets	Supply enzymes that strengthen digestion and help break down proteins; peppermint is a stimulant for stomach acid secretions and aids digestion. Peppermint also acts as a stimulant and can help keep you more alert.	Chew one to two tablets before and after meals.
Whole-leaf aloe vera	The aloe vera plant is one of the most widely utilized healing plants; not only is it a good remedy for external applications to soothe burns, but internally it also works to soothe irritated tissues, cleanse the bowel, and provide concentrated nutrition such as many B vitamins, 18 amino acids, vitamin C, and selenium.	Add a capful daily to water or juice, or drink straight.
Ginkgo biloba and/ or gotu kola	Both are brain tonics; ginkgo is used in Germany to treat Alzheimer's disease, and gotu kola helps rebuild energy, stamina, and memory. Studies show noticeable memory improvements within four to six weeks.	These two herbs can be used together or separately. Take according to directions. A tea can be made, but a standardized product will be found in a pill. Take caution if you are on prescription blood thinners, as both of these herbs can thin the blood. See your physician and your holistic practitioner before taking any herbs if you are on medications.

Herbs that can benefit us as we age and also that can prevent us from age-related health problems include:

➤ Herbs that support the digestive and intestinal tract

➤ Herbs rich in minerals (many people get structural weakness, such as osteoporosis, arthritis, and other bone disorders in old age—and sometimes sooner if the proper nutrients are not furnished in the diet)

➤ Herbs that feed and support the brain and that tone the senses

As you've read in this chapter, it's never too late or too early to begin taking herbs. So what are you waiting for? More thyme?

The Least You Need to Know

➤ Some herbs help cleanse the body before pregnancy and others can be used as nourishment for a healthy pregnancy.

➤ Herbs can alleviate many pregnancy-related ills.

➤ Children respond quickly to herbs and need smaller doses than adults.

➤ Used responsibly, herbs can enhance the health of children, pregnant women, pets, and the elderly.

➤ Herbs can be used to counteract the effects of aging.

Part 2
When You're Bugged by Illnesses A–G

Don't you wish that one herb was your cure-all for any ailment starting with the letters A through G? Well, there's not!

But we will cover about four to six ailments in each chapter that begin with these letters, and then I'll give you some herbal remedies that have been used to help. So, let's proceed with the first third of the alphabet, beginning with a very common ailment, so you can sing "A, B, C, D, E, F, G; now I have an herbal rem-a-dee!"

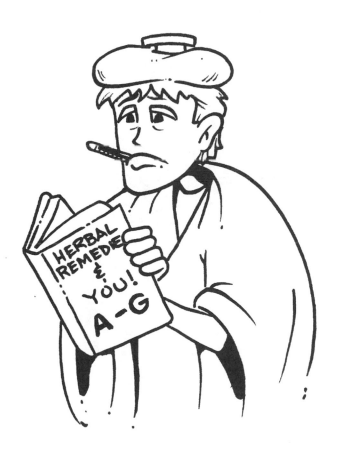

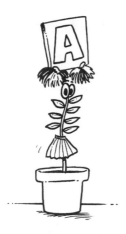

A Is for Ailment

Starting with this chapter, you'll find information on particular ailments and some herbal remedies that can help. Along the way, you'll also get some insight on what may be causing your problem in the first place. This is to help you make smarter choices that will facilitate a quicker recovery. Using the quick reference chart at the end of each chapter might get you quick results, but read the chapter thoroughly for more insight on how to help yourself maintain and prevent your problem from recurring.

Acne: Squeezing Out a Cure

Acne is a condition of the skin in which oil produced by your glands just below the skin gets trapped, producing inflammation—and usually infection. Unfortunately, acne commonly occurs on the face, making it an unsightly problem that needs to be cleared up once and for all.

Keeping the face clean is certainly important when suffering from acne, but a dirty face is not usually the core problem. Acne occurs because of overactive glands, usually hormonally induced. In addition, excess toxins usually are present in the blood and are being eliminated through the skin, causing skin conditions such as acne, pimples, and/or rashes.

Botanical Bit

Acne is a condition of the skin in which the sebaceous glands become inflamed and usually infected. This condition commonly occurs on the face and is more common in adolescents.

Adolescent Acne: An Herbal Cure Is Zit!

As if being a teenager isn't hard enough, now you have pimples to deal with! No doubt this condition is annoying, but before you cancel your engagements for the rest of your life, read on to see how herbs can help.

The liver is instrumental in filtering away excess hormones. In the teen years, our body fluctuates its hormone production—sometimes wildly. Therefore, when our liver (which is responsible for filtering excess hormones from the blood) can't keep up with this pace, we find the excess hormones in the blood showing up as acne or pimples on the face.

Making up for the insufficient liver-filtering function by cleansing the blood and liver is an effective approach toward clearing up the problem. Additionally, cleansing the bowel helps get rid of toxins through the intestinal system instead of the skin—a nicer way to go!

Burdock Root: Cleaning the Blood

One of the best-known blood cleansers to herbalists is burdock root. Burdock (*Arctium lappa*) not only cleanses the blood of excess wastes, but it also helps your glands regulate hormonal balance. Burdock seems to be very politically active—it is against everything! Burdock is anti-fungal, anti-bacterial, anti-inflammatory, and anti-tumor. These qualities make it helpful for anti-acne, too.

Burdock seems to work well for cleansing the liver, kidneys, and bowel, and is therefore helpful for clearing up associated symptoms. Soak a cotton ball in a burdock fomentation or tea and apply to your face for a toning effect.

Herb Lore

In Russia, the use of burdock root can be traced back through many generations as a food and as a medicine. The parsnip-like roots of this plant can be boiled as a vegetable and the leaves steamed. Medicinally, burdock has been used in Russia as a remedy for gout, rheumatism, and dropsy. The inventor of Velcro is said to have been inspired by observing the curved hooks of the burdock burrs under a microscope.

Burdock has also been used to ease anger, irritability, cancer, eczema, chicken pox, measles, and mumps. It has been used as a hair rinse for dandruff, and the juice has been drunk to rid the body of mites. Burdock also may serve as a mild aphrodisiac.

Females who need a little more help regulating those hormones can add extra herbs that support balance for the glands, such as black cohosh, red raspberry, dong quai, and evening primrose oil. Adolescent males need balance, too, and can take sarsaparilla in addition to burdock root for a glandular balancing act. Sarsaparilla has been referred to as a "cowboy tonic" because cowboys used to order sarsaparilla (root beer) in the late 1800s and believed it to be a cure for syphilis.

On the Surface

Topically, keep your face clean and apply tea tree oil to infected pimples. The tea tree oil is very drying, so use it topically to help dry up infection. Be careful that you don't apply it so often that it makes your skin dry and flaky, however. A tea tree oil soap is very effective for washing and drying up infection at the same time. Tea tree oil is antiseptic and anti-fungal, prevents infections, and even acts as a local anesthetic to reduce pain.

A little sunshine on your face will not only help you get some vitamin D, which helps the skin, but will also help to clear your acne condition. But of course don't overdo the sunshine!

You've Heard This Before

Finally, stay away from junk food! Excess caffeine, sugar, and oily fats overburdens the liver and defeats your goal. Drink plenty of pure water; adding some lemon to your drinking water will help, too—vitamin C content in the lemon will help cure skin problems, and lemon is a good tonic for the liver.

Sage Advice

Pumpkin seeds are a good source of natural zinc, which aids in wound healing and helps clear up any skin condition, especially acne. Eating pumpkin seeds is a safe way to supplement your body with zinc—provided that you enjoy pumpkin seeds, of course!

Adult Acne: A More Mature Approach

If you are a female adult and you suddenly begin to break out with pimples, my first suggestion would be to get a check-up by your obstetrician or gynecologist. Have the doctor check for any type of reproductive organ problems, growths, or any other problems. If you are on any type of hormonal replacement therapy or any medications that have an effect on your hormones, have your dosage checked. A sudden acne or pimple problem can mean that your hormones are fluctuating—and you need to know why! If your doctor finds no problem, regulating your hormones with the use of herbs can help calm them down or tone them up, whichever may be needed.

Herb Lore

A 28-year-old client couldn't take her birth control pill without terrible break-outs. A combination of red clover, pau d'arco, yellow dock, burdock, sarsaparilla, dandelion, horseradish, cascara sagrada, buckthorn, peach bark, barberry, stillingia, prickly ash, and yarrow—along with two cascara sagrada pills each night and four acidophilus pills each morning—cleared her up right away. (As a side benefit, her bowels were stimulated into action!) She decided after her face was all clear to stop her herbal program. Within one week, the acne was back. The program worked for her until she discontinued the birth control pill. She still occasionally takes cascara sagrada to keep things moving, and she continues to have beautiful, clear skin.

Note any changes in your diet or facial products that could have caused a temporary break-out. Some adults who pick up coffee drinking as a new habit will quickly be burdened with new blemishes; the oil from the coffee beans may be the cause of a break-out. What? No more afternoon cappuccinos?

Burdock and Red Clover: Your Pimple Problems Are Over

Adults with acne can follow the same herbal advice for teenagers by using burdock root to cleanse the blood. For men or women, red clover (*Trifolium pratense*) taken internally has been an excellent herb for cleansing the blood and clearing up skin ailments such as acne. You can support the liver (which filters excess hormones from the blood) to get to the source of your problem. Take two to three tablets of either burdock, milk thistle, red clover, or dandelion two to three times daily to help your face clear up.

Red clover has been used for centuries as a key herbal ingredient in fighting cancer because of its effect on cleansing the blood and liver and assisting with protein assimilation. See Chapter 8, "C's for a Common Cure," for a more detailed look at red clover.

Both men and women can take supplemental zinc, vitamins A and D, and niacin. All have proven helpful for acne. Zinc helps in skin healing of any kind, vitamins A and D feed the skin, and niacin helps flush built-up wastes from the circulatory system.

Poison Ivy

Be warned that when taking niacin, you may experience a temporary hot rash or lightheadedness known as a niacin flush. Some believe that the more you flush, the more you need it. You might want to talk to your doctor or vitamin expert before taking niacin because it has been used as an adjunct therapy for high cholesterol levels.

Inside and Outside

To cleanse the bowel, colonic irrigations or Ivy's colon cleanse (see Chapter 4, "Herbs Are Not Just for Hippies Anymore") should prove helpful almost right away, although the red clover or burdock root may act as a mild laxative for you. You can utilize a periodic herbal cleansing to assist your body with any ailment, and it will make you feel better and healthier and clear up your skin. A cleanse doesn't need to be harsh to be effective. A gentle, slow-cleansing action can be obtained by adjusting your herbs accordingly. Red clover, in fact, acts as a slow detoxifier. See your herbalist to find a cleanse that is right for your body. Otherwise, give Ivy's cleanse a try.

Herb Lore

The key in 80 percent of all health problems, including skin conditions, begins in the bowel. Here's how the whole mess gets started: When our digestion is not optimum (learn more about that in Chapter 12) the intestines get loaded up with undigested proteins, hardened feces, mucus, and parasites. When this happens, the symptoms and ailments we face are endless. Since the blood has the job of carrying assimilated nutrients from the intestines to the rest of the body via the blood, it also picks up the toxins and distributes them throughout the rest of the body. The skin is an elimination channel for the blood wastes, and toxic blood can equal poor skin conditions!

Tea tree oil may be used topically to help dry up the condition (see the previous section, "Adolescent Acne: An Herbal Cure Is Zit!"). Don't forget to get a little sunshine on your face, too.

Allergies Bee Gone

In general, allergy symptoms are miserable. Some people suffer from different types of allergies; however, whether you are allergic to hay, pollens, molds, animal dander, or things that irritate your skin when you come in contact with them, the irritating symptoms are all quite common.

Most allergy symptoms (not including food allergies, which will be addressed later) include one or more of the following symptoms:

➤ Itchy throat, nose, eyes, and ears

➤ Watery eyes

➤ Runny or stuffy nose

➤ Tightness in chest

➤ Sneezing, coughing

➤ Fever

The good news is that your body is still working by giving you a runny nose, watery eyes, and generally making you miserable. As irritating as these symptoms are, they are mechanisms that are protecting your body from accepting what it believes to be a toxin. Helping your body get rid of these toxins is better than plugging them up with medications and having the toxins settle back into your tissues.

Herb Lore

The root cause of many allergies is a taxed immune system. When the body is dealing with an abundance of toxins, the immune system is already busy. When another pollutant is then introduced, the body can react very strongly to rid itself of the allergen. I have seen allergies clear up time and time again in folks who have cleansed their systems and then strengthened their immune systems using herbs.

Your body will need a little rest and some cleansing if you are experiencing any type of allergies. Fortunately, some herbal remedies can help alleviate some symptoms and boost your immune system, which can raise your tolerance level for new allergens. Let's take a look at which ones!

Bee Pollen: Bumbling to Get Some

If I had my choice of only one herb for hay fever or any allergy, I would have to utilize bee pollen. Bee pollen has proved to be one of the best foods/herbs that will help with allergies of any kind. Bee pollen is exactly what it sounds like: not a substance made by bees, but a substance collected *from* bees. It is usually gathered by gently scraping off the hind legs of the bees after they return home from a day of feeding on flowers and plants. Beekeepers set up special homes for bees that squeeze the collected pollen into a container when the bee enters the hive.

When the bee drinks from a flower, he is naturally dusted with the flower pollen. He spreads this pollen to the next flower or plant he feasts on and, in turn, is instrumental in the reproductive life of plants. When the bee returns home, the beekeepers save up the pollen and bring it to you for your allergies. Bee pollen is rich in many nutrients. Just a few include these:

➤ Zinc

➤ Vitamin A

➤ Vitamin C

➤ Calcium

➤ Potassium

➤ Iron

➤ B-complex vitamins

➤ Enzymes

You can consider bee pollen a survival food because it contains every substance needed by the body to maintain life. Bee pollen is most effective when taken before your typical allergy season begins. If you know when your most intensive suffering season is, begin taking bee pollen three months beforehand, and slowly increase your dosages as the season hits. Maintain dosages during the entire time, or increase as needed.

Some believe that bee pollen is more effective if you get local pollen from local beekeepers, but I have seen local and non-local bee pollen work for all types of allergies. If you have severe allergies, a local pollen may cause more reaction at first. Bee pollen works by slowing helping your body to build a resistance to the allergens. Taking it is like inoculating yourself against allergies. Because bee pollen strengthens the entire body by nourishing you, any bee pollen you can obtain should prove helpful, but your best bet is to begin with small doses and work your way up slowly.

Sage Advice

Herbalist and nurse Elaine Nerland of Arlington, Washington, offers this advice when first taking bee pollen: Take one granule of pollen and see how you react to it before taking more. Place one tiny granule on the tip of your tongue and let your body absorb it. Wait at least 20 minutes to monitor your reaction before taking more.

Poison Ivy

If you have an allergy to bees, you might not want to use bee pollen. Every once in a while, a bee stinger will be found in the bee pollen, which might cause an allergic reaction. Ask your doctor if you suspect an allergy to bees before taking it, and give barley green juice powder a try instead.

More Supplements Not to Sneeze At

Many good herbs for the respiratory system exist, such as horseradish, which can clear out your sinuses immediately. Horseradish is a very strong herb (and condiment) and should be used carefully, as it might burn sensitive tissues. You can find horseradish usually combined with other herbal combinations for the respiratory system, such as fenugreek, mullein, fennel, and boneset.

Vitamin C and pantothenic acid (one of the B vitamins) sometimes have helped to arrest or slow down the allergy attack, and these should be considered in severe cases. Both of these vitamins are water-soluble, which means that excess will leave your body and will not cause a toxic build-up like a fat-soluble vitamin can.

There's no way to eliminate the airborne allergens from the outside, but here are some tips you can use to change your home environment:

Sage Advice

Eucalyptus oil is the essential oil gathered from the leaves and twigs of the eucalyptus tree. It has been used for many ailments, especially those of the respiratory system. The pure oil contains strong antibacterial, antifungal, antiviral, and antiseptic properties.

➤ If you are allergy-free during hay fever season but have symptoms at other times of the year, you could be allergic to mold spores, dust, or other airborne particles. Pinpointing exactly what you are allergic to will be helpful in your recovery, but there is no harm in taking all my suggestions here.

➤ Clean all linens, bedding, and pillows thoroughly. These tend to harbor dust mites, which can irritate the respiratory system and add to your sneezing. When washing, add a few drops of eucalyptus oil to the wash water. This natural oil kills dust mites and other pests and will help purify the wash. Allergenic pillowcase covers and other protective covers can be put over your existing bedding to protect your sensitive sinus passages. These can be found in many different natural health product catalogs.

➤ If you are allergic to dust and live in a dry climate, a humidifier will help keep the dust particles from flying around shamelessly. Pure essential oil of lemon or other citrus fruit oil will help purify the air you breathe. If you are allergic to molds, a humidifier may not be the best choice. But if you live in a moist climate and have mold and fungus spores, try diffusing tea tree or eucalyptus oil (both anti-fungal remedies), which can help keep the mold count down in the room you are diffusing.

➤ For eye irritants, make an herbal eyewash from a tea made from golden seal, bayberry, eyebright, and red raspberry, or any mixture of the four. Be sure to strain all the herbs from the tea. Once it is cool, use a dropper and administer as eye drops for itching, swollen, or infected eyes. This will help tone the eyes and take the itch out. Refrigerate tea, and do not keep for longer than two to three days at a time.

➤ Lemonade with capsicum is a cleansing drink that can be taken every day to help cleanse the body and push out irritants from the system. Make some homemade fresh lemonade, and add a pinch of cayenne pepper. The combination will taste sour and hot at the same time, an interesting combination. Try it—you'll like it!

Food Allergies

Many different symptoms can be linked to or caused by food allergies or food intolerance, including these:

➤ Respiratory ailments

➤ Skin reactions and rashes

➤ Mood swings

➤ Restriction of bronchials

➤ Migraines or headaches

➤ Racing heart or palpitations

➤ Copious mucus production

➤ Fatigue

➤ Flatulence and belching

➤ Heartburn

➤ Diarrhea or constipation

Sometimes food intolerance is created over the years by eating a food every day. For instance, allergy to wheat is one of the most common food allergies. Wheat can be found in almost everything these days, including pasta, breads, crackers, and cereals. It's not that wheat is bad, but eating a food over and over can deplete our body's enzymes for breaking down that particular food. This can lead to improper digestion of the food, and when improperly digested food particles pass into the blood stream, they are unrecognizable to your immune system. As a result, your body considers these particles foreign bodies that should be attacked. This attack of your immune system may be experienced as allergy symptoms.

The best way to find out if you are intolerant or allergic to a food is to eliminate it from your diet completely for a couple weeks. Watch the signals your body gives you as you abstain. Sometimes you will drool, have wild cravings, get grouchy, or have headaches for the first few days. This withdrawal is a good indication that you might have had a food allergy. After a couple weeks, eat a small portion of the food again. You should be able to tell right away if you are experiencing any negative effects from the food. You can also take a pulse test to see if you might have a food allergy.

Once you know what you are allergic to, you will need to eliminate it while you build up your

Sage Advice

To self-test for possible food allergies, take your pulse just before eating a suspect food and then again 20–30 minutes after you eat the food. If your pulse rises significantly (15 beats per minute or more), this could indicate a food allergy. More conclusive tests can be taken by an allergist.

enzyme reserves in the body again. The most common food allergies are to wheat, corn, eggs, peanuts, dairy, citrus fruits, MSG and other food additives, chocolate (oh no!), and vegetables of the nightshade family (tomatoes, chili peppers, eggplant, potatoes).

Can You Stomach It?

Supporting your digestion with raw foods and supplemental enzymes will help in all food allergies and food intolerance. As I explained earlier, proper digestion is a key factor in eliminating food allergy symptoms. Let's take a look at the digestive process so you can understand why digestion is so important.

Digestion begins in the mouth. When we chew our foods, food particles are mixed with enzymes in the saliva called amylase. Then the partially digested food gets swallowed and enters the stomach. The stomach churns the food and secretes hydrochloric acid to sterilize the food and break it down further. The stomach relies on enzymes contained in raw foods to help break down the foods we eat. If the food was processed or cooked, it will be devoid of enzymes, so the pancreas and liver have to kick in to produce enzymes to aid the digestion process. After all this takes place, the food (now called chyme) enters the small intestines where it begins the process of being absorbed by tiny protrusions inside the intestines called villi.

Sounds good, you say? So what's the problem? Plenty of things can go wrong along the way, and here are a few:

➤ If the stomach did not have enough hydrochloric acid available to digest properly,

➤ If the liver and pancreas couldn't come up with the right amount of enzymes to properly break down the food, and

➤ If you didn't start off your digestive process correctly because you wolfed down your meal, inhibiting the proper amount of amylase enzyme needed to do a complete job, then troubles begin.

This inefficient digestion (caused by improper food and improper eating habits) will leave us vulnerable to undigested food particles passing through to the blood stream. The blood stream is the vehicle the body uses to distribute nutrients to the rest of the body. When food is properly broken down to its correct size, the immune system politely acknowledges it just as a friendly police officer would tip his hat to a law-abiding passerby, and expresses no need for concern. However, when a big ol' food particle passes through, and doesn't fit the profile of a properly digested particle (i.e., law-abiding citizen), the body recognizes it as an invader and sends off the alarms for the immune system (our internal police) to go into attack mode!

When the immune system is trying to get rid of foreign invaders, you will usually experience some type of allergy-type symptom. This is what makes it so important to supply the body enzymes with the cooked foods we eat and to chew thoroughly. It not only will help your digestion, but will aid in calming an overly stimulated immune system and will help put your allergies to rest.

Mamma Mia: It's Papaya

Papaya fruit (*Carica Papaya*) is one of the best ways to supply enzymes for better digestion. The papaya is a fruit that is commonly made into a supplement and is taken (usually chewed) to support digestion. This is because its active enzymes help break down foods, especially proteins.

To improve digestion, chew two capsules before every meal. Sometimes papaya is combined with mint and will serve as a perfect after-dinner papaya mint!

Sage Advice

In many tropical countries, natives serve papaya fruit before every meal as a custom and because the enzymes aid in digestion.

More to Digest

Juicing raw fruits and vegetables will load you up with plenty of raw enzymes that can help strengthen digestion. In addition, other herbs and supplements support the digestive process, including marshmallow and pepsin. Pepsin is a protein digestive enzyme used to clear the accumulated protein waste from the intestinal walls, allowing the villi to absorb nutrients better. Marshmallow is a soothing digestive aid that carries the pepsin where it needs to go and then soaks up and carries bowel toxins out of the body. Marshmallow and pepsin definitely work as a synergistic team. Four of these capsules, or one each if you are taking individually, after each meal will clean your digestive tract and eliminate mucus from your system, which will make your allergies better.

Safflowers also aid digestion by stimulating the stomach to produce hydrochloric acid (HCl). One tablespoon of raw apple cider vinegar before or after meals helps many digest better, too.

A good combination of herbs to support the immune system that will help lessen the allergic reactions also includes:

➤ Rose hips (rich in vitamin C)

➤ Ginseng

➤ Parsley

➤ Red clover

➤ Wheat grass

➤ Horseradish

The real bottom line with all allergies is to eliminate the allergen if possible and aid your immune system by addressing any digestive troubles that could be an underlying cause of lowered immunity. Then support your immune system after you have taken care of the source of the problem. You can achieve much of this using herbs. Look for the summarized program in the table at the end of this chapter.

Environmental Allergies

Environmental allergies (that is, being environmentally sensitive) is an unusual but terrible condition. In these cases, the liver, one of our great filters of toxins, has usually been damaged by some exposure to a pesticide or poison that damaged its ability to filter toxins. In many cases the kidneys (also serving as filters for toxins) have also been damaged. The body becomes so sensitive that a walk into a hardware, department, or even grocery store that stocks detergents and other chemical products can cause a person migraine headaches, mood swings, vomiting, or dizziness that can sometimes last for days.

Work with a qualified professional to help you detoxify and support your liver and your entire body if you suffer from environmental allergies.

Milk Thistle: This–tle Do

Liver- and immune-supporting herbs are certainly called for if you are environmentally sensitive. Milk thistle (*Silybum marianum*) will help rebuild the liver and has even been shown to assist in the repair of already damaged liver cells. This tall green plant with a bristly purple flower on top is a common herb usually referred to as a weed—especially to those of us who happen to brush up against its prickly body! Much research has been done on this valuable weed to support its merit as a liver protector. This herb even has regenerative powers for liver cells as well.

Herb Lore

Renowned author Jean Carper writes in her book *Miracle Cures* about a Hungarian study done in 1992 on over 2,600 workers in a chemical plant who had been exposed to toxic vapors for years. All the workers showed liver damage, and their symptoms included nausea, lack of appetite, abdominal bloating, and fatigue. Some were given milk thistle, and after only 30 days, liver function tests found a definite improvement in the herb-takers, and enlarged livers returned to normal size.

Other Helpful Supplements

Liquid chlorophyll is another excellent remedy. The green pigment from the alfalfa plant is usually used to make liquid chlorophyll, a green wonder food that helps purify the blood and liver and that filters out toxins we come in contact with before they have a chance to harm us. See more on chlorophyll in Chapter 7, "B Well."

Combinations of herbs to detoxify the body from environmental pollutants include sarsaparilla, milk thistle, red clover, dandelion, yellow dock, burdock, marshmallow, pepsin, fenugreek, ginger, echinacea, and cascara sagrada.

Also make sure you do not bring any new items into your home that are not environmentally safe. Chemicals used to make paints and glues, and even fabrics used to make furniture, clothes, and other items can out-gas poisonous materials that may be undetected by smell but can wreak havoc on an already compromised system. Find places that offer "safe" furniture, cleaning products, clothes, art, and tenant finish materials. For instance, my holistic health spa floor is absolutely beautiful and was done by a team of environmentally sensitive artists who cannot tolerate toxic chemicals. The floor is unique, fabulously beautiful, and the best part is that it does not out-gas toxic chemicals into my healing spa!

Sage Advice

Doctor to Gil: "I'm afraid you have a long liver condition."

Gil to Doctor: "That's not surprising; since most of my relatives have lived past 100, I come from a family of long livers!"

Your local health food store may know of a source for you to purchase environmentally safe materials. Two good sources I have ordered through are:

Seventh Generation
49 Hercules Drive
Colchester, VT 05446
800-456-1177

Natural Materials
1365 Rutina Circle
Santa Fe, NM 87501
505-438-3448

If you are having any type of remodeling done and wish to use non-toxic yet beautiful designed materials, you can certainly contact the company I used for my spa. They work globally. Check with your architect or designer if you use one, to see if they are already in contact; if not, you can contact them directly at:

Enigma Design, LLC
2417 Bank Drive, Suite B-105
Boise, ID 83705
208-381-0764
E-mail: endesign@micron.net
www.enigmapaper.com

Even if you aren't environmentally sensitive, supporting these types of environmentally friendly, non-toxic companies and their products will help create a less toxic world for everyone.

Bowel cleansing will help to detoxify your body as well. You can use Ivy's cleanse described in Chapter 4, or read up on using enemas or colonic irrigation. An excellent book on bowel cleansing including using enemas, herbs, and diet is Dr. Bernard Jensen's *Tissue Cleansing Through Bowel Management* (Bernard Jensen Enterprises, 1981). You can call your local colonic therapist and discuss the procedure, or you can even contact the school I attended to become a certified colonic therapist. They will give you the name of a graduate close to you. Contact Wood Hygienic Institute in Kissimmee, Florida, USA, 407-933-0009. Also consider steam bath detoxification. Some holistic spas will have places where you can use these safely. (Steam rooms, however, are not recommended for pregnant women.)

In addition, purchasing a juicer and juicing fresh organic fruits and vegetables is a healthy addition to any lifestyle and will be helpful to the environmentally sensitive.

Avoid overburdening your body with toxins by eating only organic foods. Some local farmers offer pesticide-free foods; buy from a source you trust.

Sage Advice

You can make a detoxing bath by adding a handful of Epsom salts to the water. Soak in this tub for an hour or until the water cools. Don't be surprised if you see a thick ring of sludge around the tub when you are through!

Alzheimer's: Don't Forget to Take Your Herbs

Alzheimer's disease is a progressive degenerative disease that negatively affects a person's memory. The disease strikes predominately in the elderly, but can begin any time in adulthood.

Botanical Bit

Alzheimer's disease is a progressive form of dementia occurring in middle age or later for which there is no medical treatment. It is associated with severe degeneration of the brain.

Some known and suspected causes of Alzheimer's disease include:

➤ An excess of aluminum in the body: Sometimes aluminum can build up from high aluminum content in the drinking water, aluminum from personal health care products, and even some over-the-counter medications. Read all labels carefully! Get a hair mineral analysis to find out if you might have excess aluminum. Ask your local holistic practitioner about this procedure.

➤ Dental work: Some people believe that fumes from silver fillings (which contain mercury) cause dementia over time. Discuss the possibility of having your fillings replaced with a composite material if this is a concern. For a biologically or holistically oriented dentist, contact the Environmental Dental Association at 800-388-8124 or 619-586-1208, or The International Academy of Oral Medicine and Toxicology at 407-298-2450.

➤ Poor circulation: Make sure there are no circulatory problems when it comes to Alzheimer's disease, as any lack of oxygen and blood supply to the brain can affect thinking. Consider herbs such as ginkgo and gotu kola to improve brain circulation.

Ginko Biloba: Did I Mention That Already?

Prevention is best when it comes to Alzheimer's disease, but in Germany this condition is treated with a wonder herb called ginkgo biloba. Ginkgo biloba (*Ginkgo biloba*) is a heavily studied herb from China that has proven over and over again its positive effects on the brain and the circulatory system. The ginkgo tree is one of the oldest living trees in China, and some have used its leaves in books to prevent bookworms!

The best results for Alzheimer's disease can be seen after several months of steady use, although some improvement can be noticed sooner. Ginkgo has been shown to greatly slow down the degeneration caused by Alzheimer's disease and even to restore a better memory to others. Ginkgo increases blood supply to the brain, which helps bring the brain needed nutrients such as oxygen and glucose. If I had only one herb to use for any type of memory problems, it would have to be ginkgo. To fight Alzheimer's take 240 mg of standardized ginkgo twice daily, before meals. If you are not suffering from the disease, but want a memory boost, 40–80 mg two times a day should be sufficient.

Sage Advice

Studies on ginkgo shows that a positive effect in brain wave activity can be detected in humans within 20 minutes after ingestion of the herb.

Food for Thought

Gotu kola (*Hydrocotyle asiatica*) is another excellent brain food herb that can be combined with ginkgo for added effect. The gotu kola leaves are used in Ayurvedic (Indian) medicine especially for nervous system disorders. Author and Master Herbalist Louise Tenney says that "Two capsules a day will keep old age away." For more on gotu kola, see the section "Tinnitus (Ringing in Ears)" in Chapter 21, "T: Terrific Solutions."

Other brain foods you can take in supplement form are lecithin, zinc, B-complex, and vitamin E (which helps with circulation). Remember this zinc rhyme, "If you drink, take zinc; if you stink, take zinc; if you need to think, take zinc." Zinc should be taken in an herbal form, such as herbal pumpkin. If you are taking a zinc pill, do not exceed 45 mg per day without supervision. Too much or too little zinc can lower your immune system. Make sure you are getting the right amount for you.

Just a Reminder

Also keep your brain active by reading (there are plenty of *Complete Idiot's Guides* out there that will interest you!). Make changes in your life that help you think in new ways. Practice or play memory games, and if you are beginning to be forgetful, think about working preventatively with herbs right away.

Herbal Remedies for Common Ailments

Acne, Adolescent Female

Best Single Herb: Burdock root

Best Combinations: Golden seal, red raspberry, black cohosh, ginger, queen of the meadow, blessed thistle, dong quai, marshmallow, capsicum, althea; burdock root

Other Helpful Supplements: Zinc; beta carotene

Possible Causes: Junk food, especially oily foods and caffeine; constipation—answer when nature calls!

Complementary Help: Use tea tree oil topically; drink lots of water with lemon; get plenty of sunshine

Acne, Adolescent Male

Best Single Herb: Burdock root

Best Combinations: Sarsaparilla; burdock root

Other Helpful Supplements: Zinc; beta carotene

Possible Causes: Hormonal adjustments, junk food, constipation, sluggish liver

Complementary Help: Use tea tree oil externally; drink lots of water with lemon; eat lots of pumpkin seeds (rich in zinc, which helps heal skin); get plenty of sunshine

Acne, Adult

Best Single Herb: Burdock root

Best Combinations: Red clover, pau d'arco, yellow dock, burdock root, sarsaparilla, dandelion, horseradish, cascara sagrada, buckthorn, peach bark, barberry, stillengia, prickly ash, yarrow

Other Helpful Supplements: Zinc; vitamins A and D; niacin

Possible Causes: Dirty bowel; sluggish liver; hormone medications too strong/weak; hormonal changes

Complementary Help: Tea tree oil used externally; bowel cleansing; sunshine

Allergies, Hay Fever

Best Single Herb: Bee pollen

Best Combinations: Boneset, fennel, fenugreek, horseradish, mullein; bee pollen

Other Helpful Supplements: Vitamin C; pantothenic acid

Possible Causes: Lowered immune system; need for rest and strengthening therapies; exposure to allergens

Complementary Help: Fresh-squeezed lemon juice with pinch of cayenne pepper (drink twice a day); bowel cleansing

Allergies, Molds, Dust, Pollen

Best Single Herb: Bee pollen

Best Combinations: Burdock, golden seal, parsley, althea, ephedra, capsicum, horehound, yerba santa; bee pollen

Other Helpful Supplements: Pantothenic acid; vitamin C

Possible Causes: Lowered immune system, need for cleansing and strengthening therapies

Complementary Help: Cleanse bowel; use diffuser or humidifier where applicable; clean bedding; use an herbal eyewash

Allergies, Food

Best Single Herb: Papaya

Best Combinations: Marshmallow and pepsin to support digestion; rose hips, ginseng, parsley, red clover, wheat grass powder, and horseradish to support the immune system

Other Helpful Supplements: Food enzyme tablets with hydrochloric acid

Possible Causes: Low enzymes for particular foods

Complementary Help: Juicing broccoli, cabbage, carrots, and all raw fruits and veggies; find out which foods you are allergic to by rotating your diet

Allergies, Environmental

Best Single Herb: Milk thistle

Best Combinations: Sarsaparilla, milk thistle, red clover, dandelion, yellow dock, burdock, marshmallow, pepsin, fenugreek, ginger, echinacea, cascara sagrada

Other Helpful Supplements: Liquid chlorophyll; acidophilus; antioxidants; olive leaf extract

Possible Causes: Liver damage; immune system needs strengthening

Complementary Help: Cleansing bowel; juicing fresh fruits and vegetables; using only organic foods and natural home and beauty products; taking a steam bath; using Epson salt baths

Alzheimer's Disease

Best Single Herb: Ginkgo biloba

Best Combinations: Ginkgo, gotu kola

Other Helpful Supplements: Lecithin; zinc; B-complex; vitamin E

Possible Causes: Check dental work for fillings; eliminate beauty products or antacids that contain aluminum; drink only purified water

Complementary Help: Check for circulatory problems

The Least You Need to Know

➤ Finding out what is causing your ailment will empower you to apply the best remedies and will prevent you from experiencing the problem again.

➤ Bee pollen is one of the most widely used and seemingly effective remedies for hay fever and other allergies.

➤ Chinese ephedra (also known as ma huang) has been used successfully by asthma sufferers but is too strong for some and illegal in some states. Use lobelia instead if either of these apply to you.

➤ Most allergies are a response to an overburdened immune system; sometimes brought about by improper digestion. Strengthening the immune system with herbs will therefore help your allergies.

➤ Studies show that Alzheimer's disease can be arrested—or at least slowed—with the use of ginkgo biloba.

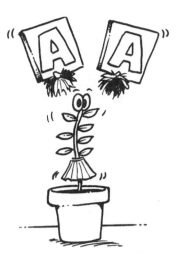

Chapter 6

Give Me Another A!

In This Chapter

➤ Calm anxiety with herbs

➤ Breathe better using herbs for asthma

➤ Use herbal applications for arthritis

➤ Find the root cause of your ailments

I once said that having a problem and just reaching for an herb to cure you is never as good as working toward total health by prevention with a diet of whole raw foods, pure water, fresh air, sunshine, positive mental attitude, daily affirmations, exercise, weekly reflexology treatments, monthly massages, worry-free relationships, a bright, happy spouse who cooks and cleans for you, and a perfect home surrounded by all the luxuries you could ever imagine—well, okay, you'd better reach for those herbs!

Here we continue with ailments beginning with the letter A, and we cover anxiety, asthma, and arthritis, and some possible causes and herbal remedies to help prevent and alleviate these things. Now sit back, relax, and let's talk about anxiety.

Anxiety: Panic Not—Herbs to the Rescue

Anxiety is a common and normal part of life, especially when trying to find the best herb for your needs in a hot, crowded health food store with hundreds of people shoving past you wildly grabbing herbs to stockpile for the year 2000 crises! Just kidding.

An *anxiety attack* is also commonly referred to as a *panic attack*. Either is brought on by excessive fear and can be characterized by the following:

➤ A rapid heartbeat

➤ Shortness of breath

➤ An out-of-control feeling

➤ Shaking

➤ Uncontrollable crying

These attacks are more common in women than men and are usually related to some psychological factor. Too much change at one time, family- or work-related stresses, or anything that makes you feel overwhelmed can trigger an attack.

Other factors that could trigger or disguise themselves as panic attacks are:

➤ Food stimulants, such as caffeine or sugar.

➤ Any foods to which you could be allergic.

➤ Chemical food additives such as MSG (mono sodium glutamate), aspartame (commonly known as NutriSweet®), and the like could also make you have what you believe to be a panic attack.

If these attacks are a recurring problem, it is helpful to take notes and record what you have eaten, drunk, or even chewed before each of your attacks. A daily journal can give you feedback on the big picture and will help you pinpoint patterns.

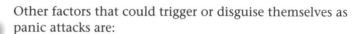

Botanical Bit

An **anxiety attack** or **panic attack** involves pervasive fear dominating the feelings and can be characterized by a rapid heartbeat, shortness of breath, an out-of-control feeling, shaking, or uncontrollable crying. These attacks are more common in women than men and are usually related to some psychological factor.

Valerian: Nature's Valium

For panic attacks in progress, or to help prevent attacks when you feel vulnerable, take a few capsules of the herb valerian root (*Valeriana officinalis*). Valerian root is nourishing and soothing to the nervous system and can ease hysteria. It contains calcium and magnesium and calms without the sedative side effects of prescription drugs. The energetics of valerian seem to work best on folks who are in a "cold" condition (refer back to the discussion on energetics in Chapter 3, "What to Expect with Herbs"), which means that they might look pale, have cold extremities, or feel clammy to the touch.

Poison Ivy

Although valerian acts as a sedative for most people, those with low thyroid activity should not take this herb because its effects can be stimulating.

This herb also has been used in folk medicine to promote sleep. As a sleep aid try two to three capsules before bed. In northern England, the dried root is added to meats as a preservative. To obtain the best medicinal effects from valerian, it should be dried because it gets stronger with age.

Don't Worry—Be Hoppy

For panic attacks with a "hot" condition in the body, hops (*Humulus lupulus*) is a better choice over valerian. You will know when you or someone is having a hot-type attack because the face becomes flushed and the person is more actively hysterical.

Hops are mild herbal downers and are used in making beer. This may be the reason that some folks like to wind down with a few beers after work or on the weekends—they just may be craving the soothing effects of the hops. Ironically, hops have been used to ease DTs (effects from alcohol withdrawal), and they support the nervous system and can help you calm your anxiety. Take two hops capsules before bed if you are having trouble sleeping, a cup or two of chamomile and hop tea will work as well, plus the chamomile makes the tea taste good.

Neither valerian nor hops should be used consistently over long periods of time, however, because they can bring you down too far. Use them during times of change or stress that can trigger anxiety, or as a safe relaxing aid.

Lettuce Relax with Some Herbal Combinations

Wild lettuce leaves contain properties that can serve to ease anxiety. Many times wild lettuce will come in the form of a tincture and needs refrigeration. A well-known combination of herbs used for general stress management includes a mix of chamomile, passion flower, hops, fennel, marshmallow, and feverfew.

Other supplements that feed the nervous system include the B-complex vitamins. Magnesium also serves as a muscle relaxant and can help in tension that accompanies high anxiety. Other

Sage Advice

Don't worry if you cannot correctly assess the nature of the hysteria between a hot or cold condition. If you don't know which one and are feeling anxious, it will not hurt to take both hops and valerian root. Many mixtures combine both these herbs since they can be used together to soothe the nervous system.

Sage Advice

To induce a good night's sleep, try making your own herbal eye pillow. Find some crushed velvet or other soft material, and sew it into a small rectangle. Fill it with the aromatic leaves and flowers of chamomile and lavender. The herbs will smell wonderful, and you will get the calming benefits when you lay back and place the pillow over your eyes or forehead.

stress-management ideas are psychotherapy, meditation, body work, quiet time for journaling, taking a bath, and playing calming music. All will help you calm yourself by refocusing your energy.

Asthma: It's So Wheezy to Fix

Asthma is a disease characterized by shortness of breath, wheezing, and coughing due to bronchial constriction. In severe cases, a person may pass out from oxygen deprivation, and sometimes emergency trips to the hospital are required. *Bronchodilator* medications are used by many asthmatics to force open their air passageways.

Many causes are linked to asthma, including allergic reactions, emotional issues, adrenal gland imbalances, spinal misalignment, environmental pollutants, and dehydration. It's best to understand what is causing your attacks in the first place and use herbs to correct the problem. However, for a quick fix, the next herb we'll talk about can force open the air passage ways and allow you to breathe easier right away.

Botanical Bit

Asthma is a disease characterized by shortness of breath due to bronchial constriction. Most asthma is treated with **bronchodilators**, which are inhaled steroid substances that force the airways open to allow more air to pass through.

Ephedra: A Remedy That Won't Take Your Breath Away

The Chinese have used Chinese ephedra (*Ephedra equisetina*), also known as ma haung, for centuries as a wonder herb for many different uses. One of its greatest attributes is the bronchodilator effect it has on the body, but it may also be used in herbal preparations designed for weight loss. This herb is a strong heart and nervous system stimulant and therefore is not suitable for everyone.

Herb Lore

Ephedra is illegal in some states because it has been mixed with caffeine or caffeine-rich herbs (such as kola nut) by unscrupulous or ignorant herbal manufacturers to create an herbal high for the consumer. Some consumers abused this combination for the high, instead of using herbs responsibly. This resulted in a few reported deaths and the subsequent ban of ephedra altogether in some states. It's a shame that such a helpful herb has been taken away from some of us simply because a few unscrupulous manufacturers offered inappropriate mixtures. You can help keep this from happening by choosing to purchase your herbs only from responsible herbal manufacturers or working with a competent herbalist.

Epinephrine, the medication used in over-the-counter asthma and allergy medications such as Sudafed®, Contac®, and Primatene Mist®, has very similar chemical properties to ephedra. For an asthma attack, one capsule of this herb can be effective right away, but make sure you are not sensitive to ephedra before taking any more than that.

Getting All Choked Up over Lobelia

If you live in a state where ephedra is banned, or if you have high blood pressure and are sensitive to ephedra products, another excellent and old-time remedy for clearing the lungs is the herb lobelia (pronounced *low-beel-ya*). Lobelia (*Lobelia inflata*) is used for many afflictions, including asthma, because of its *expectorant* abilities—this means that it helps the body clear out toxins and mucus. As a member of the lobeline family, lobelia acts in a similar way on the nervous system as nicotine does—in fact, it was once smoked by Native Americans instead of tobacco. Even today, supplementing with lobelia has been useful in supporting those who want to stop smoking (see Chapter 21, "T: Terrific Solutions").

Be warned, however, that lobelia is both an *emetic* and an *expectorant*, so taking this herb along with cigarettes may make you very queasy after smoking. This nauseating effect has helped many associate their sick stomach feeling to cigarettes and has made quitting easier.

Lobelia also serves to calm the nervous system and is another reason why nervous smokers might like lobelia. For asthma, lobelia works to relax constricted bronchials, making it much easier to breathe.

Small doses work best with lobelia—taking too much at once (even if you are not a smoker) might make you nauseous or even cause you to vomit. However, once this passes you should feel better than ever because the toxins have been expelled. Start out with one capsule of lobelia and see how you do before taking more.

Botanical Bit

An herb that serves as an **expectorant** has properties that help the body expel phlegm or mucus from the lungs and sinuses. An **emetic** herb can induce vomiting.

A Combination to Offer a Breath of Fresh Air

One particular combination used to support lung function includes marshmallow, Chinese ephedra, mullein, passion flower, catnip, horehound, and slippery elm. Many of these herbs have nourishing and mucilaginous qualities, which means that they serve to moisten the tissues of the body. If the lungs are all dried up, as Dr. Batmanghelidj's research seems to prove, these herbs will help put moisture back into them.

Dr. Batmanghelidj's research on healing with water suggests that asthma is nothing more than a disease brought on by dehydration. The lungs lose water every time we exhale, and he describes this as a drought condition in the body, similar to hard, cracked moisture-lacking soil. Drinking more water will help replenish that water for the lungs—and it could just be your least-expensive remedy!

Also consider having your blood sugar checked if you have asthma, as plummeting blood sugar levels can often trigger asthmatic reactions.

Sage Advice

The lungs are where we tend to hold grief. If you have lost someone dear to you and then began experiencing asthmatic symptoms shortly thereafter, consider counseling to help you release the emotions that could be causing your problem.

Botanical Bit

Arthritis is an inflammation of one or more joints characterized by swelling, redness, and warmth of the overlying skin; restriction of movement; and pain in affected areas.

Furthermore, take note if you are having trouble breathing when you haven't eaten in several hours; then note whether your shortness of breath comes after you have ingested sugary foods. Licorice root is one of the best herbs to take to help bring blood sugar up and keep it steady throughout the day. Try two to four capsules between meals. Also take note if you tend to get short of breath when dealing with a certain person. If so, you might need to get to the core of the emotional issue before any herb can help.

Consider eliminating milk, dairy products, and sugary foods that can increase mucus in the lungs and sinuses and make your asthma symptoms worse. Ginkgo and grape seed extract have also been added to herbal programs designed to combat asthma. Both help by decreasing the sensitivity to allergens and lowering the histamine response.

Arthritis: A Flexible Treatment Plan

Arthritis is an inflammation of one or more joints. Many different diseases can cause arthritis, including rheumatoid arthritis, osteoarthritis, gout, tuberculosis, and other infections. Arthritis involves painful symptoms, but the good news is that many have gotten relief by using herbs to heal the core problem. Many herbalists believe the main problem is linked directly to a lack of minerals or improper absorption of minerals due to weak digestion.

Alfalfa: Good for Darla

The alfalfa plant (*Medicago sativa*) should be the first herb you think of when you think arthritis. The Arabs first discovered alfalfa's beneficial uses and referred to it as the Father of All Foods. Alfalfa is very rich in organic minerals: Its deep roots penetrate the earth and find the minerals it needs to thrive; in turn, it provides us with generous amounts of minerals and vitamins when we consume it.

Your dosage will vary depending on how minerally deficient you are; start with the dose recommended on the bottle and work your way up. You can take plenty of alfalfa without doing any harm.

Alfalfa has been used to neutralize uric acid in the body (arthritis sufferers are commonly over-acidic in body chemistry due to weakened digestion). In addition, alfalfa seems to prevent cholesterol accumulation in the veins, cleans deep in the cells, provides enzymes for better digestion and assimilation, rebuilds decayed teeth, and helps relieve pain and inflammation. What a helpful little rascal alfalfa turns out to be!

Herbal Combinations: A Joint Effort

The blood of the alfalfa plant is sometimes used to make liquid chlorophyll, which helps keep your body from losing calcium. A combination of herbs and supplements to help with arthritis symptoms includes bromelain, hydrangea, yucca, horsetail, celery seed, alfalfa, black cohosh, catnip, yarrow, capsicum, valerian, white willow, burdock, slippery elm, and sarsaparilla.

Other supplements that support digestion and that have been helpful to my own arthritic clients have been B6 supplements and food enzymes with hydrochloric acid.

If you have arthritis, consider these complementary treatments as well:

➤ Externally, you can apply pure birch essential oil to painful areas to increase blood supply to the area and help ease pain.

➤ Sodium-rich foods are helpful when suffering from any type of arthritic or structural problem. Juice and drink daily raw carrots, celery, parsley, and okra—all sodium-rich foods used to help relieve or correct arthritis.

➤ Getting and keeping the circulation flowing will help maintain or bring back flexibility in the joints. Reflexology offers great relief for arthritic feet and hands by stimulating circulation and lymphatic movement. Massage also helps all joints and circulation, along with lymphatic flow. Massage and reflexology might be slightly painful at first but will usually bring relief shortly into the treatment.

Sage Advice

Did you know that the highest concentration of sodium in the body is in the lining of the stomach and in the joints? Most people with arthritis had or have digestive troubles—could this be due to a lack of organic sodium in the diet? Juicing fruits and vegetables that have been vine-ripened will feed you organic sodium to pass on to your stomach and joints.

Herbal Remedies for Common Ailments

Anxiety

Best Single Herb: Valerian (best for "cold" conditions) or hops (best for hot, flushed conditions)

Best Combinations: Chamomile, passion flower, hops, fennel, marshmallow, feverfew; wild lettuce

Other Helpful Supplements: B-complex; magnesium

Possible Causes: Change; food allergies; caffeine

Complementary Help: Meditation; reflexology or other relaxing bodywork; a warm bath with tangerine oil or lavender oil in the tub; chamomile tea; space for quiet time; dim lights and candles

Asthma

Best Single Herb: Chinese ephedra, lobelia (ephedra is illegal in some states and is not suitable for everyone)

Best Combinations: Marshmallow, Chinese ephedra, mullein, passion flower, catnip, horehound, slippery elm; licorice root (if low blood sugar); lobelia

Other Helpful Supplements: Beta carotene; magnesium; pantothenic acid

Possible Causes: Dehydration might cause asthma because the lungs are all dried up—drink more water than your share; also pent-up emotions, grief, and low blood sugar could have an effect

Complementary Help: Counseling; blood sugar testing

Arthritis

Best Single Herb: Alfalfa

Best Combinations: Bromelain, hydrangea, yucca, horsetail, celery seed, alfalfa, black cohosh, catnip, yarrow, capsicum, valerian, white willow, burdock, slippery elm, sarsaparilla; licorice root; alfalfa

Other Helpful Supplements: Food enzyme tablets with hydrochloric acid; vitamin B6

Possible Causes: Improper digestion, lack of circulation; lack of minerals or poor mineral absorption

Complementary Help: Bodywork for help with circulation; external application of birch essential oil to sore joints; sodium-rich foods; juicing carrots, celery, parsley, and okra (all rich in sodium)

The Least You Need to Know

➤ Valerian is nature's valium and can come to the rescue for high anxiety.

➤ Asthma has been helped by the proper use of Chinese ephedra for its beneficial effects on opening up the bronchials.

➤ Lobelia helps to relax the bronchials and also serves to help the body rid itself of mucus from the lungs and sinus passages.

➤ Alfalfa helps arthritis by supplying an abundance of organic minerals and supporting digestion.

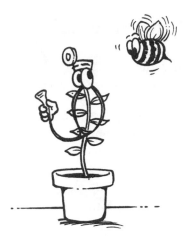

B Well

"Here's good advice for practice: Go into partnership with nature; she does more than half the work and asks none of the fee." —Martin H. Fischer (1879–1962) *Fischerisms* (Howard Fabing and Ray Marr)

Nature can provide many answers indeed. If we would all follow nature's lead closely instead of trying to out-do her, we would probably be more balanced mentally, physically, and emotionally. Take a look at the wild animals, for instance. When an animal is injured it fasts, it only eats when hungry, and then stops when it has had the proper amount of food. Most animals stretch after sleeping and before walking around again. The female animal chooses her mate very carefully before mating and creating offspring. Don't we all have something to learn from nature?

This chapter will address some imbalances such as high and low blood pressure, bladder infections, bronchitis, and more, and then will show you what nature has to offer as the balancing remedy.

Bad Breath (Halitosis): A Refreshing Remedy

You don't have to eat onions to have bad breath. And you don't need to be a rocket scientist to realize that if everyone around you backs away when you talk to them you probably need an oral odor eater! Local infection such as gum disease (also known as gingivitis) harbor bacteria and can give a foul odor to your breath. (See Chapter 12, "G: Great Remedies," for more help with gingivitis.) Sinus drainage can be another localized factor. If no localized problem exists, and if you haven't had onions or garlic lately, bad breath is probably a result of a toxic bowel or sour stomach.

When bad breath is due to a sour stomach, food enzymes will help support your digestion and get to the cause of the problem. Enzymes will also help you break down your foods better so that you are eliminating more efficiently. Enzyme tablets are best taken before meals.

Remember our zinc rhyme? If you stink, take zinc. A client told me once about a friend's son's feet that smelled terrible all the time. His mother took him to a naturopath, who told him to take zinc. After taking zinc for two days, the smell was gone!

Activated charcoal is another absorbing remedy that will absorb toxins and their smells from the body. Charcoal is used for other things as well, such as filtering harmful pollutants from drinking water. Taken internally, charcoal helps neutralize your bad odors, including body odor.

Chlorophyll: Nature's Deodorizer

Chlorophyll, the green pigment of the plants, works as one of the best natural deodorizers for the body. Liquid chlorophyll can be swallowed straight, put in water or juice, or taken in capsule form. Liquid chlorophyll takes the smell out of the body and neutralizes acids in the body that can make you smell. It's also good for helping to cleanse the bowel, which is where many waste materials are harbored.

Liquid chlorophyll has been used for various conditions and has been useful in:

Sage Advice

I met a couple who fed chlorophyll to their female show dog when she was in heat and they didn't plan to breed her. They claimed that the chlorophyll deodorized the dog enough to keep the neighborhood male dogs from sniffing around—and it kept them from being a spectacle during dog shows!

➤ Deodorizing the body
➤ Building up blood count in cases of anemia
➤ Stopping bleeding when applied externally to wounds
➤ Supporting the digestive system
➤ Restoring minerals in the body after depletion
➤ Clearing up skin conditions
➤ Providing energy
➤ Easing sore throats when used as a gargle
➤ Speeding the healing of canker sores

Gee, Your Breath Smells Terrific

Until the chlorophyll and charcoal kick in, you can use a dab of pure peppermint oil on your tongue to refresh your breath. Peppermint is stimulating and will give you a little lift, too. I like to carry a small bottle of peppermint oil with me wherever I go because I like it so much; I put a dab on my finger and rub it on my gums so my whole mouth feels refreshed.

Peppermint also is an activating herb that is used as a flavoring in hard candy. Not only does it aid digestion by stimulating digestive juices, but it also has been useful in stimulating mental alertness.

Bites and Stings: Those Nasties with Wings

Ah, the great outdoors: fresh air, rustling leaves, sunshine, and—ouch! whack!—bugs! From flies to mosquitoes to stinging bugs, there's not much we can do about living with these things. Bugs are part of our environment, and I remember my parents telling me that all creatures on earth have a purpose. (I still cannot figure out what purpose biting flies serve, however, except to help humans create new curse words!) Read on for some herbal help on keeping some bugs at bay. And to fight off allergic reactions to bites and stings, a mixture of blessed thistle, pleurisy root, skullcap, and yerba santa will help you through. Another mixture rich in organic minerals includes alfalfa, marshmallow, plantain, horsetail, oatstraw, wheat grass, and hops. For allergic reactions, I also recommend taking pantothenic acid and high doses of vitamin C. Activated charcoal will help internally and externally as well.

Poison Ivy

Although peppermint serves as great breath freshener and pick-me-up, sometimes the strong smell of peppermint can smell like alcohol on your breath! Make sure that you have your little peppermint oil bottle visible so that any suspicious folks can put two and two together. Either that or start slurring your words like a drunken sailor and at least entertain yourself by watching others react!

Sage Advice

In a pinch, chewing on a fresh sprig of parsley can help beat garlic or onion breath.

Shoo Fly, Why Are You Bothering Me?

Flies are attracted to dark colors, so try wearing nice white slacks next time you go camping. Just kidding, but remember the tip when you are packing your camp gear—bugs truly are less attracted to lighter-colored clothing.

Blood-sucking bugs such as mosquitoes seem to be attracted to the sweet smell of your blood, so put away those M&M®'s to fully enjoy the great outdoors. Also make sure you don't wear any sweet-smelling perfumes or personal care products, which can attract way too much attention. In fact, pumping up your body with herbs that smell offensive to bugs—such as garlic—will offer your best prevention.

Sage Advice

Eating garlic or taking high-potency garlic tablets can change the smell of your blood and keep mosquitoes and other biting bugs at bay.

Black Cohosh: De-Bugging the Simple Cure

Black cohosh (*Cimicifuga racemosa*), known to some as snakeroot, can be used internally or externally for bites of all kinds—especially snake bites, which is how this herb got its nickname in the first place. Used also as a female tonic, black cohosh will help relax the nerves and bring on menstruation. However, this is a very strong herb and should be used in moderation; too much can make you nauseous.

Compressing the Situation

Make sure you remove any stinger from the skin before applying any external applications. You can make a compress out of activated charcoal or black cohosh mixed with some aloe vera and place it on the affected area. For multiple stings, take a bath with activated charcoal in the water to draw out poisons from skin.

To prevent being bitten in the first place, I use a mixture of essential oils on my skin that works like a charm. Remember that your skin is an organ, so it also absorbs into the body what you apply to it. I like to use natural products whenever possible. Mix up a batch of equal parts of the following pure essential oils: citronella, lemongrass, lavender, and melaleuca (also known as tea tree oil). You can add these to olive oil, store in a dark glass bottle, and apply as needed. If your oils are pure, they contain enzymes that will eat through plastic containers, so make sure you store any oils you mix in glass. These oils are natural and not harmful to your body, and best of all, bugs hate them!

Botanical Bit

A **bladder infection** (**cystitis**) is a painful inflammation of the bladder usually caused by a bacterial infection. Symptoms include feeling the need for frequent urination, but with a voided bladder, and painful or burning urination. The bladder may be so irritated that blood will be detected in the urine. Infection can be caused by the bacterium E. coli.

Bladder Infection Correction

A *bladder infection* (*cystitis*) is a painful inflammation of the bladder. Its symptoms include an urge to urinate frequently, even when bladder is empty, and painful or burning urination. The bladder may be so irritated that blood will be seen in the urine.

Bacteria found in the bowel can cause a bladder infection, so good old bowel cleansing is a great helper in reducing the possibility for future infection.

Herb Lore

Many holistic practitioners believe that any ailment can have an emotional link that can cause or worsen your symptoms. And some believe there is a relationship between specific organs and different emotions. The liver is believed to be where we hold anger. Physically, anger is a chemical reaction. When the feeling leaves us our liver is left to filter out those chemicals. (I have helped clients through herbal liver cleanses who have had attacks of rage during the process!) Other examples include the heart, where we hold love or feelings about being loved or heart broken, and the lungs, where we hold grief.

An emotional link to bladder infections can literally be interpreted as "pissed off." If you are getting reoccurring infections, you might want to ask yourself who you're really angry at. Letting go of this anger might or might not help, but at least you will feel better emotionally!

Cranberries to Make You Feel Bladder

Cranberries are Mother Nature's aid to our bladder. These berries are very acidic and help to alter bacteria in the urine. In fact, studies have shown that a special factor in the juice of a cranberry seems to make harmful bacteria less likely to cling to the surface of cells in the urinary tract and can be your best preventative solution against bladder infections. Cranberry concentrate can be found in powder form in capsules; drinking cranberry juice is good, too, but sugar-sweetened cranberry juice is not your best choice because the sugar can serve as food to harmful bacteria. Most health food stores carry cranberry juice sweetened with fruit juice—cranberries alone are very astringent and will make you pucker without some type of sweetener.

You may also juice and/or eat raw celery, watermelon, cucumbers, parsley, and kale to help heal and soothe inflamed, internal mucus membranes in the bladder during or after a bladder infection.

Buchu root (*Barosma betulina*) is another excellent herb to aid the bladder, and cranberry and buchu work very well together as a remedy for preventing

Sage Advice

A clinical study (*New England Journal of Medicine*, October, 1998) on cranberries has identified a key component that helps in urinary tract infections. This component, proanthocyanidins, has been shown to successfully prevent E. coli bacteria from attaching to urinary tract walls. Other berries of the same family, including blueberries, also contain proanthocyanidins and demonstrated similar properties.

bladder infections or any urinary tract infections. Golden seal can be used to help fight the infection as well; uva ursi is another bladder tonic, and cornsilk nourishes the bladder and can serve as a diuretic. These herbs can all be used together or separately for any type of bladder problems. And don't forget to drink copious amounts of water when you have a bladder infection—water will help flush out your infection.

Unmentionable Mentionables

To all you gals suffering from reoccurring urinary infections of any kind, I'd like to give you some kind advice that you might not have learned elsewhere. Typically bladder infections occur because of outside contamination. This can occur two ways. First, make sure that you wipe from front to back after urination. Second, urinating after intercourse will help flush away extra bacteria and any rectal bacteria that can contaminate the vaginal area. You might want to use non-scented or non-dyed toilet paper because the chemicals used to make these pretty patterns and smells can be irritating to your sensitive parts.

Also, "holding it" can weaken the bladder and make you more vulnerable to future infections. When nature calls, be sure to answer!

Blood Pressure: Easier to Deal with Than Peer Pressure

Blood pressure is the measurable pressure exerted by the blood against the walls of the arteries. Blood pressure can vary depending on the flexibility and strength of your blood vessel walls, your heartbeat, and the volume of the blood. Neither too high nor too low is ideal—like Goldielocks, you want it just right. Get your blood pressure checked by your doctor; many times pharmacies and even shopping malls have machines where you can check your blood pressure for free. For more accuracy, home units can be purchased and are fairly inexpensive.

The following chart contains general guidelines for what your blood pressure should be at different ages. Numbers well above these can indicate over-activity in the glands; numbers well below these figures could indicate glandular under-activity.

Normal Blood Pressure Ranges

Age	Systolic/Diastolic
10	100/70
20	120/80
30	122/81
40	126/84
50	130/86
60	135/89
70	166/91

How High I Am—and Why

So, you don't understand what could be causing your high blood pressure? You eat right, get plenty of exercise, and still the doctor tells you that your numbers are too high? Let's take a look at some reasons for why you might have this condition.

Many factors can cause high blood pressure, including:

➤ High cholesterol (because of the thickening of the blood)

➤ Hardening of the arteries

➤ Abuse of stimulants, such as caffeine

➤ Stress

Think about your stress level—maybe your heart is telling your body something about how you are managing your life. Use herbs that calm, and choose a stress-management therapy.

I'll give you some more advice on other things to consider, but for now let's talk about one of the best herbs for blood pressure: garlic.

Garlic: Help from a Bulbous Friend

Good old garlic (*Alium sativum*) is great for so many things, and it seems to have an affinity for helping the circulatory system, too. In fact, this would be my choice if I had only one herb to help bring blood pressure into balance.

Garlic is high in phosphorous, potassium, sulfur, and zinc, and it has an affinity for the lungs, sinuses, circulatory system, and digestive system. It has been known to dissolve cholesterol, which can contribute to high blood pressure, and helps remove it from the arteries. If you have high cholesterol and begin to take garlic, you should also add milk thistle and a bowel cleanser (a mixture of psyllium hulls and cascara sagrada works well), to help the cholesterol exit the body through the bowel. Garlic also is a natural antibiotic, and it makes a great remedy for killing parasites and fungus.

Garlic capsules can be taken if you'd rather not chew on raw cloves. Some are coated with chlorophyll to help odor, and some are enterically coated, which means that the capsule or tablet will break down in your intestines, not your stomach. The oil of garlic contains the same properties and can be rubbed on the chest for respiratory infections. Take enough pills to equal at least three cloves daily when fighting hypertension. Unfortunately, much of garlic's medicinal effects are

Sage Advice

Raw garlic is best for hypertension: Three to five cloves a day have helped many, although it may have killed the dating game! Parsley helps neutralize the garlic odor.

contained within the compound that gives it its strong odor. If you don't have a raw garlic capsule, make sure the manufacturer did not remove the allium. If they did, your garlic won't be effective.

More Pressure, More Supplements

Beating high blood pressure involves many factors, so you might want to take several herbs and remedies to bring it back down. Here are a few to try:

➤ A mixture of hawthorn, capsicum, and garlic will support the entire circulatory system.

➤ Cornsilk will support the kidneys, which are usually involved in high blood pressure.

➤ Chamomile will sooth the nerves and stress usually associated with the problem.

Non-herbal support that works to balance the blood pressure includes coenzyme Q_{10} (CoQ_{10}), which is a co-enzyme factor (a compound that works together with your body's enzymes to help them function) essential to the health of all human tissues. Its purpose is to increase the efficiency of cellular metabolism.

Trace minerals are often lacking or out of balance in people who have high blood pressure. Try a trace mineral supplement, or take alfalfa or liquid chlorophyll for natural supplementation. Daily Omega-3 oils and a B-complex vitamin are also useful in bringing down the pressure.

How Low Can You Go?: Low Blood Pressure

At the other end of the pendulum swing is low blood pressure, which is not the best thing to have, either. Low blood pressure can signify hormonal under-activity, and many people with this condition have thyroid problems. Symptoms of a low thyroid include fatigue, depression, cold hands and feet, and coarse hair or skin.

Please Kelp Me—I'm Fallin'

If the thyroid is underactive, it may need nourishment. The thyroid likes iodine, and one of the richest foods in iodine is kelp. Kelp grows in our oceans and is packed with many trace minerals from the sea. Other tonics for the glandular system include licorice root, which helps tone the adrenals, and ginseng, which is an all-around tonic for the entire body.

Ginkgo biloba and hawthorne both work well together to bring blood pressure back up into balance. Add a trace mineral supplement and some capsicum, and you

Sage Advice

If you are a salt lover and have low blood pressure because of an underactive thyroid, you can keep bulk kelp powder in your salt shaker and sprinkle it on your foods to taste. If your thyroid is low, the kelp will help feed it and will give you energy. But beware, kelp is very salty!

will have a remedy to boost you. All these foods and herbs will also help feed your entire circulatory system; a weakened heart can be the cause of low blood pressure.

Other Things You Probably Already Knew

Exercise will help get your blood moving and your heart pumping, which can have an effect on overall blood pressure. Deep-breathing exercises help to bring more oxygen into the blood stream and can help regulate many disorders of the body. Here's a breathing exercise to try. This might make you dizzy, which is why I suggest you try it sitting down.

Breathing Exercise:

1. Sit up straight.

2. Breathe in through your nose, open up your throat to get more air, and concentrate on the air filling the bottom of your stomach first, then your abdomen, then your diaphragm, and, finally, the lungs, from the bottom up. (This full inhale should take approximately 8–12 seconds to complete.)

3. Hold this full breath for as long as you can.

4. Then push the air out of your body forcefully in three or four exhales; repeat.

Try this exercise, and take your blood pressure before and after to see if it makes a difference for you. I find it energizing and stimulating, especially when I have been at my computer writing all day!

Bronchitis: Coughing Up a Solution

Bronchitis is an inflammation of the mucus membranes of the bronchi, tubes that branch off the trachea leading to the air sacs of the lungs. Symptoms include spastic mucus-filled coughs usually accompanied by a general sick feeling, a fever, and general lethargy. An airborne virus or bacteria causes bronchitis.

Bronchitis is generally caused by inhaling toxic vapors including cigarette smoke. A cold or other upper-respiratory infection can also lead to bronchitis. If you are prone to bronchitis, don't smoke, avoid chemical exposure, smog, and traffic pollution and beware of breathing in cold, wet air (not an easy option for skiers, is it?).

Keeping the bowel clear is always helpful when you are suffering from any type of respiratory congestion; make sure you are not constipated. Use herbs to relieve constipation (see Chapter 8, "C's for a Common Cure"), or use an enema to fix

Botanical Bit

Bronchitis is an inflammation of the mucus membranes of the bronchi, tubes that branch off the trachea leading to the air sacs of the lungs.

this problem. Enemas work well for small children, too. Let me briefly explain how a clogged bowel can hinder your respiratory system functions. The lymphatic system is a small filtering system running alongside our arteries and veins and runs throughout the entire body. This filtering system will dump its excess waste materials into the bowel, but if the bowel is clogged, there is no room for the lymph to dump. Since it is overflowing, its waste materials will be squeezed back into your mucus membranes—creating more mucus and making you vulnerable to future infection. Cleaning the bowel will not only help when you have respiratory congestion of any kind, but will help prevent a problem in the first place.

Herb Lore

A helpful old home remedy for bronchitis is to use an onion poultice on the chest. To make, chop up a strong, white onion. Pour some honey in a pot (a double boiler works best if you have one) and add the onion. Warm up this mixture on the stove until the onion's essential oil has mixed well into the honey. Apply warm mixture to the upper chest area; cover with plastic, a towel, and a hot water bottle. Eating the leftover honey may also help.

Diffuse pure eucalyptus oil in your room to help with recovery and help protect others from the airborne viruses and bacteria.

Fenugreek: Nothing to Get Choked Up About

Fenugreek (*Trigonella foenum-graecum*) has been an excellent remedy for bronchitis because it not only kills infections and fights against viruses, but also works as an expectorant to help push mucus out of the body. For that reason, fenugreek is great for any type of mucus condition of the respiratory tract.

Fenugreek works well with thyme to discharge mucus from the lungs and fight infections. Thyme is also thought to be good for the thymus, which is the seat of your immune system. In addition, lobelia and mullein can work to ease bronchial spasms and eliminate mucus and coughs. Beta carotene feeds lung tissue and will help boost your immune system and soothe lung tissue. Magnesium is helpful because it is a muscle relaxer to the body and can help lessen a coughing. Zinc boosts the immune system, and vitamin E may assist in the fight against bronchitis.

Foods That Can Help or Hinder

When dealing with a condition involving an excess of mucus, such as bronchitis, it is wise to remember that sugary foods and dairy products cause excess mucus production in many people. If you are one of these people, avoiding those products until you are well again may aid your battle.

My most revered teacher, Dr. Bernard Jensen, says that carrot juice is one of the best foods to eliminate mucus from the body. It works great for me, and carrots are rich in beta carotene, which feeds the skin and soft tissues of the body, too. Drink your carrots!

Sage Advice

With all ailments involving congestion (and for that matter, for overall better health) remember that you have Five White Enemies: white flour, white sugar, white rice, white milk, and white salt. Nature doesn't produce natural foods that are this pure white. These foods have been stripped of nutritional value. Overconsumption of any of these products can lead to ill health. Make sure your diet is colorful!

Burns: Now You're Cookin'

Burns can result from chemicals, electrical accidents, or fire—including the fire from too much sun! For best results, take care of the burn immediately. Sometimes getting burned is a careless accident because you weren't paying attention or were lackadaisical about safety. Burns can serve as a wake-up call to pay more attention to your well-being and make you more aware of your movements and actions.

Aloe Vera: Nice to See You!

The best remedy for burns of all types is aloe vera (*Aloe vera*). Aloe can be taken internally as well as externally to soothe and heal tissues. It contains special ingredients that work together when applied directly to burns to produce a pain-relieving effect.

In addition, vitamin A feeds the skin, and vitamin E taken internally and also applied directly to skin can reduce scaring. Zinc helps in wound healing, and vitamin C strengthens collagen, which is helpful in all skin healing. Calendula (usually found added to a cream) has been helpful in soothing skin irritations when applied externally.

Other Great Home Remedies for Your Skin

Always protect your skin from sun exposure with sunscreens and hats to keep sun off your face when outside. Air pollution is causing our earth's atmosphere to break down, which also breaks down our protection from the sun's damaging rays.

Honey has been used as a beauty aid applied to the skin. I use Dr. Jensen's honey facial when I want to spruce up my skin. Here's the procedure, honey:

Dr. Jensen's Honey Facial

1. Wash your face.
2. Lay a hot washcloth on your face to open up pores.
3. Splash your face with cold water to close pores and increase circulation.
4. Apply raw honey to your face.
5. Let the honey cool down a bit, and gently pat the honey all over your face and neck.
6. Rinse.
7. Splash your face with cold water and pat dry.

Your skin will look renewed and glowing!

Honey (as well as pure vanilla) is also useful as an external application for burns—if nothing else, you will smell edible! Vitamin E oil can be used externally to prevent scarring from burns; a capsule may be punctured with a needle and squeezed onto the burnt or scarred area.

Herb Lore

Applied topically, the essential oil of lavender is an excellent natural burn remedy and is healing for skin ailments of all types. A French cosmetic chemist working in his laboratory discovered this when he burned himself and instinctively plunged his burnt hand into a cold vat of lavender oil. It is said that the lavender oil alleviated his pain instantly and he had no scarring, and the benefits of lavender was born.

Herbal Remedies for Common Ailments

Bad Breath (Halitosis)

Best Single Herb: Liquid chlorophyll

Best Combinations: Liquid chlorophyll, spearmint

Other Helpful Supplements: Activated charcoal; food enzymes; zinc

Possible Causes: Sour stomach; constipation; gum disease (gingivitis)

Complementary Help: Dental check-up; peppermint oil; extra liquids; bowel cleansing

Bites and Stings

Best Single Herb: Black cohosh

Best Combinations: Black cohosh; alfalfa, marshmallow, plantain, horsetail, oatstraw, wheat grass, hops; blessed thistle, pleurisy root, skullcap, yerba santa

Other Helpful Supplements: Activated charcoal; pantothenic acid; vitamin C

Possible Causes: Sweet-smelling blood from sugar consumption

Complementary Help: Using a compress made from charcoal and aloe vera to draw out poisons; taking a charcoal bath; placing ice on the area to control spread and swelling; removing the stinger; preventing stings through external use of essential oil of citronella to keep mosquitoes and flies away

Bladder Infection (Cystitis)

Best Single Herb: Cranberries

Best Combinations: Cranberry and buchu root; golden seal; uva ursi; cornsilk

Other Helpful Supplements: Acidophilus

Possible Causes: Constipation; improper toilet habits; not emptying the bladder when you have the urge; unresolved anger and frustration

Complementary Help: Bowel cleansing; tea tree oil applied to entrance of the urethra

Blood Pressure, High

Best Single Herb: Garlic

Best Combinations: Hawthorne, capsicum, garlic; cornsilk (kidney support); chamomile (to calm nerves); milk thistle or dandelion (for liver)

Other Helpful Supplements: CoQ_{10}, trace mineral supplement; vitamin C; Omega-3 fatty acids; B-complex vitamins with extra niacin

Possible Causes: Stress; high cholesterol or hardening of arteries; abuse of caffeine; mineral imbalance; kidney problems; constipation

Complementary Help: Stress management; bowel cleansing; drinking more water

Blood Pressure, Low

Best Single Herb: Capsicum

Best Combinations: Ginkgo and hawthorn; kelp (if thyroid-related); licorice root

Other Helpful Supplements: Trace minerals

Possible Causes: Glandular imbalance; thyroid problems; weak heart

Complementary Help: Physical exercise; deep-breathing exercises

Bronchitis

Best Single Herb: Fenugreek

Best Combinations: Fenugreek and thyme; lobelia; mullein

Other Helpful Supplements: Beta carotene; magnesium; zinc; vitamin E

Possible Causes: Pollution; constipation

continues

Herbal Remedies for Common Ailments (continued)

Bronchitis (continued)

Complementary Help: Cleanse bowel; avoid dairy, wheat, fruit juices, and other sugary foods and drinks; use an onion-and-honey compress; diffuse eucalyptus oil in the room

Burns, Minor

Best Single Herb: Aloe vera

Best Combinations: Slippery elm; aloe vera (whole leaf is best)

Other Helpful Supplements: Vitamins A, E, and C; zinc

Possible Causes: Lack of attention to self or care for well-being; distracted manner

Complementary Help: External applications: honey; pure vanilla extract; essential oil of lavender; vitamin E capsule, punctured and squeezed onto area

---

The Least You Need to Know

➤ Bad breath is usually an internal problem and can be helped by chlorophyll.

➤ Bugs like the smell of sweet blood but are repelled by the smell of garlic in the blood.

➤ Cranberries are one of nature's best remedies for fighting bladder infections.

➤ Fenugreek helps in bronchitis because of its infection fighting abilities and its assistance in pushing mucus from the respiratory tract.

➤ Aloe vera is a healing and soothing remedy for burns.

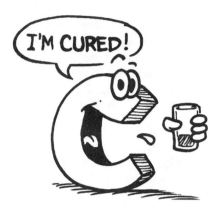

Chapter 8

C's for a Common Cure

> **In This Chapter**
>
> ➤ Fight cancer with more than just herbs
>
> ➤ Herbs and supplements for high cholesterol
>
> ➤ Fast-forward your cold symptoms using herbal remedies
>
> ➤ Herbal cold sore help
>
> ➤ Relieve constipation with sacred herbs
>
> ➤ Herbal help to dissolve cysts

This chapter deals with some common ailments beginning with C. I hesitated to add cancer here, as this is serious business, and it's best to work with your doctor and a reputable herbalist or holistic practitioner so that you get the best of both practices. However, I was inspired to share with you not just herbs that have been historically used to beat cancer, but, more important, the attitude that those who beat cancer possess. I want to share a different way to look at illness, which can be a big part of your recovery. Of course, if you don't have cancer, you can incorporate some of these immune system-supporting herbs and philosophies into your life to help keep you strong.

Beyond that serious subject, we'll cover the less pressing ailments such as common colds and constipation. First, though, let's get cancer out of the way.

Cancer Answer: Some Philosophical Support

The greatest challenge I have in working with anyone who has had cancer is the panic factor. Most people who find out they have cancer are, understandably, in shock. On top of that, the medical treatments are usually initiated immediately, which can also put someone in a state of shock or trauma. When I see people who decide to investigate natural therapies, I see them bombarded with information from helpful friends and family members suggesting what they should and shouldn't do. They're routinely offered all sorts of suggestions for some miracle remedy or therapy.

As if you weren't already in a state of shock, this overwhelming information—mixed with the urgency factor that cancer brings because of its typical aggressive nature—can put a person over the top, so to speak. Motivated by fear, a person may jump from practitioner to practitioner, each one offering a different program, contradicting each other, and making the patient feel lost and helpless. Stop! I'll try to take away some of that panic by explaining a few things that I believe will help you see cancer a little differently and empower you to truly help yourself.

Sage Advice

Even if everyone in your family has cancer, that doesn't mean you will have it yourself. Cancer is a possibility in every one of us, and if it runs in your family, you need to start living preventatively. Get with a good practitioner who can get you on a preventative program, and listen to other's inspirational stories on how they overcame their own battles.

First of all, you are in charge of your body. If you are diagnosed with cancer, go home, sit down, and think. Do not panic immediately (yeah, sure). Realize that you were not born with this disease—you walked into it by doing something over a long period of time, or perhaps *not* doing something over a long period of time. In most cases, it is very possible to walk back out of the disease by figuring out what those things were and then correcting them. That's not to say that the walk will be a walk in the park, of course, and it's not to say that surgery won't be required in many cases, but surgery is not the total answer to a cancer-free rest of your life. In other words, consider more than just surgery to treat cancer.

You need to understand how you wound up with cancer in the first place—and then don't repeat your mistakes. Remember that you are in control of the choices that you make. You can choose health, or you can choose to do things that have negative consequences.

This list details some helpful things you can do to deal with the panic factor that comes when diagnosed with cancer. Engrain these thoughts in your heart and mind; they will help you understand the situation you are in and will empower you to make a choice.

Herb Lore

One of my first herb teachers put it very well when she recently described cancer surgery to me by saying: "Removing cancer via surgery is like cutting off the moldy part of the cheese." I thought, wow, she's right—the mold grew for a reason. Does just cutting off the mold protect the cheese from growing more? Does it change the nature of the cheese? No. You need to change your whole inner environment so that you need no more mold cut off!

Some thoughts for cancer patients:

➤ Do not take your doctor's diagnosis as a voodoo curse. Think of all the hundreds—and maybe thousands—of people who have been given a certain amount of time to live and have contradicted the doctor's diagnosis by beating the cancer and living cancer-free beyond their doctor's allotted time.

➤ Decide whether you are going to beat the cancer or whether you will let it beat you. You have a choice to make.

➤ Remember that your body works to keep you healthy and that you just need to provide the opportunity. Cancer did not fall out of the sky and attack you—you harbored it by lifestyle. Avoid blame, and just get prepared to make some changes.

➤ Remember that you are in control. Stay focused. We all have inherent intelligence when it comes to nutrition and nature's laws. If you are getting advice from a natural health practitioner that doesn't make sense to you, do not follow it; seek someone else. (Word-of-mouth referrals are usually the best.)

➤ Do not jump from practitioner to practitioner—you will confuse yourself. Find a good holistic nutritionist or herbalist and a good medical doctor, and use their skills and caring to help you heal yourself. Sometimes your medical doctor will be open and willing to write a prescription to see your natural health care provider. This prescription might help you get reimbursed by your medical insurance for your natural health care.

➤ Your body is constantly being rebuilt, cell by cell. In fact, you have a whole new body every seven years. Give your body what it needs to start rebuilding the good cells today!

➤ If you are spiritually connected (or want to be), pray. God answers prayers; pray for the right help to come to you, and pray that you will recognize it when it does.

➤ Read inspiring books by people who have fought cancer naturally and won:

Sir Jason Winters Story: From Deadly Cancer to Perfect Health by Benjamin Roth Smythe and Jason Winters, 1997

Beating Cancer with Nutrition: Clinically Proven and Easy-to-Follow Strategies to Dramatically Improve Quality and Quantity of Life by Patrick Quillin and Noreen Quillin (Contributor), 1998

You Can Heal Your Life by Louise L. Hay, 1987

➤ Remember that attitude is 90 percent of anything. Enhance your attitude of gratitude for the good things you have in your life.

➤ Have faith. Don't worry about money, time, or anything else. Focus on healing yourself, and the universe will provide you with what you need.

➤ Be open to learning a whole bunch about yourself in a short period of time. Old thought patterns that do not serve you will be busted up during your true healing process. Many times we realize we are harboring negative emotions that fester as a cancer in the body. This is your opportunity to make your peace with yourself and others.

All these things might sound naive, but, this is how most people overcome any potentially life-threatening disease. Once you are on the other side of the battle, you will be a whole new person—literally cell by cell!

Cancer is given the opportunity to grow in our body when our immune system is lowered. This can happen by being overexposed to things that cause damage to the body. The list of these things, from toxic chemicals to radiation and sun exposure, is so long that it would be too cumbersome to list them all here. Besides eliminating the overexposure to the damaging substances that are overloading your body with toxins, it is imperative that your immune system is strengthened. Your immune system is the system that goes to war for you to fight off anything in the body that shouldn't be there. It also keeps cells that are potentially cancer-causing under control.

Sage Advice

If you are going to beat cancer you must address every factor that effects the immune system including nutrients, stress, environmental toxins and pollutants, heavy metals, insufficient mineral levels, adequate amounts of sleep, exercise, and water, to name just a few.

Fighting cancer is like helping your body fight an internal war. To win the battle you must first supply your troops with the tools they need to fight and secondly, eliminate your enemies' food source. Sometimes the food source is pesticides, smoke, sugar, built-up toxins in the body, negative thoughts, and radiation. You can weaken the enemy cells by depriving them of what gives them strength.

Cancer thrives on low oxygen environments. A clogged up system where mucus, bowel wastes, and a dirty lymphatic system exists leaves little room for revitalizing oxygen to nourish the cells. Exercise and deep breathing as well as nutrients will help flush toxins out of the body and bring oxygen back into cells.

On the other side of the battlefield, your good guys need your support. You can support them by feeding them immune system-building foods, herbs, and thoughts. This is how you begin to tip the scales in your favor.

Eliminating the Opportunity with Red Clover

A myriad of herbs and supplements exist to boost your immune system and detoxify the system. For simplicity's sake, I have had to choose a best single herb for each ailment. In this case, it would have to be red clover.

The purplish flowers of this common clover plant have been used medicinally to cleanse the blood, liver, and lymphatic system. Red clover is a tonic and is believed to help cancer patients because of its ability to aid protein assimilation. Red clover is rich in calcium, potassium, vitamin C, and magnesium.

Red clover is an excellent blood cleanser and is used for a host of ailments, including acne, athlete's foot, bronchitis, leukemia, psoriasis, skin cancer, skin diseases, and whooping cough.

> **Sage Advice**
>
> Red clover's properties for fighting cancer have been studied by the National Cancer Institute, which has found that the herb does contain anti-tumor properties. Red clover contains high amounts of a chemical found in vitamin E, shown to prevent breast tumors in animals.

Combinations for Feeding Your Body's Army

Because the cancer-fighting battle is a serious one, you are going to have to use more than just one herb or supplement to boost your immunity, cleanse the body, bring oxygen into the cells and balance the hormones. Best combinations are listed in the chart at the end of this chapter and include other blood cleansers such as pau d'arco, a bowel stimulator such as cascara sagrada, and a combination called Essiac formula or tea. Essiac formula is a Native American formula used to fight cancer. It was passed down from the Cherokee tribe to a Canadian nurse in the early 1920s and was used successfully by hundreds over the years. ("Essiac" is the nurse's name spelled backward.) Some refer to this tea as "E tea."

> **Botanical Bit**
>
> **Antioxidants** are substances known to fight oxidation and protect the body from free radical damage. Antioxidant vitamins include vitamins C, A, and E and help neutralize free radical scavenger cells.

Other supplements that can aid you in your fight include all the *antioxidant* vitamins that help fight free radical damage. (See Chapter 4, "Herbs Are Not Just for Hippies Anymore," under herbs for the elderly for more on free radicals.) Some antioxidant vitamins and supplements include vitamins E and C, beta carotene, grape seed, pine bark extract, zinc, shark cartilage, reishi mushroom, germanium, food enzymes, acidophilus, and fish oil lipids known as Omega-3 oils or Omega-3 fatty acids. These are designed to help your body digest proteins (many people with cancer have poor protein assimilation), cleanse the bowel, and build immunity.

In addition, it is imperative to eat primarily organic fruits, vegetables, and animal products. Pesticides and chemical fertilizers found on non-organic foods can only add to your enemy cells. Take the energy required for digesting solid foods, and juice your organic fruits and veggies. Your body can utilize the extra energy to get well.

If your cancer is hormonally induced (involving the reproductive organs), it is a good idea to stay away from animal products unless they are organic. The hormones given to non-organic cows and chickens can be passed on to you through their flesh or products, and this can unbalance your own hormones. That's not to mention that the pesticides put in the feed for these animals could be lingering in the animal products you ingest. Soy products contain substances that block receptor sites for hormones and may help balance your own hormonal levels. See your physician or holistic practitioner before you begin a soy supplement.

Complementary help includes bowel cleansing. You can administer your own enemas at home or see a colonic irrigation specialist. Laughter also is good medicine. Watch uplifting movies and read inspirational books, and avoid negative situations while you are battling cancer—or at any time, for that matter!

The thymus gland, a butterfly shaped gland that sits at about the top of the breastbone at the bottom of the throat, is responsible for making immunity cells. Tapping this area with your fingers is called thymus thumping and may help stimulate T-cell production. Eating 10 raw almonds a day has also been recommended for folks with cancer. Eat them between meals to help balance blood sugar level.

Coping with Chemo

Chemotherapy is a radical chemical therapy that kills cancer cells in the body. The bad news is that it kills good cells, too—you can think of it as a big bomb being

Sage Advice

Bovine Growth Hormone (BGH) is given to dairy cows to increase their milk production. A recent Canadian study has shown that BGH does pass through the human gut and can increase human cell growth seven fold. You don't want to add any hormones that helps your cancer grow! Avoid products with BGH.

Sage Advice

If you are taking chemotherapy as a cancer treatment, you will want to protect the good cells as best you can with the same herbs used for fighting cancer, especially antioxidant vitamins and herbal supplements.

dropped on the battlefield. Chemotherapy can make some people very ill and can even make hair fall out. Consider using herbs to do your best to protect your body from the side effects of chemotherapy, and discuss these things with your doctor also.

Some controversy has arisen about antioxidants during chemotherapy. Some believe that the antioxidants will lessen the effect of the chemo by removing it from the body. I believe that anything that you can do to protect the good cells that you have will strengthen you. You will have to discuss this with the health care professionals you work with and must make up your own mind. Bee pollen and coenzyme Q_{10}, have also been used to help combat the side effects of chemotherapy treatment. Talk to some folks who have gone through chemotherapy using antioxidants with success, and see what you think.

Herb Lore

My good friend's mother took chemotherapy treatments for a bowel tumor and underwent a customized herbal program that my friend and I helped her with. She also took fairly large doses of antioxidants throughout her treatments. Not only did she not get sick, but she also never lost her hair. Her doctor told her to keep doing whatever she was doing, and five years later she is still cancer-free.

Recovery: Pumping You Up for Prevention

Once the battle is over, the healing can begin. You will need to rebuild your body after the destruction so that you can maintain your health and live preventatively. Hopefully you will have added the good things to your diet and lifestyle that have helped you win and recover, and it will serve you to keep those good habits for prevention for the rest of your life.

Maintaining your health with nutrients such as alfalfa (rich in minerals), bee pollen (nourishment for the body), antioxidants, acidophilus, enzymes, and red clover will keep your good cells strong and will serve as your preventative program.

High Cholesterol: Cutting Through the Fat

Basically, having a high cholesterol level means that you have a lot of fat in the blood. When the fat begins to adhere to the walls of your arteries, this can lead to hardening of the arteries, or coronary artery disease—and that can give you a heart attack. The good news is that plenty of great herbs can help emulsify that blood fat and protect you from heart diseases.

Eating too much saturated fat, such as deep fried foods, fatty meats, cheeses, and other dairy products, can sometimes cause high cholesterol. The liver is responsible for synthesizing all this fat and can use some support and cleansing. Stress also has been found to be a factor in raising blood cholesterol levels, too.

The Guggul Advantage

Guggul (*Commiphora mukul*) is a plant resin extract found in India that contains properties similar to niacin and fish oils—it supports and cleans the circulatory system. Some have described guggul lipid as the most powerful cholesterol-lowering herb known. It is best to try to find a standardized product to ensure that the beneficial part of the plant (guggulsterones) are present in each pill.

Once the guggul cleanses the fat from your arteries, you will need to help your body eliminate the fat. Let's see what other herbs you can use to support this process.

Herbs for a Sticky Situation

A good way to support eliminating dissolved cholesterol from the body is by taking a fiber supplement daily with your guggul. Psyllium hulls, apple pectin, and oat bran are all excellent fiber supplements alone or in combinations to help absorb fat and remove it from the body via the intestinal tract. Then speed up the process with a couple capsules of cascara sagrada at bed time each night. This will increase the bowel's peristaltic action and help to push out all that grabbed fat by morning.

Furthermore, capsicum sprinkled on foods in place of salt will boost circulation and encourage arterial cleansing. Some osteopathic doctors will offer *chelation therapy* or can provide a good reference for you. Chelation therapy is a practice administered intravenously to strip built-up fat from arterial walls. Keeping the bowel clear to make room for the harmful fat to leave the body will speed recovery; the use of fiber supplements will help this along.

Colds: A Cure for All Seasons

Sometimes a cold is just your body's way of doing its spring cleaning. Throwing off toxins that have built up throughout the long winter months can show up as a slight fever, runny nose, aches and pains, and sneezing. You can help this process along by speeding up the elimination of toxins with herbal support.

Sage Advice

If you have high cholesterol, you should begin cleansing the liver with herbs like milk thistle, dandelion, or turkey rhubarb. Beware however, when cleansing, your blood cholesterol reading will shoot up before it drops back down, which is part of the cleansing process. Stay clear of cholesterol screenings for at least three months to save your or your doctor's panic. You should also work with an herbalist or holistic practitioner to help you with this goal.

Sage Advice

Garlic also has been used to lower cholesterol levels, whether taken in pill form or eaten raw. For garlic breath, chew on some parsley sprigs, which is also good for your urinary tract.

Echinacea: The Cold Remedy

Echinacea (*Echinacea augustifolia,* or *Echinacea purpurea*) is a flower that has been discovered to be a mild healer and an excellent support herb for cold and flu symptoms. Different types of echinacea are available, and some are not useful in fighting a cold. Try to obtain echinacea purpurea, which is more effective than echinacea angustifolia. Echinacea helps boost your body's white blood cells, which are important in fighting infection. Echinacea works somewhat mildly in the body, so you might have to take it often. You can take two capsules every two to four hours when fighting off a cold. Echinacea also has an affinity for the respiratory system and helps to dry up a runny nose. This herb is safe for both adults and children.

Cold Combinations

Fighting a cold using combinations will show quicker results. Echinacea mixed with golden seal makes an excellent formula, and rose hips contain vitamin C, known for its power to boost the immune system. A good synergistic combination to fight off cold symptoms includes rose hips, chamomile (calms), yarrow, golden seal, myrrh, peppermint, sage, slippery elm (also eases sore throat), lemon grass, capsicum (stimulates), yerba santa, mullein, and astragalus.

Sage Advice

Some health practitioners utilize a method called chelation therapy to clean the circulatory system directly, and many use this for high cholesterol. The process involves intravenously injecting a formula of chemicals and substances that claw away heavy metals, artery fat, and other debris from the walls of the arteries.

Herb Lore

A sweat bath might help you fast-forward a cold or sickness. For a sweat bath, take a few capsules of capsicum or ginger internally, and run a hot bath. Empty a few capsules of either herb (or both) into the bath water, and soak in the hot tub. You should begin to sweat profusely, which will purge your body of toxins and help you to burn out any bad bacteria you are harboring. When finished, wrap yourself in warm sleep wear and go to bed with the blankets piled high. You should sweat all night and wake up feeling like a new person!

Of course, good old garlic is always a good remedy anytime your immune needs a boost. Throat lozenges with zinc, licorice root, vitamin C, and slippery elm also are helpful for coughs and sore throats.

Begin using any or all of these remedies after exposure to anyone contagious. Drink plenty of water to help your body flush out the cold, stay warm, and try a sweat bath.

Sage Advice

If you believe you have been exposed to cold germs, taking rose hips right away may help you experience less severe symptoms if you get the cold.

Cold Sore No More (Herpes Simplex)

Cold sores, otherwise known as fever blisters, are the result of the herpes virus, known as herpes simplex. Cold sores usually show up on or around the lips, and can even show up on the nose or face. The ailment is painful and unsightly—and is highly contagious. The virus lives in the body and manifests itself only when we are under stress and have a lowered immune system. Fighting the herpes virus needs to be approached from the inside, although external application will help the area heal after the virus has been fought.

Prevention is the best remedy for this ailment. Many factors can trigger cold sores, including an imbalance of amino acids or a lack of l-lysine (an essential amino acid provided in foods), too much stress, and overexposure to sun. To protect yourself, always wear a sunscreen on your face and lips when outdoors, and keep it on continuously.

Some trigger foods that can cause an outbreak include almonds, peanuts, citrus fruits, and chocolate. Also keep your immune system up by getting rest. If cold sores are reoccurring, find out why your immune system is so low, and deal with that problem.

Evening Primrose Oil: Fighting from Within

If I were stuck on a desert island with my choice of one herb to fight cold sores, I would have to choose evening primrose oil. Among its many healing properties, evening primrose oil contains essential fatty acids similar to essential amino acids that cannot be manufactured by the body. Evening primrose supports the immune system and helps reduce inflammation.

Evening primrose may help fight the progression of the herpes virus by boosting the immune system. It has been helpful for a variety of other diseases as well, including allergies, asthma, hormone imbalance, multiple sclerosis, obesity, skin and hair problems, eczema, and hyperactivity in children.

Combinations Sore to Help

White oak bark has astringent qualities that help contract tissues and that may help the swelling associated with cold sores. L-lysine or a combination of amino acids containing lysine have helped many not only during time of break-out, but also daily as a preventative measure. Acidophilus is important in the intestinal system because this good bacteria will help keep viruses at bay. Finally, zinc boosts the immune system and aids in skin healing.

A mixture of Chinese and western herbs designed by Chinese herbalist, Sabudi Darmandanda, has been used successfully by many for both cold sores (herpes simplex) and genital herpes (herpes complex). The mixture includes: dandelion root, scute root, purslane herb, pinellia rhizome, indigo herb and root, ginseng root, thlaspi herb, cinnamon twig, bupleurum root, and licorice root. Begin taking this combo at the first sign of an outbreak.

Tea tree oil, vitamin E oil, colloidal silver, and a topical cream called Super Lysine Plus+®, which contains lysine and other healing ingredients for the lips, have all been useful for arresting an outbreak and helping the area heal. (Lysine Plus+ is manufactured by a company in Eugene, Oregon, and is found in most health food stores.)

Sage Advice

Colloidal silver has served to kill viruses in petri dishes, and some say it will kill a virus if taken internally. Use as you would an antibiotic, only for 10 days in a row. Then supplement with acidophilus again. A friend claims that when he applies colloidal silver to an emerging cold sore, the cold sore disappears.

Constipation: All Dressed Up and Nowhere to Go

Constipation is a problem that most everyone suffers from at some time or another, whether they know it or not. Indeed, most of us are not as bowel-conscious as we ought to be. But how could we be constipated without knowing it? Well, the bowel is a tube that can stretch to many times its normal size. We can harbor old fecal matter, undigested foods, parasites, and other things that are compacted on the sides of the colon walls. I consider this condition of the bowel to be constipated because the feces is still compacted in the bowel, even though there may be a tunnel of space through the middle allowing the person to pass some waste material through. This means that a person can still be eliminating daily wastes through the bowel, however, not all the waste is being dislodged.

To illustrate, when a client comes to me and they don't believe that they are constipated, although my assessment shows that they are, I will discuss with them a cleansing diet and herbs designed to eliminate the backed-up wastes. Some will even take colonics or enemas to speed the process. When they follow the program and see that they are actually eating less than normal, and evacuating up to six times their normal amount of waste, they are absolutely amazed. Not to mention, usually lighter! The point is that the bowel can store up material on the sides of the colon walls and in bowel pockets, although you might be eliminating daily. See Chapter 4 for information on bowel cleansing and Ivy's daily cleansing drink recipe.

So what is the profile for the ideal bowel function? Ideally, you should eliminate once for every meal eaten. (That's thrice daily for you three-meal-a-day people!) The stool should be approximately 2" in diameter, a light brown color, soft in consistency (but formed), usually remaining in one piece from 6"–12" in length, and should come out without strain. The total evacuation time should require no longer than one minute, and should not leave a foul odor (really!). So how do you match up? If you are one of those who needs to take a novel to the pot with you, then you are probably constipated! (Note: As a general rule, while on a cleansing program, you will eliminate more than once for each meal eaten.)

Some factors that contribute to constipation include these:

➤ Lack of water

➤ Ignoring the call of nature (not going when you feel the need)

➤ Nervous tension that keeps the bowel tense

➤ Lack of exercise can help the bowel get lazy

➤ Side effects of many medications that make constipation a problem

➤ The five white enemies: white flour, sugar, milk, salt, and rice

It's best to learn the cause of your constipation and correct that first. For cleansing purposes and to stimulate things into action, though, herbs make a great remedy.

Cascara Sagrada: Make Like a Tree and Bark!

Cascara sagrada (*Rhamnus purshiana*) is Spanish meaning "sacred bark." Its medicinal value comes from the dried and aged bark of the herb rhamnus purshiana. This bitter herb has been used for centuries and is one of the best and safest herbs to stimulate a laxative effect for chronic constipation (bitter-tasting herbs are notorious for their bowel-stimulating properties). Cascara is so bitter, in fact, that some have used a cascara sagrada tincture applied to their fingernails to help break the habit of chewing on their nails!

Cascara has also been used to restore tone to a relaxed bowel. Remember that the bowel is a muscle and needs strength for proper function; a lazy bowel is a constipated bowel. Cascara is also useful for the stomach, liver, gallbladder, and pancreas, and can be used to help expel worms from the bowel. It stimulates bile flow, which in turn stimulates bowel peristalsis.

A few capsules given to an herbal non-believer before bed will make a true believer out of him by the next morning!

Fiber: Moving Right Along

For some, cascara is too harsh. Other wonderful herbs with laxative effects on the bowel include flax seed, psyllium hulls, chlorophyll, and aloe vera juice. A wonderful combination to cleanse the bowel, blood, and entire digestive tract includes cascara sagrada bark, barberry bark, buckthorn bark, turkey rhubarb root, licorice root, couch grass herb, capsicum fruit, red clover tops, and ginger root.

Of course, we already mentioned that a lack of certain things can cause constipation, such as lack of water, fiber, and exercise. Other things besides herbs that can get things moving for you include reflexology treatments, acupuncture, figs, and prune juice. Go lightly on the prune juice, as some can have explosions of relief! But it is always something to consider in an emergency if you cannot obtain herbs.

Cysts—No, I Insist

Cysts usually result from stagnant energy where toxins in the blood build. Blood cleansing is the best remedy for cysts: I have seen plenty of tumors and cysts disappear with the use of herbal blood cleansers.

Cysts are benign growths caused by an excess growth of fat cells created by internal toxicity and infection. You should not only use herbs to help melt the cysts, but also use digestive herbs and enzymes to assist your body in breaking down fats. Let's take a look at a well-known herb that has a reputation as a cyst dissolver.

Pau D'Arco to Dissolve the Problem

Pau d'arco (*Tubebula avellanedae*) (pronounced *paw dee-arc-oh*) and also commonly referred to as Taheebo tea, is the bark of a tropical tree found mostly in Brazil and Argentina. The tree is known for its ability to resist fungus growth even though it exists in a tropical (and, thus, ideal for fungus) area. Used by the Inca Indians as an immunity tonic, pau d'arco has served many well in fighting cancer and melting tumors.

Pau d'arco also has antioxidant properties that work to fight free radical scavengers in the body. It has been used to fight lung, prostate, and colon cancer, and is believed to increase red blood cell production and decrease blood sugar.

One particular client of mine had a cyst on her right leg for 14 years. In fact, she had it for so long that it was like a cyst-ter to her (groan). Anyway, after only one week on an herbal program that included two cups of pau d'arco tea daily, four burdock root capsules, six red clover capsules, and two cascara sagrada at bedtime, she claimed her cyst completely disappeared. It has been several years now and the cyst has not returned.

In–Cyst on Blood Cleansers

Other blood-cleansing herbs include red clover tops and burdock root; when taken together, these make a great blood-cleansing tonic. Other useful

Sage Advice

A chemical contained in pau d'arco known as lapachol may inhibit tumor growth by preventing the tumor from utilizing oxygen essentially suffocating the tumor.

Sage Advice

Cysts may be activated or aggravated by hormones found in non-organic animal products. Try eliminating these, or eat only non-hormone-induced dairy or animal products.

supplements include reishi mushroom, shark cartilage, Essiac formula (especially for cancerous cysts), and vitamins A, D, and E.

Working from the outside in, the external application of an ointment or poultice made from chaparral herb, lobelia, comfrey leaf, golden seal root, plantain root, red clover herb, mullein herb, marshmallow root, chickweed herb, and myrrh gum in a base of olive oil, beeswax, pine tar, and vitamin E oil has proven helpful.

Because most cysts are the result of stagnant energy, moving energy with therapies such as reflexology, acupuncture, or acupressure may help get your energy un-stuck and flowing smoothly again. Daily dry skin brushing will also improve circulation and stimulate lymph flow. Use a natural bristle skin brush and brush your body (avoid your face) before you get in the shower each morning. Lymphatic massages will help move stagnate lymphs also.

Herbal Remedies for Common Ailments

Cancer

Best Single Herb: Red clover

Best Combinations: Essiac formula; pau d'arco; cascara sagrada; red clover

Other Helpful Supplements: All antioxidant vitamins; shark cartilage; reishi mushroom; germanium; food enzymes with hydrochloric acid; acidophilus; Omega-3 oils

Possible Causes: Lowered immune system; overexposure to carcinogens

Complementary Help: Laughter; exposure to positive influences; thymus thumping; eat raw almonds (10 a day); drink carrot juice; eat only organic foods; avoid junk foods; cleanse the bowel; do not overtax the body

Cholesterol, High

Best Single Herb: Guggul lipid

Best Combinations: Psyllium hulls, oat bran, apple pectin; guggul lipid; garlic; milk thistle; cascara sagrada

Other Helpful Supplements: Omega-3 oils; niacin; lecithin

Possible Causes: Sluggish liver; stress; high-fat diet

Complementary Help: Chelation therapy; cleansing the bowel; using capsicum as a seasoning

Colds

Best Single Herb: Echinacea

Best Combinations: Golden seal, echinacea; rose hips, chamomile, yarrow, golden seal, myrrh, peppermint, sage, slippery elm, lemon grass, capsicum, yerba santa, mullein, astragalus; garlic

Other Helpful Supplements: Vitamin C; zinc lozenges (licorice root and slippery elm added to lozenges help coughs and sore throat)

Possible Causes: Natural detoxifying process; built-up mucus and toxins; lowered immune system

Complementary Help: Rest; sweat bath

Cold Sore (Herpes Simplex)

Best Single Herb: Evening primrose oil

Best Combinations: Dandelion root, scute root, purslane herb, pinellia rhizome, indigo herb and root, ginseng root, thlaspi herb, cinnamon twig, bupleurum root, licorice root; alfalfa, marshmallow, plantain, horsetail, oat straw, wheat grass, hops; white oak bark; evening primrose or black current oil

Other Helpful Supplements: L-lysine or combination of all amino acids; colloidal silver; acidophilus; zinc

Possible Causes: Overexposure to sun (use lip balm consistently); trigger foods such as peanuts, citrus, almonds, and chocolate; high body temperature; Candida or other problems lowering the immune system; stress

Complementary Help: Externally, some of the following have been helpful: vitamin E oil; colloidal silver (internal and externally); tea tree oil; Super Lysine Plus+®

Constipation

Best Single Herb: Cascara sagrada

Best Combinations: Cascara sagrada bark, barberry bark, buckthorn bark, turkey rhubarb root, licorice root, couch grass herb, capsicum fruit, red clover tops, ginger root; flax seed; psyllium hulls; chlorophyll; aloe vera juice

Other Helpful Supplements: Food enzymes

Possible Causes: Dehydration; tension; poor diet; not enough exercise; some medications

Complementary Help: Bowel cleansing; exercise; reflexology; acupuncture; prune juice

Cysts

Best Single Herb: Pau d'arco

Best Combinations: Red clover tops, burdock root; pau d'arco

Other Helpful Supplements: Reishi mushroom, shark cartilage, Essiac formula; and vitamins A, D, and E

Possible Causes: Hormonal imbalances

Complementary Help: Bowel cleansing

119

The Least You Need to Know

➤ A healthy philosophy about cancer can help you overcome the battle.

➤ Red clover contains properties that may prevent and fight cancer.

➤ Help your body fast-forward through a cold with herbs; it may just be your body doing its own spring cleaning.

➤ Cascara sagrada is one of the best herbal remedies for chronic constipation.

➤ Blood-cleansing herbs can help dissolve cysts in some people.

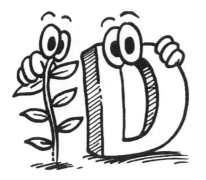

Chapter 9

D Best Herbal Solutions

In This Chapter

➤ Deal with dandruff herbally

➤ Fight depression the herbal way

➤ Herbal supplements to help prevent diabetes

➤ Herbal rescues for diarrhea

"As soon as he ceased to be mad he became merely stupid. There are maladies we must not seek to cure because they alone protect us from others that are more serious." —French novelist Marcel Proust (1871–1922) *A la recherche du temps perdu: Le Cote de Guermantes*

This chapter will take you through some common ailments beginning with the letter D and you'll be introduced to several more herbal cures. We'll start out by discussing dandruff, so stop scratching your head and read on!

Dandruff: Not Too Tough

Have you been accused of being flaky? Do your co-workers wonder if it's snowing outside when they first see you arrive? Do you get asked where the parade was or what celebration you just came from? If so, you could be suffering from dandruff. Dandruff is a common problem characterized by small flakes of dead skin that fall from the scalp and tend to accumulate on a person's shoulders. This can be quite embarrassing when wearing dark garments.

Sage Advice

Silicon gives skin, hair, and nails strength and resiliency, so nourishing the skin with herbs rich in silicon is a good idea when dealing with dandruff. Herbs rich in silicon include horsetail, alfalfa, cornsilk, and oatstraw.

Poison Ivy

Rosemary can raise blood pressure, so consider using a different herb internally for dandruff if you also have high blood pressure.

Well, before you go wearing all white, let's take a look at what can cause dandruff in the first place. You'll see how herbs used topically and internally have helped many get rid of their dandruff right away.

Poor circulation, nervous disorders, or a combination of both may cause dandruff. When there is poor circulation to the scalp, the skin cells die from lack of nourishment and shed in large flakes. You should improve circulation to help bring nutrients to the top of the head, and you also should decrease stress. Herbs can assist in both of these areas.

Rosemary: Dealing with Flakes

Rosemary (*Rosarinus officinalis*) is an herb used topically for dandruff, but it may also be taken internally. Rosemary should be taken in small doses for internal use to help improve circulation and aid in digestion. Rosemary leaves are rich in minerals such as calcium, magnesium, phosphorus, sodium, and potassium, all of which are needed by the nerves and the circulatory system. Rosemary has a mild sedating effect on the body and can calm frazzled nerves.

Rosemary oil also can be rubbed into the scalp and rubbed onto the temples for relief of tension headaches. You can also make rosemary leaves and flowers into a tea and use it as a hair rinse for treating dandruff.

Jojoba's Witness to Cleaning Up Dandruff

Topically, jojoba oil is one of the best herbal remedies to help your dandruff problem. When applied to the scalp at night and shampooed out the next day, the oil of the jojoba plant will nourish your skin and eliminate dandruff. Some people like to add a drop or two to styled hair for extra shine.

Sometimes dandruff is just your scalp's way of telling you that your skin needs nourishment. A great combination of herbs to feed the skin, hair, and nails includes dulse, horsetail, sage, and rosemary. Dulse supports the thyroid, and horsetail is rich in silicon to nourish hair, skin, nails, and even teeth. Sage contains zinc and B vitamins that nourish the brain. And we already talked about rosemary's usefulness for treating dandruff. When combined, these herbs make a great combination for dandruff.

Your blood carries nutrients to all parts of your body, and an excellent herb to increase blood supply to the head area is ginkgo biloba. This herb is great for memory loss, too (see the section "Alzheimer's: Don't Forget to Take Your Herbs," in Chapter 5, "A is for Ailment," for more information).

If your dandruff is caused by stress, a B-complex vitamin can help you with that. Other nutrients include beta carotene, vitamin A, and lecithin. Lecithin is a good brain food as well and is used to help the circulatory system.

With any problems affecting the hair, you also might want to have your thyroid checked. The thyroid takes part in regulating the metabolism, and problems with the thyroid can cause hair loss and other symptoms. Also make sure that you do not have high cholesterol, which could interfere with proper circulation. If you do, see the section "High Cholesterol: Cutting Through the Fat," in Chapter 8, "C's for a Common Cure."

Depression Suppression

Depression can be a serious illness—as with all these ailments in this book, see your health care provider for any medical problem. For the purposes of mild to occasional depression, we will discuss some herbs used to give a temporary mental lift; however, you should also concentrate on what is causing your depression if it seems to be ongoing.

If your goal is to wean yourself from your depression medication while your nervous system responds to your consistent use of herbal remedies and other supplements, you can work toward that goal. However, this should ONLY be attempted under supervision! Do not base your efforts solely on the suggestions given to you here! Do yourself a favor and work with your physician and a qualified herbalist to guide you in your goals.

Otherwise, for occasional "down times" and if you are not already on antidepressants, try the suggestions given here to lift your sagging spirits.

St. John's Wort: A Saint for the Depressed

St. John's wort (*Hypericum perforatum*) is a pleasing-looking yellow flowering herb used by many as a mood enhancer and a stress reliever. This herb has become very popular in the media and among consumers in the United States lately. Of course,

Sage Advice

Occasional depression is a normal part of life and growth, and we can use these periods to reflect on ourselves. Used wisely, short periods of depression can make us better people by giving us the opportunity to reflect and set goals to improve our life.

Poison Ivy

St. John's wort should not be taken if you are on any other type of antidepressant medication. It is also not recommended for pregnant or nursing women. St. John's wort can also cause nausea in some. If this happens to you, try taking some ginger to subside this symptom.

Germans have known about its positive effects on depression for some time, and doctors there write more prescriptions for St. John's wort than for antidepressant drugs. (Maybe they are on to something there.)

Other Things to Cheer You Up

A wonderful combination of Chinese herbs used to beat mild depression that seems to linger over your head like a dark cloud is a combination containing perilla, saussurea, gambir, bamboo, bupleurum, pinellia, aurantium, zhishi, ophiopogon, cypreus, platycodon, ligusticum dang gui, panax ginseng, hoelen, coptis, ginger, and licorice. This combination will work on decongesting the liver which can help lift depression. Another good single herb to use along with this Chinese combination is milk thistle. (See more on milk thistle's work on the liver in the section "Environmental Allergies," in Chapter 5.)

Herb Lore

Depression can indicate the need to strengthen or cleanse the liver. Because the liver is where we hold our emotions of anger, cleansing the liver physically with herbs can sometimes bring about a purging of strong and sometimes angry feelings. I have seen this happen over and over—don't ask me why or how it works, but be warned that during liver cleansing, you might have a few days of unexplainable anger! Afterward, you should feel uplifted and happy, even though those around you might not be so happy!

Besides stemming from a burdened liver, depression can be brought about by other physical factors, including nervous system or chemical imbalances, thyroid problems, or circulatory problems.

Herbs and supplements that feed the nervous system can be found under the section "Anxiety: Panic Not—Herbs to the Rescue," in Chapter 6, "Give Me Another A!" The B-complex vitamins can help combat stress and should always be considered when depressed. Zinc is another mineral crucial to mental health, and a zinc deficiency should not be overlooked with serious depression.

You might want to consider some extra steps as well if you cannot seem to snap out of depression:

➤ Find yourself a good counselor/psychiatrist/psychologist.

➤ Get some exercise.

➤ Temporarily change your environment to help stimulate a change in your mood.

➤ Act happy! The saying goes that if you act happy, you will eventually be happy. Smile and tell me you're cranky, try it!

➤ Remember the big picture, and get philosophical. Things don't seem so glum when you realize that there is a universal order and that everything happens for a reason.

➤ Try helping someone else who's worse off than yourself. Remember that we all have something to offer the world. So don't be sad—be glad you have something to offer!

➤ Give your cat some catnip and watch her play!

Herb Lore

Do you remember your dreams? Dream recall is a normal, healthy event. Studies have found a link between mental illness and the inability to have dream recall. In fact, supplementing with zinc and vitamin B6 helped people remember their dreams and improved their psychiatric health. Herbs rich in zinc include bee pollen, scullcap, capsicum, spirulina, garlic, sage, eyebright, bilberry, buchu, and gotu kola. Herbs rich in B6 include alfalfa, slippery elm, ginseng, spirulina, sarsaparilla, peppermint, papaya, parsley, gotu kola, and hops.

Diabetes: How Sweet It Isn't

Diabetes mellitus, commonly referred to as diabetes, is another serious illness and should be supervised by your medical doctor. It is an illness where the body loses its ability to utilize *insulin*, a chemical our pancreas makes to control the level of *glucose* in the blood. There are actually four types of diabetes, but we will discuss the two main types, Type I and II, in more detail.

Botanical Bit

Diabetes mellitus is a blood sugar disorder caused by the lack of or inability of the body to utilize a pancreatic hormone known as insulin. **Insulin** is a hormone produced by the pancreas to regulate glucose in the blood. **Glucose** is the term for blood sugar. Symptoms of diabetes include excessive thirst and production of large volumes of urine.

Type I diabetes tends to run in families and is the more serious form of the disease. Type I diabetes is also called insulin-dependent diabetes, juvenile-onset diabetes, brittle diabetes, or ketosis-prone diabetes. This type most often develops during childhood, although young adults also can develop this form. In childhood and in Type I diabetes, coma from not enough insulin is a constant danger.

Type II diabetes is also called non-insulin-dependent diabetes, adult-onset diabetes, ketosis-resistant diabetes, or stable diabetes. Type II often develops in overweight adults. Insulin tablets are sometimes used for Type II diabetes, although insulin is given in injections in more severe cases. The kind and amount of insulin given varies with the person's condition, and stress of any kind may require a change in the dose.

Herb Lore

Diabetes is the third leading cause of death in the U.S. One in five adults will develop adult-onset diabetes. It is a contributing factor in heart disease and stroke. It has been highly associated with a chromium deficiency (a trace mineral), largely due to a top soil deficiency where our foods are grown. Statistics show that 90 percent of Americans are deficient in chromium. Herbal sources of chromium include: kelp, licorice, and spirulina. Sugar and refined foods deplete chromium.

Type II diabetes is a condition usually brought on by lifestyle factors such as lack of exercise and too much sugar or carbohydrates in the diet. Because it is lifestyle-related, this condition is easier to control and may even be reversible with natural remedies. Let's see how we can work to reverse this problem by using nutritious herbs.

Golden Seal: The Golden Healer

Poison Ivy

If you are a diabetic and decide to try golden seal, make sure that you notify your doctor and get regular check-ups to monitor your insulin requirements. Too much insulin can cause hypoglycemia (low blood sugar), which can be just as damaging as having high blood sugar levels.

One herb that would most benefit the management of diabetes (of any type) alone would be the herb golden seal (*Hydrastis canadensis*). Golden seal is a bitter herb that has an antibiotic effect on the body and is used by many to fight infections. Its use for diabetics may have been overlooked, as this herb also lowers blood sugar levels.

In fact, some borderline diabetics have tried golden seal with success before using insulin to lower their blood sugar levels. Insulin is a substance produced by the pancreas to lower our blood sugar level. This substance is insufficient in diabetics. When using golden seal to lower the blood sugar, you will decrease your insulin requirement, so please work with your doctor to have your insulin requirement checked regularly. I have seen many utilize golden seal and other herbs in combination to make it possible for my clients to eliminate the need for insulin. This is just another wonderful benefit of using herbs for health.

Herb Lore

Golden seal's yellow color made it useful to the Native Americans as a dye for cloth. The Cherokee tribe recognized that those who wore cloth dyed in golden seal rarely became ill, which may have been how this herb was discovered for its medicinal uses. The Native Americans were responsible for teaching European settlers about golden seal's beneficial properties for uses as an eye wash and for treating skin wounds and ulcers.

A combination of any of the following herbs will help to bring down and regulate your blood sugar: cedar berries, burdock, horseradish, golden seal, and Siberian ginseng. Psyllium hulls are also an excellent bulk fiber to use when suffering from diabetes. The fiber swells in the digestive tract and slows the absorption of sugars, which helps keep blood sugar from spiking up and down rapidly. Taken before each meal, psyllium hulls are a positive addition for diabetics, especially those who lack fibrous foods in their diet.

Trace minerals and zinc are other helpful supplements for diabetics of either type. With more advanced diabetes, circulatory herbs such as cayenne pepper are useful; the glands need to be balanced, the circulation improved, and the kidneys strengthened in someone with diabetes. Please refer to other chapters in this book on herbs for the kidneys, herbs that nourish the eyes, and herbs that improve circulation to help complete your herbal program.

Sage Advice

Zinc is an important nutrient to diabetics because this mineral influences the digestion of carbohydrates in the body. Pumpkin seeds are one of the richest sources of zinc from nature.

Take a Hike

Exercise lowers blood sugar levels as well. Incorporating a regular exercise program into your life is important whether you are diabetic or not, but it's especially important if you have high blood sugar. Work with a specialist who can help design a program for your needs. If you can't do that, take a walk. Walking is the most natural and comfortable form of exercise; it gets the circulation moving, cleanses the lymph nodes, increases the heart rate, gets the lungs pumping, and is a wonderful and safe exercise that everyone can enjoy.

Diarrhea: Some Gripping Advice

Diarrhea can be caused by different factors, which may include:

➤ A parasite infestation. A parasite is any organism that lives as a guest in your body and that contributes nothing to your well-being. Parasites can include fungus, bacteria, viruses, protozoa, and worms. Any of these can be contracted through contaminated food, commonly referred to as food poisoning.

➤ Stress and anxiety. The bowel is intimately connected with your nervous system and can react negatively to nervousness.

➤ Intestinal infections or inflammation can be brought on by other diseases, such as Chrone's disease.

Knowing what might be causing your diarrhea will help you to treat it with the best remedy and to eliminate the source of your irritation.

Poison Ivy

If you or someone you are responsible for has a bad bout of diarrhea, you can utilize the herbs and supplements described to stop the diarrhea. If diarrhea persists, however, you should contact your physician to make sure that the person does not suffer the complications associated with dehydration.

If you catch a bug (whether a parasite or bacteria) foreign to your body, your body reacts to eliminate the invader by stimulating peristaltic action of the bowel. This creates a forceful movement of the bowels, which can manifest itself as diarrhea. In this case, diarrhea is really a protective mechanism your body is activating to rid itself of a toxin.

Due to the loss of fluid, salts, and nutrients that accompany diarrhea, dehydration is a concern—severe dehydration can cause brain damage or death if not treated. Therefore, it is important—especially for the elderly and children—to counteract the dehydrating effects of diarrhea through the intake of plenty of liquids. Make sure that the water supplied is filtered water and is not the source of possible contamination that could be causing the problem.

Bayberry: Berry Good for Diarrhea

For diarrhea caused by any condition, an astringent herb can be used to contract tissues and slow things down. A good single herb used to combat the problem is bayberry (*Myrica cerifera*), not to be confused with barberry (*Berberis vulgaris*). For its best use against diarrhea, bayberry should be made into a decoction or tea. If bayberry cannot be found, blackberry tea also works very well. Taking either of these herbs in a capsule form is helpful as well; however, the results may take longer in a pill form because the capsules require digestion.

Bayberry has special properties that act as germicides and that can destroy harmful bacteria and help the body get rid of mucus and toxins. It contains a rich amount of vitamin C and calcium, which makes it a very nourishing herb.

Bayberry has also been used to stop profuse menstruation and bleeding gums, and it has been useful in helping fight infections, cholera, colitis, dysentery, hemorrhoids, and jaundice.

Other Herbs on the Run

For the prevention of diarrhea caused by food poisoning, bacterial infections, or parasites, food enzymes with hydrochloric acid supplements should be used before every meal, especially when dining out or traveling. Hydrochloric acid (HCl) is an acid normally produced by the stomach to kill off parasites when we consume foods that are contaminated. As we age, our stomach produces less and less of this acid, which can leave us more vulnerable to infections caused by ingested foods, drinks, or anything that enters through the mouth. Supplementing with these can help protect us from getting diarrhea in the first place.

Acidophilus is the good bacteria normally present in our digestive tract. These bacteria keep other harmful bacteria and viruses in our body at bay. They also eat up other foreign substances that enter through our digestive tract and serve as another form of protection against invaders. Substances such as caffeine, carbonated beverages, and antibiotics can kill off these good bacteria temporarily, leaving us vulnerable to infections. Acidophilus or bifidophilus supplementation can help replenish our body with these helpful bacteria. Take four to six capsules on an empty stomach every day for best protection against picking up bugs and to stop diarrhea. Acidophilus will fight against any existing bacterial infection going on in your system.

Other herbs that can help slow things down include psyllium hulls or oat bran. Psyllium acts like a bulking agent in the colon and will help absorb excess water.

For children suffering from diarrhea, red raspberry in a liquid extract is an excellent remedy.

Sage Advice

Garlic is one of the best-known herbs to kill parasites. Eating raw cloves of garlic will help fumigate any parasitic infection you may be contaminated with. For serious parasitic infections, however, you might need more than garlic. See Chapter 19, "O, P, and Q: Obvious Painful Questions and Answers," for more information on fighting parasites.

Herbal Remedies for Common Ailments

Dandruff

Best Single Herb: Rosemary
Best Combinations: Dulse, horsetail, sage, rosemary; ginkgo biloba
Other Helpful Supplements: B-complex, vitamin A, or beta carotene; lecithin
Possible Causes: Thyroid problems; nervous disorders; poor circulation
Complementary Help: Jojoba oil or rosemary oil (both used externally)

continues

Herbal Remedies for Common Ailments   (continued)

Depression

Best Single Herb: St. John's wort

Best Combinations: Chinese combination perilla, saussurea, gambir, bamboo, bupleurum, pinellia, aurantium, zhishi, ophiopogon, cyprerus, platycodon, ligusticum dang gui, panax ginseng, hoelen, coptis, ginger, licorice; milk thistle

Other Helpful Supplements: B-complex, zinc

Possible Causes: Weakened liver; nervous system problems; thyroid problems; circulatory problems

Complementary Help: Counseling; exercise; change of environment

Diabetes

Best Single Herb: Golden seal

Best Combinations: Cedar berries, burdock, horseradish, golden seal, Siberian ginseng; psyllium hulls

Other Helpful Supplements: Chromium; zinc; trace minerals

Possible Causes: Dehydration; poor diet

Complementary Help: Exercise

Diarrhea

Best Single Herb: Bayberry root

Best Combinations: Psyllium hulls; blackberry root, or bayberry root

Other Helpful Supplements: Bifidophilus or acidophilus

Possible Causes: Parasites; food poisoning; stress

Complementary Help: Prevention with food enzymes with hydrochloric acid and acidophilus, especially when traveling

---

The Least You Need to Know

➤ Rosemary and jojoba oil are two excellent topical applications for the treatment of dandruff.

➤ St. John's wort is a popular herb to fight mild to moderate depression, but it should not be taken with other antidepressant medications.

➤ Golden seal helps lower blood sugar levels and is a helpful supplement for diabetics.

➤ Blackberry root or barberry root tea makes an excellent remedy to arrest diarrhea.

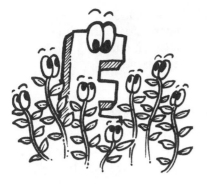

Chapter 10

E: Everywhere an Herb, Herb

In This Chapter

➤ Fight ear infections with herbal remedies

➤ Get relief from eczema using herbs

➤ Herbs that may reverse endometriosis

➤ Nourish the eyes with herbs

"E" might stand for "everywhere you look you see herbs," but it also stands for an "end to your ailments." If all else fails with your medical care, or if you are deciding to go au natural, herbs may be the missing link that will help you on your road to recovery. This chapter will show you how herbal remedies can nourish your eyes, ease the pain in your ears, and clear up eczema and endometriosis. This is a good way to ease into using herbs and hopefully e-rase your pain!

Earaches

Oh, your aching head! Earaches are painful ailments usually brought on by an infection and can not only be painful but also cause dizziness. Many times earaches are a common childhood complaint caused by allergies; make sure that there are no foreign objects in the ear before using herbs topically.

Some ear infections start with the growth of fungus on the ear drum. This can happen especially in warm, moist climates or when a person swims frequently. The following remedies will help you or your child fight the infection causing the earache and also help fight the fungus or infection locally.

Some infections can be aggravated by excess mucus production, and testing for food allergies is a good idea. Common food allergies involve wheat and sugar, so it will be helpful to eliminate these foods completely from your diet while fighting an infection.

Mucus and ear wax can harden in the ear canal, leaving you vulnerable to earaches, infections, and dizziness. Sometimes a lack of essential fatty acids is the culprit in the excess production of ear wax. Consider supplementing with an Omega-3 oil, lecithin, or flax seed oil supplement to help emulsify some of that wax build-up. A capsule or two daily of any of these is useful.

Echinacea: 'Ears to Its Infection-Fighting Ability

We have already talked about echinacea being a great remedy for colds, allergies, and other ailments. This is just one of those all-around safe herbs that is helpful for all types of infections. Echinacea can dry up excess mucus and can serve to heal earaches that are due to excess mucus in the sinus cavities.

Herbal Synergy and Supplemental Support

Other herbal combinations you can take with your echinacea to help fight infection include garlic and a mixture of parthenium, yarrow, myrrh, and capsicum. These all work synergistically to kill infection and lessen mucus; the capsicum acts as a stimulator to increase the effectiveness of all herbs.

After infection is over, an herbal calcium supplement will aid your body in rebuilding tissues that need healing. Think of calcium as the "knitter" in the body; it helps wounds heal by supplying the ingredients your body needs to rebuild. Herbs rich in calcium and silicon (silicon is also food for the structural system) include oatstraw, horsetail, dulse, and rosemary.

Herbal Ear Drops and Other Home Remedies

Going right to the source with herbal infection fighters and pain relievers can speed up the healing process. Two to three drops directly into the ear using lobelia, garlic, mullein, or tea tree oil has been used with success for earaches for adults and children alike. However, please avoid placing any drops in ears that have had tubes surgically inserted. Warm the oil up slightly by placing the oil bottle in a hot pan of water for a minute or so first. This makes it feel better and makes the oil less viscous, helping it slide easily into the ear canal. These will all serve to soothe the canal and fight infection locally.

Another home remedy helpful for ear pain involves a large onion. Here's the remedy:

1. Bake the onion until soft.

2. Cut the onion in half.

3. Let the onion cool until you can stand to place your finger into the center.

Poison Ivy

Ear coning should not be done at home by yourself. Ask around your health food store, or ask your favorite herbalist or natural health practitioner—they will usually have a source where you can have it done.

4. Lay the flat side of each half on each ear, and wrap the onion snugly around your head (you can do one at a time if you keep the other half of the onion warm).

5. Keep on until the onion cools.

Not only does this help to relieve pain, but it can clear mucus congestion, too.

Eliminate toxins from the body with bowel cleansing to help any ailment. Enemas for both children and adults can bring relief fairly quickly. Add some garlic to the enema water to give an extra bacterial-fighting boost to the body and speed recovery time.

Herb Lore

Ear coning, also known as candling, is an ancient Egyptian healing practice still used today to clear the head of congestion and mucus, to ease the pain associated with ear infections, and to remove excess ear wax and debris from the ear canal. Some believe it helps clear psychic congestion as well. Ear cones are hollow tubes made from gauze dipped in beeswax. The cones are lit at one end, and the other end is placed gently in the ear. As the cone burns down, it sucks excess debris from the ear canal. When the smoke enters the ear canal, it has a healing or soothing effect on the tissues. Some ear cone manufacturers add mullein, echinacea, and other respiratory herbs to the wax mixture.

Ear coning is used by some to get sinus and ear ache relief. Do not attempt ear coning alone, however. It is wise to have an experienced practitioner do this for you, or have someone teach you and your partner how to do it for each other.

Eczema: Getting Under Your Skin

Eczema is described as a superficial inflammation of the skin, an itchy red rash often accompanied by small blisters that weep and become encrusted. Typically, eczema will be treated medically with locally applied steroid hormones to help reduce inflammation; however, since drugs can do damage to the body, try these safe herbal remedies first.

To help yourself get the best treatment possible you will need to understand which type of eczema

Botanical Bit

Eczema has several different categorizations, but the disease is divided into two general categories based on the suspected cause. The first is caused by external factors, and the other has no known external cause (presumably, it comes from within).

you are exhibiting. Knowing this will help you better understand what your cause might be and will govern the approach to your treatment. Like I say over and over, finding your cause is a big part of finding your cure. Some eczema is caused by allergy, some by lack of circulation, and some by something from the outside that your skin is contacting.

For the sake of simplicity, we will work with an herb or two that serves to cleanse the blood via the liver and the lymphatics. Remember that the skin is always as clean as the blood is.

Some of these herbs will work to help your body chemistry balance, which will eventually cause your symptom to disappear. Once you find out the root of this problem, you can add herbs or make lifestyle changes to help you with the cause. For instance, if you have eczema related to a lack of circulation in the legs, incorporating an invigorating exercise program along with taking herbs that stimulate circulation will get to the core of your problem.

Oregon Grape: A Grape Remedy for Eczema

Oregon grape (*Berberis Aquifolium*) is probably the most widely used and accepted herbal remedy for chronic skin conditions such as eczema, dermatitis, and psoriasis, all skin inflammation diseases. Its best use for helping eczema is in a liquid extract or tea, and it can be used internally as well as externally.

Oregon grape goes to the liver and lymphatics, helps purify blood, and serves as a mild laxative. It contains a powerful natural antibiotic similar to golden seal and has been used to clear up skin conditions of all kinds.

Herb Lore

It is said that Oregon grape got its name from the pioneers traveling the Oregon Trail, which runs through the western United States. These pioneers gathered the herb for its use as a food and medicine along the trail where it grows abundantly, although at one time it was almost extinct near populated areas because of its popularity in trade. Settlers would make the herb into tea and drink it for the prevention or treatment of scurvy, fever, and upset stomach. Oregon grape is rich in vitamins C, D, and E; manganese; silicon; sodium; and zinc.

Oregon grape is also used for acne, dandruff, and detoxification. It gets to the source of skin problems because it helps regulate bile flow, decreases liver congestion, promotes the digestion of fats, and helps relieve constipation, all of which contribute to skin ailments.

The Beauty of Herbs: Not Just Skin-Deep

Combinations used together to cleanse the blood and feed the skin include burdock root, Oregon grape, pau d'arco, vitamins A and E, and zinc. Because you will either make or purchase Oregon grape in a liquid form, it will be easy to apply to affected areas on the skin. Apply to a test area, such as the back of your hand, for several days each day, and watch how it works for you. You may want to apply it straight, or you can add it to your natural shampoo for eczema in the scalp. Externally, you can also add the herb calendula (from marigold flowers), known for its soothing effects on the skin. Mix it with some aloe vera, and apply as a paste to affected areas.

If you do not yet know the source of your eczema, eliminate any possible causes of skin irritants, such as toxic and industrialized chemicals. Make a note if you have changed any of your soaps or laundry detergents.

Some eczema can be triggered by allergies, so make a food diary and eliminate all things that show up on your food list more than every four days. Eliminate red meat, citrus fruits, and sugar from your diet, and see if your problem clears. This will help you learn what might be triggering this condition, too. Cleanse the bowel for quicker relief of all skin ailments.

Herb Lore

While I was writing this book, I came down with an ugly eczema-like rash on the back of my hand and wrist. Of course, I used all the remedies that I told you about here. Although the rash did not get worse, it did not get better, either, until I added evening primrose oil to my program. Within one week, the rash disappeared. Evening primrose was my cure, and I think I was supposed to share this with you so that you. Try the same if the remedies listed here don't work for you. See more on evening primrose oil under the section "Cold Sore No More (Herpes Simplex)," in Chapter 8 "C's for a Common Cure."

Endometriosis: A Growing Concern

Endometriosis is a female concern involving the presence of tissue similar to the lining of the uterus located (and usually growing) at other sites in the pelvis. Symptoms include painful menstruation, infertility, and, if left untreated, adhesions which attach themselves to other pelvic areas, such as the fallopian tubes, ovaries, uterine muscles, colon, and bladder. These adhesions pull pelvic organs out of alignment and cause other painful problems. Many women have hysterectomies for relief of this problem.

Possible causes of this overgrowing tissue may be linked to hormonal imbalance, especially excess estrogen production, that cause tissue to grow wildly.

Estrogen dominance can be caused by an improper diet, prescription medications, xenoestrogens (plastics and petroleum products), and dioxins (herbicides and pesticides).

Botanical Bit

Endometriosis is the presence of uterine-like tissue in abnormal places, usually in the pelvic cavity. Symptoms are usually painful menstruation and may exacerbate related menstrual symptoms.

Poison Ivy

Dioxin is used to bleach coffee filters white. This poison is then be released into your coffee or tea. Who needs white coffee filters anyway? Unbleached coffee filters work just as well, are available at most stores, and are almost always found at health food stores. Avoid using dioxin-laden products whenever possible, especially if suffering from endometriosis or any other ailment.

Pau D'Arco Power to the Rescue (Again)

Pau d'arco is utilized by many women as a blood cleanser and to dissolve cysts, as you might remember from Chapter 8. Use pau d'arco to help in all ailments that are related to abnormal growths, such as cysts, cancer, tumors, and endometriosis.

As always, combinations of herbs—and sometimes supplements—can speed your recovery. Use sarsaparilla and pau d'arco at the same time. Pau d'arco aids in dissolving cysts and tissue overgrowth while sarsaparilla aids your body in progesterone production—which will help balance estrogen levels sometimes related to endometriosis.

For extra benefit, and more hormonal balancing effects, add the following combination along with your pau d'arco and sarsaparilla: golden seal, capsicum, ginger, uva ursi, crampbark, squawvine, blessed thistle, red raspberry, and false unicorn. Extra vitamin C can enhance this herbal program. Soy estrogens from plant sources are known as phyto-estrogens and offer a very mild form of estrogen. They bind the estrogen receptors, making it difficult for "bad" estrogen to be effective. This makes soy valuable in helping to balance estrogen levels, especially when those levels are in excess.

Other Things to Do (or Not to Do)

As with anything of a hormonally induced nature (this includes supplemental, over-the-counter hormones such as melatonin or DHEA supplements) do not take hormones unless you first discuss it with your doctor. It might also be wise to consume only animal products that are labeled hormone-free or organic.

Herb Lore

Growth hormones that are given to cattle, pigs, and other animals raised for meat help them weigh more and produce more litters. However, these hormones also may be passed onto the consumer when eaten. An alarming case was reported involving children as young as four and five who had developed breasts, pubic hair, and other signs of puberty presumably because of their consumption of animal products from hormonally injected animals. Dr. Carmen Sanez, a physician in Puerto Rico, reported this case in the *Journal of the Puerto Rico Medical Association* in 1982 and found that when the children stopped consuming milk, poultry, and beef, most of their symptoms usually regressed.

Eyes Got an Herb for You

The eyes are the windows to the soul, and sight is one of our most valued senses, however sometimes we take it for granted until we begin to lose our perfect vision. Most often it is some type of malnourishment that causes our eyes to loose focus. Sometimes it is a symptom of another progressive disease. But for the common eyesight degeneration, I have seen people reclaim their good vision several months after incorporating an herbal program into their life. I have also seen people who have worked on their core problem with herbs improve their eyesight as a side effect of taking herbs and supplements.

You can use herbs to tone the eye muscles, relieve and nourish stressed or irritated eyes, and bring circulation to the eyes. All this can help restore better vision and increase the general health of your eyes.

Eyebright: A Sight for Sore Eyes

Appropriately named, eyebright (*Euphrasia officinalis*) is an herb used to nourish, cleanse, tone, and strengthen the eyes. It contains a component that strengthens the blood capillaries, which improves circulation to the eyes. Eyebright has been used internally and externally for eye

Poison Ivy

Sometimes blood sugar imbalance—especially in diabetes—is a factor causing vision problems. Low blood sugar, known as hypoglycemia, might also be a cause of blurry vision, as well as "floaters," which look like little amoebas floating across your vision. Have your blood sugar levels checked if you are suddenly having vision problems. You should also consider liver weakness as a source of vision problems and use herbs to strengthen it.

137

problems of all sorts. For better vision take internally. Eyebright usually comes in capsules and is many times found with other astringent herbs. Its antibacterial effects make it an excellent tea to be used as an eyewash for conjunctivitis (pink eye) or sore, irritated, or itchy eyes.

To use eyebright as an external eyewash, you have two options. If you have the herb in a capsule, empty one capsule per cup of water (one cup at a time should be more than sufficient). If you are using the herb in bulk form, four heaping teaspoons equals about one capsule of powder. Then follow these steps:

1. Put herb in a cup of water, and bring to a boil.

2. Boil 10 minutes.

3. Let cool, and strain mixture well. (That's better than a sharp stick in the eye!)

4. Use a glass dropper to administer to eyes as needed. Do not touch the glass dropper to the eye, however; this will contaminate the mixture with the dropper, unless you sterilize it first.

5. Store the mixture in a glass container in the refrigerator. Do not keep mixture longer than three to four days.

Bilberry: Focusing on the Problem

Bilberry fruit (*Vaccinium myrtillus*) is a potent herbal antioxidant source. Its ability to neutralize free radicals in the brain and the eyes makes it a powerful protector for the eyes. The part used historically is the fruit, sometimes also called huckleberry or blueberry.

British pilots during World War II used bilberry to improve their vision for night flying. Some reported improved vision within two weeks of using bilberry, and long-term use of this safe herb will prove most beneficial. Bilberry's ability to strengthen blood capillaries also makes it an excellent tonic for people who bruise easily.

Sage Advice

For sore or infected eyes, a combination of golden seal, bayberry, eyebright, and red raspberry is excellent for internal and topical application.

Bilberry used with eyebright and beta carotene makes a powerful combination to nourish and protect the eyes and to strengthen vision. It also works well for light-sensitive individuals. Bilberry is also used for diabetes, diarrhea, and mild inflammation.

Zinc and vitamins E, A, and C all work well to protect our vision and are all contained in eyebright and bilberry.

Another practice you can choose to help tone the eyes is a cold water splash every morning and each night. Simply fill your sink with some cold water, cup the water in your hands, and splash your eyes. The cold will help muscles retract, will tighten capillaries, and will tone your eyes. Many find this very refreshing and strengthening to their eyes.

I Can See! A Testimonial to Herbs and Eyesight

When poor eyesight is caused by a lack of nutrients, herbs can restore eyesight safely and sometimes very quickly. My husband is a good testimonial for this wonderful herbal "side effect." When I met him he wore glasses, he had chronic sinusitis that was long standing, and he was getting shots in his nose by his allergist, which didn't seem to alleviate his suffering much. He suffered from stress because of his high-pressure job and other circumstances at the time. He also had mild digestive and intestinal distress and symptoms of fluctuating blood sugar.

The last thing I was concerned about for him was his eyesight. But I think it's interesting to note how these other problems may tie in with vision.

Here's the herbal program I put him on:

A combination for stress that included: chamomile flowers, passion flowers, hops flowers, fennel seeds, marshmallow root, and feverfew herb.

A combination for his allergies that included: burdock root, ephedra, golden seal, capsicum, parsley, horehound, althea, and yerba santa.

Bifidophilus to improve his digestion and absorption of nutrients.

A fiber supplement for his bowel that included a mixture of psyllium, oat, and apple fibers.

A soothing combo for his digestive tract that contained: slippery elm bark, marshmallow root, plantain herb, chamomile flowers, rose hips, and bugleweed herb.

Licorice root to help his body produce natural cortisone (he was getting cortisone shots in his nose, and so he thought he'd try this natural alternative). Licorice root also balances the blood sugar levels, which can have an effect on eyesight.

An enzyme designed to help him break down proteins. The enzyme also included hydrochloric acid.

And a combination to support his blood sugar levels and nourish the prostate that included: golden seal, juniper berries, uva ursi leaves, cedar berries, mullein leaves, garlic bulb, yarrow flowers, slippery elm bark, capsicum fruit, dandelion root, marshmallow root, nettle herb, white oak bark, and licorice root.

Sage Advice

It is interesting to note that bilberry was not a part of the herbal combination in my husband's case, however, by helping the body absorb nutrients and using herbs to balance and nourish the body, the body is more efficient at using nutrients consumed. Remember that all herbs contain vitamins and minerals that the body can easily utilize. Many ailments can be reversed just by supporting the areas that are out of balance and feeding the system necessary nutrients.

Within two weeks on this program, he was absolutely amazed to find that his sinuses cleared up almost entirely. Within two months he was completely Kleenex-free! His digestion improved dramatically, his stress level eased, and he became even more grateful he met me! However, after about four months using the herbs he began to get headaches. We finally came to the conclusion that his prescription glasses probably needed an update.

They sure did! A trip to see his eye doctor resulted in the recycling of his glasses because his vision had returned to 20/20! It's nice to know that herbs can fill in nutritional voids and that your body will begin to restore the undernourished areas whether you "focus" on a particular ailment or not.

That was over four years ago, my husband still takes his daily herbal supplements and continues to be sinusitis- and eyeglass-free!

Herbal Remedies for Common Ailments

Earaches

Best Single Herb: Echinacea

Best Combinations: Parthenium, yarrow, myrrh, capsicum; echinacea; garlic

Other Helpful Supplements: Calcium for healing

Possible Causes: Food allergies; constipation

Complementary Help: Internal: three to four drops of warmed lobelia, tea tree, or garlic oil in ear; garlic enema for babies; baked onion over ear; ear coning

Eczema

Best Single Herb: Oregon grape

Best Combinations: Burdock root; Oregon grape; pau d'arco

Other Helpful Supplements: Vitamins A and E; zinc

Possible Causes: Skin irritants (soaps, industrial dyes, solvents); constipation; inadequate diet or poor digestion; lack of circulation; allergies

Complementary Help: Cleansing the bowel; eliminating citrus fruits, sugar, red meat, caffeine, and fried foods from diet; using pau d'arco topically

Endometriosis

Best Single Herb: Pau d'arco

Best Combinations: Sarsaparilla; golden seal, capsicum, ginger, uva ursi, cramp-bark, squawvine, blessed thistle, red raspberry, false unicorn; phyto-soy supplement to block excess estrogen production

Other Helpful Supplements: Vitamins A, D, E (with selenium), and C

Possible Causes: Hormonal imbalance

Complementary Help: Do not take hormones (including supplements such as melatonin and DHEA) unless on a physician's advice; eliminate animal products that are not organic

Eyes, General (sight/soreness/infection)

Best Single Herb: Eyebright

Best Combinations: Bilberry; eyebright; golden seal, bayberry, eyebright, red raspberry

Other Helpful Supplements: Vitamin A; beta carotene; vitamin C with citrus bioflavonoids; vitamin E; zinc

Possible Causes: Liver weakness; blood sugar imbalances

Complementary Help: Cold water splash on eyes morning and evening

---

The Least You Need to Know

➤ Echinacea can help fight ear infections.

➤ Oregon grape has been an excellent remedy used internally and externally for eczema.

➤ Pau d'arco comes to the rescue again for the aid of endometriosis and many types of abnormal growths.

➤ Bilberry and eyebright are two top herbs to nourish and strengthen the eyes.

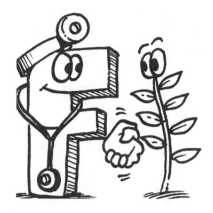

Chapter 11

F: Fantastic Healing Flora

In This Chapter

➤ Herbs that can help you break a fever

➤ Herbs that offer relief for fibromyalgia

➤ Protect yourself from food poisoning with herbs

➤ Fast-forward flu symptoms with powerful herbal remedies

They say an ounce of prevention is worth a pound of cure. Likewise, sometimes it takes a pound of herbs to give you that ounce of prevention you need. It's nice to know that herbs can help us prevent disease and ailments in the first place. However, herbs did not necessarily get their reputation by keeping people well—it was because of herbs' recuperating powers bringing folks back from their sickbeds that they gained their reputation.

So, whether you decide to reach for an herb after you already have a sickness or whether you decide to test its abilities to protect you, you will have a new and safe resource in your medicine cabinet or pantry to try.

Fever Reliever

A fever occurs when the body temperature is abnormally high. Most of the time, the body temperature rises in an attempt to burn off some type of bug or toxin. Fevers can be triggered by viral or bacterial infections of many kinds. You can think of a fever as your friend, helping you to burn off foreign invaders. Herbs will help you assist your fever and can fast-forward you to recovery.

The body temperature rises and falls an average of 1.5°F during the course of a day, based on a person's activity level, diet, anxiety, and clothing. As a guideline, you can consider the possibility of fever when your temperature reaches between 99°F and 100°F. If your temperature is 100°F or over, you can be sure it's a fever.

If you have any of the following conditions characterizing a fever, consult your physician immediately:

➤ Fever persisting more than five days could indicate a persistent or severe infection that is beyond home treatment.

➤ Fever in a child less than four months old: They are more susceptible to seizures.

➤ Fever accompanied by a sore, stiff neck could be a sign of meningitis, where an infection has entered the brain—a life-threatening condition.

➤ Fever of more than 105°F: If home treatments fail to bring down a temperature something serious may be going on that your body cannot handle without intervention.

➤ Any fever above 105°F can lead to brain damage.

Sage Advice

During any illness—but especially if you have a fever—it is imperative that you drink plenty of liquids (preferably water) to keep from becoming dehydrated. Water will also help you flush wastes from your system. If water is not appetizing, add a little liquid chlorophyll flavored with spearmint to taste.

Me and My Yarrow

Yarrow (*Achillea millefolium, L.*) is an herb traditionally used for many medicinal purposes, including lowering fevers. It is a *diaphoretic* herb and will clear even the most deep-seated fever. Yarrow has an affinity for the skin and will diffuse the blood to the surface of the skin and open up pores, letting out the inner heat and eliminating waste products that could be causing the fever. For treating fevers with yarrow, a tea or decoction is best. It is also useful in any combination of herbs used to treat colds, the flu, and respiratory ailments.

Botanical Bit

Diaphoretic is an herbal property that describes an herb's ability to increase elimination through the skin via perspiration.

Children respond well to yarrow used to break a fever, especially when the herb is mixed with elderberry and peppermint. Childhood illnesses that have been treated with yarrow include chicken pox, smallpox, measles, colds, and influenza.

Other herbs, such as an extract of catnip and fennel, can be used to break a fever. This is also a good remedy for children. And, of course, you can always take garlic, which contains anti-bacterial agents that help your body kill off an infection that may be causing the fever. Beta carotene will convert to vitamin A in the body as needed and is safer for feverish children. Vitamin E also will help protect the liver during a fever.

Bathing: Now You're Not So Hot!

Moms and herbalists alike use two good home remedies to break fevers:

1. **A sweat bath:** The sweat bath is the typical way an herbalist would handle a fever, knowing that the fever is doing the body a favor by killing infection. A sweat bath will assist your body and speed up the process.

2. **A tepid sponge bath:** It is a way to bring down a fever, but not necessarily to help the body rid itself of the cause of the fever. If you are worried about a child with a raging fever and cannot get medical care, this would be your safest home treatment.

The sweat bath will help break a fever in a similar way that the yarrow works, by opening the pores and sweat glands and pushing out wastes through the skin. For use and description of a sweat bath, go back to the section "Colds: A Cure for All Seasons," in Chapter 8, "C's for a Common Cure."

The other remedy, a tepid sponge bath, involves putting yourself or a child in tepid water to eliminate a fever by *conduction*.

Traditionally, many moms have used rubbing alcohol in the tub to help break a fever. This is because of the quick evaporating action of alcohol. However, the alcohol's fumes can be toxic. A better way to go for a tepid sponge bath is to add peppermint oil to the water. Peppermint oil also brings blood to the surface of the skin and has a cooling effect on the body. What's more, the fumes are not dangerous, and the oil leaves you feeling more refreshed. Also the bath water does not need to be cold! A more pleasing temperature (approximately 70°F) will still do the trick and can be tolerated for a longer time than colder water. A sponge bath would be a better choice than a sweat bath for very high fevers.

Either way you go, take your yarrow to help push out the inner heat and toxins through the skin.

Botanical Bit

Conduction is the process in which heat is lost to a cooler environment from a warmer environment.

Botanical Bit

A **colonic**, also called colonic irrigation or colonic hydrotherapy, is a water therapy used to cleanse the lower bowel. The colonic is administered by a trained colonic therapist, who uses equipment to administer several gallons of water to the bowel. The irrigation is not retained, as in an enema, but it leaves the bowel through a tube and is sanitary and modest when done by a professional.

Flu (Influenza): A Flu Good Herbs

Unfortunately, there is no real medical treatment for the flu or colds because they are usually caused by a virus. Antibiotics kill bacteria, not viruses. The best way to deal with the flu, therefore, is to help the symptoms fast-forward. Herbs can be a catalyst to your recovery from the flu and can help prevent you from getting complications associated with the flu. And, if taken after exposure to an infected person, these herbs just might help you bypass the flu altogether.

A colon cleansing with the use of an *enema* or *colonic* can help rid the body of waste and speed your recovery. For any infection in the body, add garlic to the enema water, and always be sure to use clean water since the bowel absorbs what is put into it.

Elderberry: Influencing Influenza

Elderberry (*Sambucus nigra*) is an excellent herb for treating acute conditions of any kind, and this is one of Europe's most widely used herbs for centuries. Different parts

Botanical Bit

An **enema** is usually self-administered at home and is a way to clean your bowels with the use of an enema bag and water. The water is retained in the bowel and then is ejected. The proper supplies can be purchased inexpensively at a pharmacy. Different herbs also can be added to enema water for different effects. Catnip tea added to the enema helps colicky babies.

of the plant are used for different medicinal purposes, including the flowers, berries, leaves, and bark. The berries are rich in vitamins A and C and potassium. Elderberry strengthens the immune system and helps it fight off viral infections. Elderberry increases mother's milk when taken by nursing moms. It can be used as a tea as a gargle and is good for head colds, laryngitis, and flu. It is best given to children in the late afternoon and evening to help break fevers.

It has been reported that research in Israel done by virologist Dr. Madeleine Mumcuouglu has shown elderberry to disarm the flu virus by neutralizing the spikes that viruses use to invade host cells.

Elderberry has been used to reduce inflammation, promote perspiration, and to serve as a laxative and decongestant. Add yarrow and mint, which will enhance the effects and make a safe remedy for children and adults alike.

Other Unpronounceables

Elderberry is a wonderful remedy, but when suffering from flu symptoms, you are likely to experience more than just what elderberry can handle for you. For stomach flu and vomiting, a mixture of ginger, capsicum, golden seal, and licorice is helpful. Vitamins C and A will help boost your immune system. As always, drink plenty of liquids and eat very lightly; your body can use the extra energy to heal you.

A homeopathic from France known as oscillococcinum (*Anas barbariae*) is claimed by many to help stop a flu dead in its tracks. Currently, Cochrane Review Group is researching whether oscillococcinum is more effective than a placebo in the prevention and treatment of influenza and its symptoms. Oscillococcinum is available in most health food stores.

Another excellent herb worthy of mention is olive leaf extract. Olive leaf is anti-fungal, and anti-viral and can be used to kill infections, cold viruses and many other ailments.

Fibromyalgia: What a Pain!

Fibromyalgia is considered a syndrome because it is a collection of symptoms with no apparent relation to each other.

You might be diagnosed with fibromyalgia if you have the following symptoms:

➤ A history of widespread pain lasting more than three months

➤ Pain on both sides of the body, above and below the waist

➤ Eleven or more established tender points that show extreme pain when pressure is applied

Other symptoms include all-over aches; insomnia; chronic aches in the hips, neck, or low back; stomach trouble; and intolerance to cold.

Fibromyalgia seems to strike after a stressful or traumatic event, such as an accident, marriage, divorce, or death of a loved one. Ninety percent of fibromyalgia sufferers are women.

Sage Advice

For best results, continue your herbs and vitamins for a few days even after you are well to protect against a relapse. Also, the body becomes used to being fed nutrients and you can shock the body by suddenly stopping your herbs and create a re-bounding illness.

Sage Advice

Researchers at the University of Alabama have uncovered proof that fibromyalgia isn't a psychological disorder, but rather is caused by abnormalities in the brain and central nervous system. They found that fibromyalgia patients have significantly less blood flow to the parts of their brains that deal with pain. The good news is, herbs like ginkgo biloba and gotu kola can help restore proper blood flow to the brain.

The true cause of fibromyalgia seems to allude physicians, but herbalists and physicians alike have theories, although much of it has been blamed on psychological disorders. Some believe it to be deep-seated stress or an immune deficiency. Because stress can have the effect of lowering the immune system, these seem to tie together. Others blame the disease on a virus. And still others believe the problem starts with poor digestion, which then leads to poor absorption, which can lead to a mineral or nutritional deficiency. What they all seem to agree on is that fibromyalgia is linked to a lowered immune system brought on by stress. When our immune is lowered we are susceptible to every disease. Here's a game plan for addressing fibromyalgia.

The best plan for dealing with fibromyalgia that I have seen work in my practice includes this set of actions:

➤ Support digestion. Using herbs such as papaya, chew properly, eat while not under stress, etc.

➤ Cleanse the colon.

➤ Eat more fruits and vegetables of an alkaline nature, which include most green vegetables, and fruits such as apples and pears.

➤ Reduce stress, if possible.

➤ Have frequent bodywork done, such as massage or reflexology.

➤ Get gentle exercise to improve circulation.

➤ Take your herbs.

Now let's talk about some herbs that have been used to help this annoying syndrome.

Uña de Gato: Clawing Your Way to Health

Uña de gato is Spanish for "cat's claw." Uña de gato is an herb that comes from a thorny vine in Peru that has thorns that are curved and resemble a cat's claw—hence its name.

Uña de gato is used by many for the pain associated with fibromyalgia. Its properties also serve to support the immune system, aid the digestive system, and feed the structural system—all of which seem to be affected by fibromyalgia. Personally, I use uña de gato combined with astragalus and echinacea for any type of inflammation. I am amazed that it works as instantly as an aspirin (within 20 minutes), and it also relieves pain and reduces inflammation. Take two or more capsules three times per day or as needed to ease your symptoms. Some relief should be felt within 20 minutes or so, if not, increase your dose.

Sage Advice

The most potent species of cat's claw (uña de gato) is uncaria tomentosa. Read the label to make sure you are getting this species because it is believed to contain the most valuable immune system stimulants.

Supplements to Ease Your Pain

When suffering with fibromyalgia, you'll need support in several different areas. This will certainly require more than one herb to help you get relief and help you to fully recover.

When dealing with fibromyalgia, you should concentrate on herbs and supplements that feed the following body systems (see the tear card in the front of this book for some top herbs that support each of these body systems):

➤ Structural system (bones, muscles, connective tissues)

➤ Nervous system (nerves, brain)

➤ Digestive system (stomach, liver, pancreas, gallbladder)

➤ Immune system (thymus, spleen, lymphatics)

Structural system: A supplement I have seen my clients benefit from is extra magnesium and malic acid. Magnesium works as a muscle relaxer in the body, and our muscles are made up of plenty of magnesium. Sometimes a pain indicates that your body trying to steal nutrients from that part of the body. Why not feed it what it might be asking for?

And, of course, any bodywork that relaxes the muscles, eases stress and tension, and improves circulation will help you feel better. Reflexology and massage are both good therapies for this. Acupressure is another therapy that has been used to restore proper health to individuals. And who doesn't need an excuse to go get a massage?

Nervous system: Lobelia may be used in small quantities to help relax nerves. In addition, make sure to add a B-complex vitamin with any conditions that could be brought on by stress. The brain utilizes a lot of the B vitamins for proper functioning, and our body utilizes a greater quantity of these important nutrients when under stress and in pain.

Ginkgo biloba can be taken to nourish the brain and help increase blood supply to the head. Since researchers have now found a link between the brain's blood supply and fibromyalgia, ginkgo might be your answer. Try one to two capsules or tablets two to three times daily. If dizziness occurs, back off slightly on dosage. This could indicate that fresh blood is being carried into the brain, and is a good sign, actually! Go slow and take your ginkgo as tolerated.

> **Botanical Bit**
>
> **Reflexology** is based on the theory that all parts of your body can be positively affected by applying massage and acupressure–like techniques to the feet and hands. Reflexology has been used for pain reduction and promotes relaxation and euphoria.
>
> **Acupressure** is an ancient Oriental art involving applying pressure to certain pressure points along your body to open energy flows, release tension, and promote balance.

Digestive system: Liquid chlorophyll and aloe vera both aid digestion and are natural bowel cleansers. If the aloe causes you too much bowel rumbling, stick to the chlorophyll. Food enzymes help the body break down cooked or enzyme-less foods, and papaya is an excellent herb to support digestion. These can be taken at the same time if digestion is very poor, otherwise, try one or the other, first.

Immune system: To boost the immune system effects of your uña de gato, you can add a combination of rose hips, Siberian ginseng, parsley, red clover, wheat grass powder, and horseradish. Beta carotene will also help boost immunity.

Food Poisoning: On the Road Again

Food poisoning is more common than you might think. In fact, food poisoning symptoms can be almost identical to flu symptoms. Many 24-hour flus may actually be the result of a bacterial food poisoning.

Food poisoning doesn't come only from restaurants; many cases come from improper food handling at home. For instance, the number of bacteria able to grow in food that is not properly refrigerated or that is not kept hot enough is staggering and can be strong enough to make you sick. Most of the bacteria that gets into our food (such as E. coli) comes from the earth that it was grown in. When fruits and veggies are not thoroughly washed, the bacteria can infiltrate the foods when we cut them. If the foods are eaten raw, we can become ill.

Poison Ivy

The Center for Disease Control (CDC) in Atlanta, Georgia, reports that 32 percent of food-borne illnesses reported to the CDC began in the kitchens of commercial eating places.

Sage Advice

You can find acidophilus or bifidophilus supplements in your local health food store. Check the refrigerated section because these bugs stay alive longer if frozen or refrigerated.

Now, I don't want to discourage you from eating raw fruits and vegetables! But I do want to encourage you to wash not only your hands but also the foods.

Some tips to avoid food poisoning:

➤ Wash hands thoroughly before handling food and eating.

➤ Wash all fruits and vegetables thoroughly before cutting.

➤ Use separate cutting boards for meats and plant foods.

➤ In a restaurant, make sure that food is very hot when served; food left to cool can harbor bacteria.

➤ Take food enzymes with hydrochloric acid and acidophilus supplements 20 minutes before eating (especially when dining out).

➤ Cook all meats thoroughly.

➤ Refrigerate foods immediately if not eaten right away.

➤ Do not keep leftovers more than 24 hours.

➤ Read the book *Poisons in Your Food,* by Ruth Winter.

Your body has ways of protecting you from these bacteria; any foreigner that enters through the mouth and makes it to your stomach usually doesn't last long.

Your stomach produces hydrochloric acid, a powerful acid that actually sanitizes the foods you eat and kills any harmful bacteria.

If your stomach acid is low and the bug makes it past this line of defense, the good bacteria in the small intestines will eat up the invader. However, low stomach acid (this becomes naturally lower as you age) along with lowered acidophilus (good bacteria in your intestinal tract that is easily killed off by antibiotics and caffeine) makes you vulnerable to invaders and can cause your body to react violently with diarrhea, vomiting, and fever. These symptoms are the body's last resort to keep you safe from poisoning.

Your best supplemental protection against food-borne illness is to supplement with food enzymes that contain a small amount of hydrochloric acid before you eat. Adding acidophilus capsules every day—especially when traveling—will also help protect you. Acidophilus is best taken in *enteric-coated* capsules so that it has a chance to reach the intestinal tract before being bombarded with your stomach's digestive secretions. This protects these critters from being killed before they get a chance to make it to your intestinal tract.

Botanical Bit

Enterically coated capsules are capsules manufactured with a coating to protect them from being digested in the stomach so that they are released in the intestinal tract. This is a more effective way of ensuring that the organisms such as intestinal flora (acidophilus) are replenished where you need them.

Lobelia: Helping You Spit It Out

In past chapters, we talked a little bit about lobelia and explored how it can serve as an expectorant to help the lungs get rid of wastes. But lobelia also serves as an *emetic*, which means that too much of it can cause you to throw up. This can come in handy if someone has swallowed any type of poisonous substance. A liquid form of lobelia would be most effective. Take your lobelia until you get the desired effect.

Botanical Bit

An **emetic** is an herbal property used to describe an herb's ability to make you vomit.

Lobelia is native to North America and is also known as Indian tobacco—and, most appropriate to its emetic quality, it is also known as pukeweed! Native Americans smoked this herb to treat asthma and lockjaw because lobelia has an ability to relax tissues and seems to soothe coughing. Because of lobelia's emetic effect, it should be taken in larger quantities only when used to promote vomiting, such as in the case of poisoning. However, many have used to lobelia to induce vomiting as a fast-forward way to cleanse.

Lobelia could be considered the best herb remedy for poisoning, but you should seriously consider utilizing other natural substances, such as those discussed in the following sections, if you have been poisoned by a contaminant.

Charcoal and Other Supplements to the Rescue

Activated charcoal capsules should be taken immediately if food poisoning or any other type of poisoning is suspected. This cannot hurt you, and in most cases you'll be much happier safe than sorry. Activated charcoal has properties that attract and absorb poisons, making them unavailable to your body and therefore neutralizing the effect a poison will have.

Poison Ivy

If you do get food poisoning, some herbal help can assist your body in getting rid of the toxin fast, but call your poison control center for small children and the elderly—sometimes food poisoning can be fatal.

Hydrated bentonite clay has a similar effect. Its powerful absorbing properties eliminate toxins, especially those in the colon, and remove them from your body.

Aloe vera and slippery elm are other herbs that have a laxative effect on the bowel. Both can be taken with any of the previously mentioned supplements to help your body quickly rid itself of wastes via the bowel.

As always, whenever your body needs to flush out poisons or toxins, drink plenty of clean water to assist the process.

Fungus Among Us?

Fungal infections seem to be more and more widespread these days and can include ring worm, Candida overgrowth (*Candidias Albicans*), yeast infections, jock itch, and athlete's foot. While some of these problems are externally contagious, such as athlete's foot and ring worm, some are caused by an imbalance of our internal environment. Just as mold and fungus need a warm, moist environment externally, bacteria and fungus need a certain environment to thrive in internally. Therefore, if we change our inner environment and make it less fungus-friendly, these problems will tend to disappear.

Some causes of internal fungal infections such as yeast and Candida include:

➤ Sugar: Sugar is bad bacteria's favorite food. Keep feeding it sugar, and it will think you want it to stay!

➤ Caffeine: Caffeine wipes out the good bacteria in your digestive tract and may allow fungal overgrowth to get a head start.

➤ Antibiotics and birth control pills: These can change your internal environment, causing it to be more fungus-friendly. If you are on birth control pills, it may be wise to supplement every day with acidophilus.

➤ Lack of cellular oxygen due to mucus in the system: Fungus doesn't like fresh air—it likes a stale environment and carbon dioxide to bathe in. Fungus thrives in or on a body that is not exposed regularly to fresh air.

By now, you're probably itching to know how to get rid of these things!

Black Walnut, Cracking Open the Cure

Black walnut (*Juglans nigra*) is an excellent herb used both externally and internally to help fight fungus, worms, and all parasites. Black walnut is a very useful plant because almost all parts of this plant are used—and all parts have different purposes.

The rinds or hulls of the black walnut are most specifically utilized for antifungal properties. Black walnut hulls will usually come in a capsule form, or you may use the powder or liquid extract of the ground hulls for external applications. Black walnut bark taken internally may have a laxative effect, but can rid the bowel of parasites and fungus at the same time.

To fight fungus overgrowth and parasites use garlic and black walnut together—these two herbs make a good pair for this purpose. You have bacteria in your body all the time; fungus or bacteria overgrowth can occur only when your internal flora is out of balance. This is why supplementing with the good intestinal flora is helpful when fighting internal fungus infections or parasites.

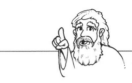

Sage Advice

The leaves of the black walnut tree can be rubbed on the skin or clothing and can serve as an insect repellent. The leaves have also been taken to treat eczema. They even have properties that help restore tooth enamel.

Pau d'arco is another herb well-known for its fungus-fighting ability. Although this tree grows in a tropical area, its bark remains fungus-free. Drink a cup of pau d'arco tea each night along with taking your garlic and black walnut supplements to fight Candida, yeast infections, parasite infestations, and fungal infections. You can use tea tree oil as a topical application for athlete's foot and ring worm; apply it directly to the area once in the morning and once in the evening. I have used a Q-tip dipped in tea tree oil for cleaning my ears to kill off an itchy fungal growth on my ear drum—in 10 days the fungus was gone. This is also effective if you dampen a cotton ball with tea tree oil and place gently in each ear. The fumes from the tea tree are effective in destroying fungus in the ear canal.

What a Fungi Can Do

This list covers some things you can do to change your inner and outer environments for treating and preventing fungus:

➤ Eat lots of brown rice, millet, veggies, and lean meats; avoid sugar, alcohol, dairy, yeast, and caffeine.

➤ Exercise brings oxygen into the body and can suffocate carbon dioxide-loving fungus.

➤ Colon cleansing helps rid the body of excess waste and mucus and allows more oxygen to revitalize the body.

➤ For yeast infections, don't wear wet gym clothes or bathing suits for long periods of time. Don't wear panty hose or nylon underwear—wear cotton undies instead.

➤ Wear rubber thongs in public showers to avoid catching athlete's foot.

➤ Always keep feet as dry as possible, and avoid wearing sweaty socks too long. Apply tea tree oil morning and evening.

➤ Take your herbs and supplements daily!

Herbal Remedies for Common Ailments

Fever

Best Single Herb: Yarrow

Best Combinations: Catnip and fennel; yarrow; garlic

Other Helpful Supplements: Beta carotene, vitamins A and E

Possible Causes: Infections; toxicity

Complementary Help: Catnip or garlic enemas; sweat bath (see Chapter 8); cool peppermint sponge bath

Flu

Best Single Herb: Elderberry

Best Combinations: Ginger, capsicum, golden seal, licorice; elderberry, yarrow, mint; olive leaf extract

Other Helpful Supplements: Vitamins C and A; oscillococcinum (homeopathic remedy from France)

Possible Cause: Lowered immunity

Complementary Help: Take a sweat bath; eat lightly; take in extra fluids; cleanse the colon

Fibromyalgia

Best Single Herb: Uña de gato (cat's claw)

Best Combinations: Uña de gato; rose hips, Siberian ginseng, parsley, red clover, wheat grass powder, horseradish; ginkgo biloba, gotu kola; liquid chlorophyll; aloe vera; lobelia

Other Helpful Supplements: Beta carotene; malic acid; magnesium stearate; calcium with magnesium; food enzymes

Possible Cause: Candida; Epstein-Barr virus; lowered immunity; digestion problems

Complementary Help: Bowel cleansing; reflexology; massage; acupressure

Food Poisoning

Best Single Herb: Lobelia

Best Combinations: Aloe vera and slippery elm

Other Helpful Supplements: Activated charcoal, or hydrated bentonite taken as soon as possible

Possible Cause: Unwashed hands when handling food and before eating; unwashed cutting boards and counters used after cutting meat; unwashed fruits and vegetables before cutting

Complementary Help: Prevention is best with enzymes with hydrochloric acid and acidophilus before every meal, especially when traveling or dining out

Fungus

Best Single Herb: Black walnut

Best Combinations: Pau d'arco; garlic; black walnut

Other Helpful Supplements: Tea tree oil

Possible Cause: Warm, moist conditions; poor diet; some medications

Complementary Help: Tea tree oil used externally; fresh air and sunshine; keeping the area dry

---

The Least You Need to Know

➤ Yarrow helps break a fever by opening up the pores and sweat glands of the skin and then pushing heat and toxins out through the skin.

➤ Elderberries are an excellent herbal flu remedy and may prove to be a natural anti-viral agent.

➤ Uña de gato, otherwise called cat's claw, is an herb whose thorns resemble claws; the herb is used by fibromyalgia suffers to relive pain and to support digestion and the immune system.

➤ Prevention of food poisoning is best, but in an emergency vomiting can be induced with the use of lobelia.

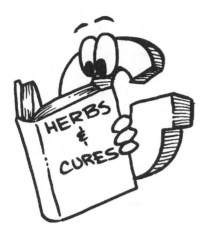

Chapter 12

G: Great Remedies

In This Chapter

➤ Get rid of gas with herbs that support digestion

➤ Herbs that help fight gingivitis

➤ Some herbal solutions for glandular balance

➤ Recover from gout herbally

"A reckoning up of the cause often solves the malady." —Roman scholar Celsus (25 B.C.–50 A.D.). *De Medicina,* Prooemium

It is true that finding the cause of your ailment is half the battle. Running around in the dark trying to treat yourself with herbs for symptoms might only leave you running into walls! So in this chapter we'll take a look at a few ailments that begin with the letter G and see what their probable causes are. Then we'll get onto the herbs that will help!

Got Gas?

Intestinal gas is funny only when we see comedians carry on about it. However, flatulence is an embarrassing symptom caused by poor digestion or constipation. I know this is no fun to talk about, but if you are one of those gaseous types, read on for herbal help. The answer to your roommates' prayers are almost over!

Our bodies create gas for many reasons. Intestinal gas is created by fermentation of wastes in the bowel, and constipation is a large part of why we have this problem.

How do you know if your gas is a result of constipation? It shouldn't be too hard to recognize, but here are a couple of clues:

➤ You have the mysterious power to clear out a movie theater without saying a word.

➤ While flying, you cause airline attendants to strap on their parachutes while passenger oxygen masks drop from the ceiling above you.

➤ Only when you sit up front during a live lecture does the speaker seem to become overwhelmed with unexplainable emotion, which causes him to go into long pauses, tightly close his eyes, and wipe sweat nervously from his brow.

But seriously, here are some reasons why you might be full of hot air:

➤ Improper combination of food

➤ Poor digestion

➤ Inadequate *mastication* of food

➤ Eating too fast (sucking wind)

➤ Drinking lots of liquids with meals

Botanical Bit

Mastication is the chewing process. Ideally, we should masticate each mouthful of food thoroughly (approximately 29 times) before swallowing. Proper mastication helps our digestive process.

Eat Here, Get Gas, Take Fennel

Have you ever seen those signs outside those rural roadside gas station restaurants? Eat here, get gas? Well, most of them don't know what a prophetic sign that is—and if they were smart, they could sell a bottle of fennel capsules to you on your way out!

Fennel (*Foeniculum vlagare*) is an herb that has historically been used to eliminate gas, colic, diarrhea, indigestion, nausea, and vomiting. Fennel has an affinity for the digestive and intestinal tract; primarily, the seeds from this plant are used for digestion. The raw seeds are served or offered in many restaurants in India and Nepal, similar to how restaurants in the United States give out peppermint candy at the end of a meal. For intestinal gas, take fennel tea or capsules right after meals. You can also chew on the raw seeds if you like their licorice taste.

Botanical Bit

A **carminative** is an herbal property that, put simply, eliminates gas from the bowels.

In herbology terms, fennel acts as a *carminative,* which makes it effective for the subject we are talking about here. For colic in babies, fennel is effective for breast-feeding moms to take. No known side effects exist for fennel, and—as far as we know—it is completely safe even in high doses.

Gas: Dispelling the Myths with the Right Herbs

Food enzyme supplements, especially those with hydrochloric added, will help your body break down foods that have been cooked. (Cooked foods kill the live enzymes in our foods, leaving our pancreas and liver to make up for the extra production of missing enzymes.) If you find a good enzyme tablet, take the tablet or capsule about 20 minutes before you eat. This gives the supplement a chance to begin breaking down in the stomach before you eat. Some people purchase food enzymes in capsules and open up the capsule and sprinkle it on their cooked foods before eating. If you forget to take your enzyme supplement before a meal, take one after or during your meal anyway.

The Answer, My Friend, Is Blowin' in the Wind

So, besides reaching for fennel and other supplements and herbs to get rid of this antisocial problem before it strikes, let's take a quick look at how and why those things that cause the problem can be handled.

Proper food combining takes a little work, but it will help your digestion. When you eat foods together that are not complementary for each other, this can be considered poor food combining.

Let's just cover the very basics of food combining:

➤ In general, do not eat starches and proteins together.

➤ Do not eat fruit on a full stomach (empty stomach only).

➤ Do not combine fruits with any other food besides other fruits.

➤ Do not eat more than one *concentrated food* (starches and proteins) at any one meal.

To demonstrate, eat only fruit in the morning. For dinner or lunch, if you have a steak or some type of meat, have a salad or other green vegetables with it, and leave out the bread and cheeses. Or, have a big salad and add a concentrated food, such as cheese *or* beans *or* meat—but choose only one.

Sage Advice

Other herbs for the gaseous include papaya, ginger, peppermint, wild yam, dong quai, spearmint, and catnip. Papaya contains enzymes that help break down foods better. Ginger stimulates digestion. All mints in the plant kingdom can help stimulate digestive juices, and catnip, wild yam, and dong quai all help relax the body. Put together, these herbs make an excellent combination when taken before, during, or after meals.

Botanical Bit

In holistic nutrition, a **concentrated food** is in contrast to a food high in water content. In simple terms, you can think of a concentrated food as a food that, when squeezed thoroughly, would produce little or no water. Foods such as cheese, meats, baked potatoes, and grains are considered concentrated foods.

Are You Masticating at the Dinner Table?

Make sure you chew your foods well. We all have enzyme activity in our saliva, which is where the actual digestive process begins. Chewing thoroughly will give your stomach and the rest of your digestion a break and should help your gas problems.

Because your body relies on digestive juices and enzymes to break down the foods you eat, don't drink liquids (especially cold liquids) in large amounts during your meals. This may dilute the digestive juices and hinder your proper digestion. Be sure, however, to drink plenty of water in between meals, as proper digestion requires a lot of water. If you must drink during meals, sip warm herbal tea. The warmth will relax the stomach and aid digestion, whereas an icy cold drink will contract the stomach and inhibit digestion.

Poison Ivy

Meat and potatoes are an example of poor food combining.

Sage Advice

Gingivitis can be one of the first signs of impending osteoporosis and other health issues. Make sure you take preventative measures to strengthen your entire structural system with herbs rich in minerals, especially if you suffer from gum disease.

Bowel cleansing will help if you have foul-smelling gas. If you have started taking a new herb supplement, such as psyllium hulls, aloe vera, or any cleansing herb, you may experience gas the first few days to a week while your bowel is cleansing. I like to think of this process as sweeping out an old, dirty basement. You stir up a lot of dust, but when you are through, you have a clean basement!

Gingivitis to Your Party?

Gingivitis (gum disease) literally means "inflammation of the gums," and it may lead to pyorrhea (periodontal disease). Symptoms of gingivitis include swollen, bright red gums that usually bleed when you brush your teeth. The whole mouth and teeth can feel extremely sore and achy. Gingivitis is usually caused by poor dental hygiene or a lack of vitamin C or calcium. Some say it is also due to an over-acidic body system caused by eating too much protein. Protein foods cause an acid base when digested.

Herbs can be used internally and externally to help tone bleeding or swollen gums. A vitamin C deficiency needs to be corrected internally, but your dentist can get rid of deposits on the teeth that can be causing the problem. Either way, you can take herbs to strengthen and tighten your gum tissue to fight infection before, during, and after dental treatment.

Myrrh: Something to Chew On

Myrrh (*Commiphora nayrrha*), a plant native to northeast Africa, serves as a disinfectant and astringent that can help tone the gum tissue. Myrrh stimulates the body to make mucus and therefore facilitates drainage. It is also used as an infection-fighter because of its ability to increase white blood cell activity. Myrrh is best teamed with golden seal, especially when taken internally to help fight infection and heal the gums.

In small does, you can take myrrh internally every few hours until inflammation stops. You can then take myrrh daily for two weeks after your dental treatment to continue your healing process. Myrrh is not suggested during pregnancy for internal use, except in very low doses.

Myrrh is great topically, but you can make a tea from myrrh and golden seal and use it as a mouthwash to treat your problem locally. Mix both with a little water and pepper-mint or spearmint oil to help hide the taste. Rinse your mouth with cold water only, which will help tighten your tissues. Myrrh resin mixed with white oak bark powder and a couple drops of clove oil makes an excellent toothpaste that can help disinfect, tone, and clean the teeth and gums. The clove oil also serves as an *analgesic* and will help relieve some of the soreness. (Read more about cloves in Chapter 21, "T: Terrific Solutions," and Chapter 26, "An Herbal First Aid Kit.")

Other topical applications of myrrh include acne, boils, bruises, cavities, halitosis (bad breath), mouth sores, pain, sore throat, thrush, tonsillitis, and wounds. Myrrh resin can be burned as an incense to repel bugs.

Botanical Bit

An **analgesic** is an herb that has an ability to help relieve pain.

Just a Pinch Between the Cheek and Gums

White oak bark is a strong astringent herb that will help shrink swollen tissues. You can moisten a little white oak bark with water or even liquid chlorophyll and pack it around your gums each night to help relieve your swollen gums. Take white oak bark internally, too, but not before meals because its tightening, drying, restricting type properties might inhibit your digestion.

Myrrh and golden seal packs can be used to pack around the gums and work just as well as the white oak bark. And don't forget your vitamin C supplementation—rose hips work as a natural vitamin C source.

If gingivitis is caused by over-acidity in the system, eliminate acidic foods such as heavy protein. Internally, green drinks such as liquid chlorophyll will help neutralize body acids.

Sage Advice

Ask your qualified health profes-sional about getting your pH levels tested.

Gland to Know You, It's Been Swell

Swollen glands are a symptom usually associated with a bacterial or viral infection. Our lymph glands are tiny glands dispersed throughout the body where white blood cells are stored and work to fight off infection. When we have swollen glands in the neck, the body is usually fighting off an infection to keep it from reaching the brain, where it could be most damaging to us.

When you have swollen lymph nodes or glands, you should try to help your immune system fight off whatever is causing the infection. Immune system herbs such as echinacea and even elderberry are both immune-boosting herbs that help do so. Otherwise, for the symptoms associated with the pain of swollen tissues, astringent-type herbs such as white oak bark make an excellent remedy for shrinking swollen tissues.

Tightening Up with White Oak Bark

White oak bark (*Quercus alba*) is the bark from the white oak tree. The great white oak tree grows up to 100 feet tall, and its wood was used to build ships because of its ability to handle moisture. Its medicinal properties are mostly astringent in their effect, making this herb very useful in tightening tissues that are loose (in energetics, this would mean a "wet" type of condition).

White oak bark can be used internally as well as externally for any inflamed tissue, and you can use it as an excellent remedy not only just for swollen glands but also for hemorrhoids, internal bleeding, gout, herpes, wounds, and gingivitis.

White oak bark is rich in calcium, magnesium, phosphorus, and zinc, all minerals involved in tissue healing. For swollen glands, use internal application along with external application until swelling subsides.

Poison Ivy

White oak bark should not be taken just before or right after meals because its tightening effect on the tissues may inhibit digestion or dry up moisture, causing constipation. White oak bark is a powerful but effective herb for shrinking swollen tissues and should be used temporarily.

Fighting the Infection with Herbs and Other Nutrients

As I've said, swollen glands are usually associated with some type of infection, and herbs should be added to your program to help your body fight the infection internally. Echinacea and golden seal work together to help fight infection; add some black walnut, althea, parthenium, plantain, and bugleweed, and you have a combination to kill infection and shrink those glands. If your white oak bark is not working for you as well as you think it should, you can add some bayberry, another strong astringent herb to your program. You should be as tight as a whistle within a few days on this combination!

Poison Ivy

It is wise to find out exactly why your glands are swollen because this condition can be linked to a serious infection such as Epstein-Barr virus or mononucleosis, both of which may require medical attention and/or a serious herbal and nutritional program.

Other things you can add are vitamin C, beta carotene, B6, vitamin D, magnesium, lecithin, and CoQ$_{10}$. These nutrients will feed your lymphatic system and help boost your circulation, which can increase your ability to fight infection and help your body rid itself of waste products in the lymph tissues.

A Poultice for a Swell Time

External applications such as an herbal poultice or compress can sometimes work immediately to shrink swollen glands, bring boils to a head, and pull toxins from the skin.

Here's what you'll need:

2 parts white oak bark powder
1 part lobelia tincture or fluid
1 part mullein
1 part grapefruit extract
Bentonite clay (as needed to create stiff mixture)

Mix all ingredients together; add water if using all dried herbs. The clay should cause the mixture to coagulate. Pack the mixture around swollen glands to help pull out the infection, reduce swelling, and soothe tissues. Let dry, and remove by splashing the area with cold water. If desired, add a heat source, such as a hot water bottle, to help the mixture seep into the glands. Remove heat source and let poultice dry before removing it.

If your glands stay swollen after you fight off any infection, you might want to seek out a massage therapist who specializes in lymphatic drainage, which will force your glands to drain and usually will reduce glandular swelling. Be sure to drink plenty of water to help you flush!

Gout of Your Mind with Acid Build-Up

Gout is a build-up of *uric acid* in the blood stream and the joints that causes damage to the joints and the kidneys. Many times there is a specific inflammation and swelling in the big toe. Stones may form in the kidneys (see herbal remedies for this in Chapter 15, "J and K: For Just the Right Kind of Cure"). Deposits also may build in the skin and ears.

Botanical Bit

Uric acid is an end product of your body's metabolism and is a component of urine. The body eliminates this acid daily via the urinary tract and the skin. With gout, crystals of uric acid are deposited in the joints, causing stiffness and pain.

163

She Wore Safflowers in Her Hair

Native to India and Iran, the yellowish-orange flowers of the herb known as safflowers (*carthamus tinctorius*) have been used historically as a remedy for digestive problems, kidney problems, and problems of the pancreas. Safflowers have the ability to neutralize and eliminate uric acid from the body, which makes them a useful herbal remedy for gout.

Safflowers are taken (usually in pill form) internally to aid digestion of oils and will help to eliminate not only uric acid, but also cholesterol from the blood. This herb is rich in potassium and sodium, both minerals needed for proper water balance in the body.

Herb Lore

The orange petals of the safflower are used not only medicinally, but also for coloring and flavoring foods such as margarine. Safflowers are used in cosmetics and to dye cloth, and you might have seen safflower oil (made from the seeds of the safflower) on your grocery or health food store shelves. Safflower is sometimes substituted for saffron because it is less expensive.

Gout to Get More Herbs

You will need more than just safflowers to change your gout condition. Other herbs that help the kidneys excrete uric acid include juniper berries, parsley, uva ursi, dandelion, and chamomile.

Make sure you take some type of food enzyme supplement unless your diet is at least 80 percent whole, raw foods to help your body break down your foods (especially proteins) more efficiently. Your diet should consist of fewer protein foods (such as meat and beans) and more vegetables—especially greens. Add the herb ginger to also help stimulate proper digestion.

Sage Advice

A high-fiber diet also helps remove bile salts from the bowel. These salts are precursors to uric acid, the cause of gout.

In chemistry, one acid can neutralize another acid. Therefore, neutralize the excess acid floating around in your gout-ridden body with natural sources of sodium. Sodium-rich foods include celery, strawberries, and parsley (see the table at the end of the chapter for more). Goat's whey is also an excellent supplementary food that is great for over-acidic conditions of the body.

Herbal Remedies for Common Ailments

Gas (Flatulence, Intestinal)

Best Single Herb: Fennel

Best Combinations: Papaya, ginger, peppermint, wild yam, fennel, dong quai, spearmint, catnip

Other Helpful Supplements: Food enzymes with hydrochloric acid

Possible Causes: Poor digestion; incorrect food combining; too much liquid with meals; eating too fast; change in food/supplements; constipation (if stinky)

Complementary Help: Bowel cleansing; better food combining

Gingivitis (Gum Disease)

Best Single Herb: Myrrh

Best Combinations: White oak bark; golden seal

Other Helpful Supplements: CoQ_{10}, vitamins C and A

Possible Causes: Poor nutrition; lack of vitamin C; poor dental hygiene; hyperacidity of the system

Complementary Help: Dental visits; white oak bark, golden seal, or myrrh pack/rinse; black walnut tincture added to toothpaste; hydrogen peroxide rinse

Glands, Swollen

Best Single Herb: White oak bark

Best Combinations: Golden seal, black walnut, althea, parthenium, plantain, bugleweed; white oak bark; bayberry; echinacea

Other Helpful Supplements: Vitamin C with citrus bioflavonoids, either separately or in combination with beta carotene; vitamins C, B6, and D; magnesium; lecithin; and CoQ_{10}

Possible Causes: Mononucleosis; localized infection

Complementary Help: Poultice made with white oak bark, lobelia, mullein, grapefruit extract, and bentonite clay place directly over swollen glands to help pull out infection and reduce swelling (add heat source if desired); lymphatic drainage massage

Gout

Best Single Herb: Safflowers

Best Combinations: Juniper berries, parsley, uva ursi, dandelion, chamomile; safflowers; alfalfa; pau d'arco; ginger

Other Helpful Supplements: Food enzymes; trace minerals

Possible Causes: A build-up of uric acid in the blood due to poor digestion

Complementary Help: Eliminate meat and beans from diet; use a dry skin brush; high-fiber diet; support digestive system; support kidneys; juice and/or eat sodium-rich foods such as celery, parsley, strawberries, spinach, Swiss chard, Romaine lettuce, red beets, and collards

The Least You Need to Know

➤ Gas is an indication of poor digestion or constipation and can be helped by ingesting fennel.

➤ White oak bark is a strong astringent and is useful for any swollen tissues, including gingivitis and swollen glands.

➤ Safflowers help your body eliminate excess uric acid, the cause of gout, and can be useful in your recovery.

➤ Myrrh and white oak bark can be packed around the gums to stop the bleeding and swelling caused by gum disease.

Part 3
Sickness from H to N

This part will continue through our alphabet and discuss remedies for illnesses from headaches to nausea. The pages will continue to fill you in and give you reasons why you may be suffering from your ailments. We will cover many, many more herbs and other natural remedies along the way.

As you learn about the best single herbs, you will also be enlightened about the herbs' many other uses, and you just might find a plant that works well for an ailment other than one that begins with the letters H to N. So happy exploring and learning!

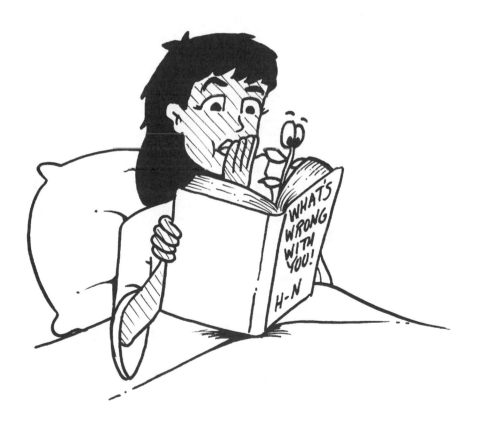

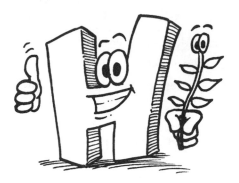

Chapter 13

H: Happy Healing with Herbs

> ## In This Chapter
>
> ➤ Ease headaches the herbal way
>
> ➤ Soothe heartburn with herbal remedies
>
> ➤ Old remedies for hemorrhoids
>
> ➤ Ease hyperactivity with nature's cures
>
> ➤ Cope with hypoglycemia using sweet herbs

"The average, healthy, well-adjusted adult gets up at seven-thirty in the morning feeling just plain terrible." —Jean Kerr, American dramatist, screenwriter, and humorist. *Please Don't Eat the Daisies,* "Where Did You Put the Aspirin?"

Hopefully you aren't one of the healthy, well-adjusted adults that Jean Kerr was describing above, but if you are, don't worry, herbs can and do change lives! In this chapter we will talk about some painful conditions that begin with the letter H, from head to toe, or rather, from headaches to hemorrhoids! Stick with me, and you'll be feeling better by morning. Read on!

Headaches: It's All in Your Head

Headaches are the body's way of letting you know something is wrong. A headache will let you know if you drank too much; ate too much; are constipated, stressed, tired, or thirsty; need to get your eyesight checked, or that your hormones are out of balance, just to name a few! All in all, we should be grateful for a headache because it serves as our alarm to pay attention and do something about it!

In a pinch, (so to speak) you can use the reflexology or acupressure point to rid yourself of a headache temporarily. Here's how to find the spot:

➤ Spread your hand out in front of you, palm facing down (either hand is fine).

➤ Locate the V between your pointer finger and thumb.

➤ Follow that V down almost to the wrist, where you can feel the two bones and muscles come together.

➤ With your other hand, place your thumb on top of your hand on the point, and place the pointer finger of your other hand on the palm side of the point. Now squeeze!

This point is usually tender if you have a headache. Hold the point firmly, as deeply as you can tolerate. The headache usually disappears within a few minutes or less. The following illustrations show you how to find the right point.

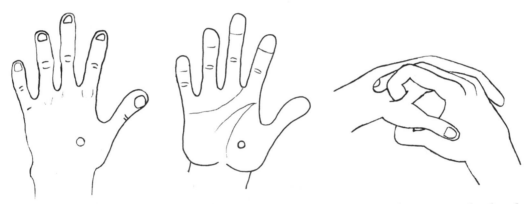

The reflex point for easing a headache shown on front and back of hand: Use your other hand to squeeze this spot, and hold until your headache subsides. You can use either hand to stimulate this area.

Oh, My Aching Head

So how do you determine which factor is giving you a headache? Let's start with the easiest first and then go to the more complicated:

➤ Many headaches are due to dehydration. Try drinking two full glasses of pure water; this should help right away.

➤ The most typical cause of headaches are from constipation. Try Ivy's Colon Cleanse, in Chapter 3, "What to Expect with Herbs," or any of the constipation remedies in this book.

➤ For headaches that may be caused by poor posture, try ergonomically designed furniture to help you with correct posture and your comfort at work. Also see your chiropractor for a spinal adjustment. Your chiropractor can offer some suggestions or inexpensive supports to add to the back of your chair or neck if you can't afford better furniture.

➤ Stress and tension can block your body's energy flow, or "chi." If this is the cause of your headaches, try acupuncture, acupressure, or reflexology to restore your flow.

➤ If your headache seems to be in the back of your head, get your eyesight checked. Your eyes could be strained, and you may need glasses or a prescription change.

White Willow Bark: Worse Than Its Bite

As you are pinpointing the cause of your headaches, a couple of white willow bark (*Salix alba*) capsules will ease your head pain. The bark of the white willow tree is used as an anti-inflammatory, antiseptic, and pain reliever. As you may remember, we talked about white willow bark originally being used to make aspirin. White willow also eases rheumatism pains and can help lower fevers in adults. Respect this herb as you would an over-the-counter aspirin, and do not exceed over 60 mg daily. Ask your physician before giving white willow to a child suffering with Reye's syndrome, since this herb is a salicylate, as is aspirin.

A combination of white willow, valerian, and wild lettuce makes an excellent remedy for a stress or tension headache. (Valerian and wild lettuce both help relax the nervous system.) A pinch of capsicum may be added as a catalyst to this remedy to speed the pain-relieving effect.

An excellent headache remedy using essential oils was brought to my attention by a client. I have used this remedy because I like the effect it promotes, stimulating and calming at the same time. Plus it smells terrific! Here's all you need:

> 6 drops pure essential oil of lavender
>
> 4 drops pure essential oil of peppermint

Drop each into the palm of your hand. Mix together with your finger using a clockwise motion. Dab a few drops on each temple and massage in gently. Rub your hands together briskly and run your fingers through your hair while massaging rest of solution into scalp. You'll be glad you tried this one!

Sage Advice

White willow bark is also useful and safe to use for children with diarrhea, cold, and flu. Other uses include nervousness, pain, rheumatism, ulceration, and eczema. White willow is rich in calcium, magnesium, phosphorus, and zinc.

Sage Advice

Magnesium and calcium supplements can help relax muscles and are helpful with many aches and pains in the body, including headaches. Be sure to drink plenty of water with your remedies, and look for the cause of your pain.

Heartburn: Putting Out the Fire with Marshmallow

Anyone who has experienced bad heartburn knows that the word "heartburn" sounds just like it feels: like a hot coal burning through your chest cavity. But heartburn is just a sign of indigestion somewhere along your digestive tract. Heartburn can indicate other more serious troubles and should be checked by your physician if it persists.

About 50 percent of the population who suffer with heartburn can track the condition to a hiatal hernia, a condition where the stomach is pushed up toward the esophagus, causing a "kink" that allows stomach acid into the esophagus causing heartburn. If you have think you have a hiatal hernia, soothing herbs such as marshmallow will serve as an excellent remedy, but you will also need to consider herbs that relax the nervous system, too (see "S-T-R-E-S-S: That's the Way We Spell Success," in Chapter 20, "R and S: Remarkable Recoveries and Super Solutions"), wear loose pants, and sip on warm herbal teas to help bring the stomach back to place. Sometimes your chiropractor will be able to mechanically "adjust" the area to bring temporary relief until the problem is healed.

Sage Advice

The stomach is where we tend to hold worry. Most people with hiatal hernias are worry worts, which causes tightness in the solar plexus area and shallow breathing. Worrying will only make your hiatal hernia worse. R–e–l–a–x, and breathe deeply from the bottom of your abdomen. Chew your foods slowly and take your mind off the worry.

Sometimes heartburn can indicate gallbladder trouble or gallstones. If you eat lots of fatty foods, tend to be constipated or don't eat enough fiber, or have a family history of gallbladder or liver trouble, you may be a good candidate for a gallbladder flush. This technique is designed to break down gallstones so your body can pass them out of the bowel. This is a three-day cleanse, but you can condense it to a single day by taking oil and lemon juice on the evening of the first day. This cleanse is for those who are not in a weakened or debilitated condition, where a cleanse would not be appropriate.

Gallbladder Flush:

Plan to have some time at home during this flush, as you will spend a lot of time in the bathroom!

Day One: Throughout the day, drink one quart (32 ounces) of unsweetened pear or apple juice, or a mixture of the two. Eat at least two cups of applesauce throughout the day. Optionally, you can add pears, apples, figs, or prunes, but do not eat any fats. For best effects, eat only fruits. If this makes you too weak, take some yogurt, soup, or brown rice to get you through.

Take the following herbs at lunch, dinner, and bedtime:

> Psyllium hulls: 3 (totaling 9 daily)
>
> Cascara sagrada: 1 (totaling 3 daily)
>
> Hydrangea: 2 (totaling 6 daily)
>
> Lecithin: 4 (totaling 12 daily)

Day Two: Repeat the same regimen as for Day One, but at bedtime drink four ounces of olive oil mixed with four ounces of fresh-squeezed lemon juice.

Day Three: By mid-morning, you should have passed little green balls known as gallstones. You can facilitate this process by giving yourself an enema.

After a cleanse or any fast, it is always wise to start back slowly into eating solid foods. If you ate only fruit for the first two days, you should eat only soup, fruit, and yogurt on the third day to ease your body back into digesting.

For occasional heartburn, an herb with a "cool, wet" energetic should be used first. The herb marshmallow (*Althea officinalis*) fits great into this category. This pretty little white flowering herb grows in marshy lands and is sweet to the taste. As you might guess, marshmallow was originally used to make those white, pillowish-looking candies we see around the campfires. As an herb, it has a soothing effect on body tissues and can be used instead of other herbs with the same qualities, such as slippery elm and aloe vera.

If we strengthen digestion, heartburn usually ceases to be a problem. Pepsin, food enzymes, papaya, peppermint, catnip, and aloe vera all help to support digestion and will help get to the root cause of your problem.

The clinical studies of Dr. F. Batmanghelidj, M.D., suggest that heartburn is a symptom of dehydration. A special mucus lining serves to protect the inner walls of our stomach and small intestines from the damage of stomach acid. Lots of water is required in order for our body to produce this special mucus; when we don't have enough water, we cannot create this protective barrier. Try drinking two glasses of water about 20 minutes before each meal, along with some marshmallow or food enzyme tablets. The marshmallow will help your body retain some moisture, and the enzymes will help you break down your food.

Sage Advice

Lecithin is a substance found in egg yolks, soybeans, sesame seeds, and other foods. This oil can be found in capsule form. Lecithin has been used as a nutrient to emulsify fat in the bloodstream, making it useful for high cholesterol and fatty stones of any kind, such as gallstones. It also aids in rebuilding brain cells and, therefore, is known as a brain food.

Poison Ivy

If you are experiencing heartburn, it is not a good idea to continue to suppress your stomach acid with antacid medications, as this can worsen your digestive troubles over time. A tablespoon of baking soda mixed in a glass of water should put out the fire, but don't rely on this remedy as a permanent cure for a deeper problem.

Hepatitis: Not in the Slightest

Hepatitis is an inflammation of the liver usually due to a virus or a toxic substance, but sometimes also a result of an immunological abnormality.

Hepatitis A is transmitted by contaminated food or drink and occurs as a result of poor hygienic practices. Symptoms include fever, yellow discoloration of the skin, and an ill feeling. The illness usually lasts about three weeks, and an infected person may be contagious during this time. The good news is that if you are infected once, your body builds a natural immunity to the disease so that you should be resistant to infection if exposed again.

Hepatitis B is transmitted via an infected person's blood or blood-soiled products, contaminated hypodermic needles, or sexual contact with an infected person. Symptoms include headache, fever, chills, general weakness, and yellowing of the skin. Some people can die from this infection.

> **Botanical Bit**
>
> **Hepatitis** is an inflammation of the liver due to a virus, a toxic substance, or an immunological abnormality. **Hepatitis A** is spread through poor sanitary habits and can be transmitted through food and drink. Infected blood or sexual contact with an infected individual transmits **Hepatitis B**.

The ABCs of Hepatitis Prevention

As you can see, prevention is definitely the best medicine for hepatitis. Here are some simple prevention tips:

➤ If you feel uncomfortable about the cleanliness of a restaurant, choose a different one.

➤ Make sure you wash your hands thoroughly before eating—and *always* after using the toilet.

➤ Stay away from any sources of contamination, such as blood-soiled products, hypodermic needles, tattoo needles, and intimate contact with infected persons.

➤ Always keep your immune system strong and your liver supported with herbs and nutrition.

Eat fruits and vegetables rich in organic iron to feed your liver. These foods are generally dark in color and include dark green vegetables such as spinach, beets, and black cherries. Pesticides must be filtered through the liver, so eating organic fruits and vegetables will keep your liver from having to work so hard.

When dealing with any liver affliction, add vitamin C, lecithin, vitamin E, and barley juice to your program.

Dandelion: Just Dandy for Your Liver

Dandelion (*Taraxacum officinale*) seems to spring up everywhere when you start talking about herbs. And if you happen to be one of those green lawn-loving types, you probably have met the dandelion personally a few times! Well, I am here to be the mediator between you and the dandelion to personally introduce you to this herb and its wide variety of uses. Maybe when you get to know the dandelion and see all the value it can bring to your life, you might not try to poison it again!

The root of the dandelion has been used for years as a tonic for the liver and to aid with hepatitis, jaundice, and gallbladder problems.

Herb Lore

Some other interesting tidbits on dandelion that you might want to remember: The white sap of the dandelion (when you break the stem) has been used topically to get rid of warts. If you want to attract wildlife to your surroundings, leave the dandelions growing—they are food for bunnies, geese, deer, and even bumble bees! Dandelion is also useful in weight-loss formulas because it can help with fat digestion.

You can pick and wash bitter leaves and eat them in a salad. The leaves are used as a blood purifier and kidney tonic and help stimulate digestion. Dandelion also contains several minerals and has been helpful in treating gout and other structural problems, such as arthritis and rheumatism. The flowers have been used to make wine and beer, and the roots can be roasted and made into a coffee. Wow—and you thought *you* were versatile! If I had only one herb to use, I would use the dandelion root to protect my liver from hepatitis. Of course, you will be seeing your doctor for help with this illness, but you can tell him that you plan to support your liver with some home remedies that will help your progress.

If you can't get to a doc, some herbs may help until you can get to see one. A mixture for the liver you can take include rose hips (for vitamin C), barberry and dandelion (both good for the liver), fennel, red beet, horseradish, and parsley. Milk thistle added to this program is especially helpful when recovering from hepatitis because it will help rebuild damaged liver cells. These are all listed in the table in the end of the chapter.

Olive Leaf, for Olive Your Liver Problems

Another special mention needs to be given to olive leaf extract as a natural herbal remedy good for fighting any form of hepatitis. In fact, olive leaf may be better for actually killing a hepatitis infection whereas dandelion is better used preventatively.

Olive leaf has now been proven to be highly effective against numerous bacteria, viruses, yeast, and parasite infections. A compound called oleuropein contains the most medicinal part of this plant. Studies show it has the ability to inhibit growth of many types of bacteria and prevent viruses from replicating in the body.

This herb is now being used to treat AIDS, arthritis, candida, colds, diabetes, Epstein-Barr, fungal infections (including toe fungus), hepatitis, high blood pressure, infections, shingles, herpes (both types), and worms.

Hemorrhoids: A Swell Solution

Hemorrhoids, also known as piles, are simply enlarged capillaries (veins) in or around the rectum. Sometimes hemorrhoids bleed after you use the bathroom, but they typically cause no pain. There are three levels of severity of hemorrhoids. The first two usually do not require medical treatment, but the third type is very painful and sometimes requires surgery to correct the problem.

Hemorrhoids are usually caused by prolonged constipation. The weight of the material in the bowel creates a pressure on the tissues, which causes a hemorrhoid to form. If you strain, you force the blood into the small capillaries and can create a hemorrhoid. Stress also seems to complicate the problem.

Sage Advice

You should never strain or push to have to evacuate the bowel. If you do, you are constipated and should consider herbs that will soften the stool and help get you regulated. A healthy evacuation is passed easily and fairly quickly; see Chapter 8 under "Constipation: All Dressed Up and Nowhere to Go," for the ideal stool.

A Remedy Amongst Piles of Herbs

Because hemorrhoids are typically caused by constipation, herbs that relieve this problem will be helpful in preventing hemorrhoids and keeping them from getting worse. Aloe vera, for one, is a soothing herb that will help act as a mild laxative. It also soothes inflamed tissues and is an analgesic, which means that it has properties that reduce local pain. You can drink the juice of aloe vera in juice, water, or straight.

Another stool-softening agent that works as a mild laxative is flax seed. Flax seed oil can be purchased in capsules or bulk in a bottle. It spoils quickly, however, and will therefore need to be refrigerated. Flax seeds can be added to foods and can be ground up and made into breads, but the oil is best for constipation.

B-complex vitamins will help feed the nervous system to ease stress-induced hemorrhoids. Vitamin C with extra bioflavonoids are helpful to strengthen blood capillaries and prevent hemorrhoids.

Sweep Away Hemorrhoids with Butcher's Broom

Butcher's broom (*Ruscus aculeatus*) is an herb used by many to counteract hemorrhoids because of its ability to strengthen tissues, tighten veins, and thin the blood. For hemorrhoids, take butcher's broom internally, although a decoction can be made from it to use as a topical application or for use in a suppository, too. In this case, you can take butcher's broom at both ends.

If you don't have butcher's broom handy, you can substitute white oak bark in its place to shrink swollen tissues. A suppository useful for painful and bleeding hemorrhoids can be made from any of the following astringent herbs:

> Witch hazel (may be purchased in liquid form at drug store)
>
> White oak bark (make into tea or decoction)
>
> Butcher's broom (make into tea or decoction)

Soak a clean piece of cotton in the solution, and insert into the rectum overnight. It will come back out the next morning with your first bowel evacuation.

Hyperactivity

Hyperactivity, also known as attention deficit hyperactive disorder (ADHD), seems to be more and more of a problem. This problem usually is first recognized in children but can be carried into adulthood as well. Hyperactivity is characterized by a wide range of disorders affecting behavior, communication, and learning ability and can include an inability to be still, outbursts of emotions, and an inability to focus.

Hurry Up and Find a Cure

Many factors have been linked to hyperactivity in both children and adults. In children, many experts say that a need for discipline is the main problem; others believe the real cause is a chemical reaction to food additives. Some chemicals in foods used as colorings, preservatives, and flavor enhancers cause strong reactions in certain people. If you are experiencing hyperactivity, or if your child seems uncontrollable, take a good look at the foods he or she is eating. See the section "Food Allergies," in Chapter 5, "A Is for Ailment," to help you pinpoint allergic symptoms.

Sage Advice

Attention deficit disorder (ADD) is associated with those who do not show the outward manifestations of being hyper. The primary issue for all people who suffer from attention disorders is that they cannot control their thought processes and are not able to focus their attention freely.

Sage Advice

Hyperactivity in children may be caused from an essential fatty acid deficiency. Supplementing with Omega-3 fatty acids, evening primrose oil, or black currant oil daily has helped many.

Poison Ivy

Kava kava is not recommended for pregnant or nursing moms. It also should not be used when you have alcohol in your system, or when you will be operating heavy equipment or driving.

Eliminate stimulants such as caffeine and sugar from the diet. A good combination that has been used successful for children includes valerian, anise, black walnut, desert tea, ginger, and licorice. Other nutrients that feed the nervous system include B-complex vitamins, calcium, and magnesium.

Kava Kava: A Quick Fix

Kava kava (*Piper methysticum*) is a plant from the South Pacific that's useful in promoting relaxation, sleep, and a mild feeling of euphoria. In Greek, kava means "intoxicating beverage," and kava kava lives up to that name: In small doses, it can calm hyperactivity, relax tensed muscles, and ease anxiety. Many people report that they remember having vivid dreams or recalling their dreams more often the next day when taking kava before bed.

Kava kava also has some pain-killing effects: Chewing on the leaves from this plant can ease pain from a toothache. In addition, the Chinese believe that this herb opens areas of blocked energy and restores better circulation and energy flow throughout the body.

Hypoglycemia: A Sweet Solution

Hypoglycemia is a condition in which a person has low blood sugar. The opposite of low blood sugar is hyperglycemia, otherwise known as diabetes. Our pancreas and adrenal glands are mostly responsible for helping the blood sugar level stay balanced. When our blood sugar drops, it signals our hunger button and prompts us to eat.

Almost every symptom you can think of can be related to hypoglycemia, which is what makes it difficult to pinpoint. Large fluctuations in blood sugar can make us feel depressed, anxious, and fatigued. Since hypoglycemia affects your brain, muscles, digestion, and glands, symptoms may also include: sleepiness, lack of concentration, memory problems, mood swings, irritability, insomnia, nightmares, blurred vision, and heart palpitations.

If a hypoglycemic gets hungry and ignores the signal to eat right away, he may experience these symptoms:

➤ Grumpiness

➤ Headaches

➤ Nausea

➤ Shakiness

➤ Sweating

➤ A spaced-out feeling

➤ Shortness of breath

Because blood sugar is the primary food for the brain, severe hypoglycemic attacks can cause a person to pass out. In some cases, an attack may even be damaging to the brain.

Hypoglycemia can usually be controlled by diet. I have managed to overcome my own systemic hypoglycemia after being properly diagnosed. I then was able to investigate the disorder thoroughly and understood what exactly was happening. As with many physical problems, hypoglycemia forces you to become more aware of your body's communication with you.

Herb Lore

Discovering what hypoglycemia is and finding the nutritional and herbal approach to its cure might answer a lot of questions about why you are suffering from other unexplainable ailments. I believe that low blood sugar can be a causative factor in migraines, irritability and moodiness, PMS, yeast infections, asthma, and overall spaciness. You can certainly use herbs and supplements to balance blood sugar. Once under control, many negative related symptoms dramatically subside or disappear completely.

Blood sugar fluctuates with the foods we eat. Learning to become conscious of the process will become routine once you understand some simple things you can do to manage the problem. Diet and herbs helped free me from attacks, and I am now able to recognize the symptoms associated with this ailment, which I'll share with you here.

Dieting for the Hypoglycemic

With hypoglycemia, it's important to manage your diet well and always make sure that you have some type of food source handy.

Avoid caffeine, which will lower your blood sugar. Also avoid sugar, which can put your own blood sugar (glucose) on a roller coaster ride and make you crash harder and faster than if you didn't eat it in the first place. If you must eat sweets, do not eat them on an empty stomach; eat sweets after a regular meal.

Other tips to manage hypoglycemia:

➤ Eat a high-fiber diet to slow digestion of foods.

➤ Eat small meals frequently to maintain blood sugar.

➤ Watch out for fruits and fruit juices. These are high in sugar content and can cause a crash just like refined sugar can.

➤ If you tend to wake up in the middle of the night, this could be an indication of your blood sugar dipping. To correct this, try a handful of cashews or other protein just before bed. Protein digests slowly through the system and will help keep you steady through the night.

➤ Eat some protein every morning—some examples for breakfast can be yogurt, a protein smoothie, or peanut butter on an apple. You can also take three capsules of the herb spirulina, which is rich in protein. It will help carry you through the day. (Read more on spirulina in Chapter 22, "U: Understanding the Power of Herbs.")

➤ Watch what you eat, and note any food allergies that may be triggering a problem.

➤ Take your supplements. The following have all been helpful in the correction or management of hypoglycemia: GTF chromium (GTF stands for "glucose tolerance factor") is a mineral that helps steady your blood sugar. L-glutamine is an amino acid useful in sugar metabolism. A combination of licorice root, safflowers, dandelion, and horseradish is helpful to the glands and digestion. Spirulina taken between meals is a rich source of protein that can help keep you nourished.

Poison Ivy

Use of licorice root is not suggested for long periods of time in large quantities because it can raise blood pressure. Also, pregnant women should not use licorice root in large quantities. Although in its pure form this herb can be used as a safe sugar substitute for diabetics, it is not usually recommended for diabetics because of its sweetness.

Licorice Root: A Sweet Choice

Licorice root (*Glycyrrhiza glabra*) is a wonderful herb that is sweet to the taste and that helps balance the blood sugar level. This herb also has been called "The Great Harmonizer" and tends to live up to its name: It has helped me steady my hypoglycemia, and I have seen it work the same for many others. Take a couple of capsules between each meal to keep the blood sugar balanced and your energy level even keel.

Licorice root is considered a tonic for the adrenal glands and will help produce adrenal hormones such as cortisone when your body calls for it. Hypoglycemia can be brought on by adrenal stress which, in turn, is brought on by poor nutrition, vigorous physical work, and mental and emotional stress. Licorice's harmonizing effects eliminate that three o'clock down-time—sometimes called the "afternoon blahs"—that you may experience, whether hypoglycemic or not.

Licorice root also soothes mucus membranes, making it a good cough remedy. It helps lower allergic responses and is also useful to bring down high cholesterol levels. By supporting the adrenal glands, licorice also provides energy—so revered an herb it is that it was buried alongside King Tut in his Egyptian tomb! In addition, licorice root is used commercially as an additive to chewing tobacco and is added as a flavoring in Guinness beer. This does not give the hypoglycemic an excuse to drink beer, however; alcohol is detrimental for low blood sugar. (Go ahead, call me a party pooper.)

Herbal Remedies for Common Ailments

Headaches (also see Migraines, Chapter 17)

Best Single Herb: White willow bark

Best Combinations: White willow bark, valerian, wild lettuce, capsicum

Other Helpful Supplements: Magnesium; calcium

Possible Causes: Dehydration; constipation; problems with eyesight; stress; spinal misalignment

Complementary Help: Bowel cleansing; acupuncture/acupressure; reflexology; chiropractic adjustments; ergonomic work furniture

Heartburn

Best Single Herb: Marshmallow

Best Combinations: Marshmallow; papaya and peppermint; aloe vera; catnip

Other Helpful Supplements: Calcium; pepsin; food enzymes with hydrochloric acid (use with caution, try an enzyme without HCl first, if no relief, try the other)

Possible Causes: Hiatal hernia; gallstones; low stomach acid; dehydration

Complementary Help: Gallbladder flush; baking soda drink

Hepatitis

Best Single Herb: Dandelion

Best Combinations: Rose hips, barberry, dandelion, fennel, red beet, horseradish, parsley (for cleansing and building); milk thistle (for repairing)

Other Helpful Supplements: Vitamin C; lecithin; vitamin E; barley juice

Possible Causes: Find and prevent source of contamination

Complementary Help: Eat only vegetables and fruit for several weeks to take a load off the liver; drink and eat dark green vegetables, black cherries, and beets

Hemorrhoids

Best Single Herb: Butcher's broom

Best Combinations: Aloe vera (eases constipation and soothes tissues); white oak bark (to shrink tissues); butcher's broom

continues

Herbal Remedies for Common Ailments   (continued)

Hemorrhoids (continued)

Other Helpful Supplements: B-complex; vitamin C with citrus bioflavonoids

Possible Causes: Stress; constipation; weakened blood capillaries

Complementary Help: Bowel cleansing; stress reduction; witch hazel suppository

Hyperactivity

Best Single Herb: Kava kava

Best Combinations: Valerian, anise, black walnut, desert tea, ginger, licorice; evening primrose oil *or* black current oil

Other Helpful Supplements: Omega-3 fatty acids; B-complex vitamins; calcium and magnesium

Possible Causes: Food allergies; emotional problems; discipline; chemical irritants in foods

Complementary Help: Check for allergies; check for parasites; eliminate sugar from diet; eliminate caffeine

Hypoglycemia

Best Single Herb: Licorice root

Best Combinations: Licorice root, safflowers, dandelion, horseradish; spirulina

Other Helpful Supplements: Chromium; l-glutamine

Possible Causes: Food allergies

Complementary Help: Diet is important: eat frequent small meals; eat plenty of protein (especially in the morning); avoid caffeine and sugar; eat a high-fiber diet

The Least You Need to Know

➤ White willow bark is effective for relieving headache pain, but finding and eliminating the cause of the headache is the best medicine.

➤ Marshmallow herb can soothe irritated tissues and put out the heartburn fire.

➤ Dandelion and olive leaf are the top herbs the liver and can help when suffering from hepatitis.

➤ Butcher's broom is one of the best single herbs taken internally to combat hemorrhoids.

➤ Kava kava is an herb that helps relax the mind and may be beneficial for hyperactivity.

➤ Licorice root is another wonder herb that has been helpful in balancing blood sugar in hypoglycemics.

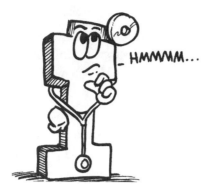

HMMMM...

Chapter 14

I: Interesting Illnesses

In This Chapter

➤ Sexually stimulating herbs for men and women

➤ Boost fertility with herbs

➤ Soothe irritable bowel syndrome

➤ Use herbs to help put you to sleep

"Sex may 'exercise' the reproductive system, but unless love is present, the mind and heart are not fed." —Dr. Bernard Jensen from his book *Love, Sex and Nutrition*

Interesting illnesses begin with I, and that includes impotency, which will be discussed in this chapter. Since we will be on the topic of love, you will also be introduced to some herbal love potions for men *and* women. And herbs for infertility so that your efforts are not fruitless! After all that sexy stuff, you probably won't need to read the section on insomnia, but it will be there for you anyway. So snuggle up with your honey and let's talk about sex, baby!

Impotence: A Very Impotent Subject

Pharmaceutical companies may have realized firsthand what a large problem male impotency has become with the explosive popularity of the new pharmaceutical drug Viagra®, a male sexual potency enhancer. But before you go experimenting with any pharmaceuticals, you might want to understand your underlying problem first. Once you eliminate some of your possible causes, I'll turn you on to a healthy, holistic approach to impotency (or frigidity, in women) along with some very stimulating herbs.

These possible causes may be affecting your sexual interest or performance:

➤ Use of drugs such as blood pressure medication, tranquilizers, and anti-depressants. Discuss these factors with your prescribing doctor.

➤ Illegal drugs, such as cocaine and marijuana, which can make a person numb to sex and may lead to impotency with prolonged use.

➤ Abuse of alcohol, which destroys important hormones and weakens sexual drive.

➤ Cigarette smoking, which can inhibit circulation to the groin area and contribute to impotency.

➤ Arteriosclerosis (hardening of the arteries due to fat in the blood, hypertension, and/or calcium deposits), which inhibits circulation to all parts of the body and could affect your sex life.

➤ Mental or emotional issues from past experiences. Traumatic events or current stress all need to be evaluated to see whether this is the core of the problem—remember that sex is also a mental process.

All of these problems can be overcome separately with the use of herbs and changes in diet. But first you'll need to consider which one(s) is most likely your contributing factor.

Sage Advice

Make sure that you address what could be causing your sexual problem, and make sure you are clear on any medical conditions that may need attention before you decide to incorporate herbs into your life. A balanced, holistic approach to the problem will be your most effective solution.

Yohimbe for Men: Hard to Find

Taking into account that many factors can be linked to impotence, I have highlighted one herb that has a stimulating effect on the male species. The herb known as yohimbe is a very powerful herb that is hard to come by (no pun intended!), for the pure stuff can sell for as high as $1.00 per capsule.

Sage Advice

Because of its expense and the possibly dangerous side effects when used improperly, many manufacturers may make yohimbe available within a combination made for men, but it is difficult to find as a single herb.

The bark of this herb contains the alkaloid yohimbine, known for its effects on the circulatory system—especially to the genitals. This tropical plant is found in West Africa and has been smoked, snuffed, and rubbed on the body for its sexually stimulating abilities. Yohimbe can cause hallucinations in high doses and is best mixed with other ingredients. See the table at the end of this chapter for a good combination you can use to heighten your senses without causing damage. Yohimbe was the first FDA-approved substance for treating impotence and is successful in 34 to 43 percent of cases. You may want to try a combination that contains yohimbe before considering the drug Viagra.

The side effects of Viagra include headaches, seeing blue, and blackouts due to a drop in blood pressure. Yohimbe used correctly and obtained from a quality manufacturer is a much safer way to add a boon to your sex life.

This table contains some general tips for men and women alike to address some common causes of impotence or frigidity (these herbs also may have a positive effect on infertility):

When problem is caused by:	Try:
Mental trauma, emotional issues, stress	Psychotherapy, B-complex, Siberian ginseng
Prostate trouble	Saw palmetto, pumpkin seeds, vitamin E, bowel cleansing, elimination of caffeine
Circulatory problems	Capsicum, garlic, hawthorn, exercise, reflexology, acupuncture
Depression	Elimination of sugar and stimulants from diet, Siberian ginseng, bee pollen

Damiana, for Cold Dames

Women occasionally can experience frigidity (lack of interest in or feeling repulsed by sex) for some of the same mental, emotional, and physical reasons that men suffer from impotency. However, some other factors may be involved for women, including vaginal dryness caused by menopause, hormonal changes, or physical problems with the uterus, ovaries, or cervix that keep sex from being enjoyable. Find out what could be causing these problems, and talk to your doctor for answers. Follow the other guidelines in the previous table that also can work for men, and then start taking damiana.

Damiana (pronounced *dame-ee-anna*) (*Turnera aphrodisiaca*) has served both men and women as a sexual stimulant. This plant comes from Mexico and the West Indies and has been used historically to tone the nervous system and stimulate testosterone, predominately a male hormone. (Women have a little in their system, too.) Herbs will help balance out the body, so don't worry—you shouldn't start growing facial hair!

You ladies will also find damiana useful for hot flashes, depression, vertigo, PMS, and constipation.

Poison Ivy

Yohimbe is a strong cerebral stimulant and should not be taken with alcohol or antidepressants (MAO inhibitors). Also steer clear of this herb if you have diabetes, hypertension, heart disease, or schizophrenia. Women should not take yohimbe, as it can reduce fertility.

Poison Ivy

Damiana should not be used if you have urinary or liver disease. No more than two capsules a day should be taken by the average person.

It has been used to strengthen kidneys and ease menopausal symptoms. Some have even smoked damiana before making love (not recommended here!).

Infertility: From Humility to Virility

Many frustrated wannabe parents are turning to science more and more to help them conceive with in vitro fertilization, fertility drugs, and the like. However, most insurance companies do not pay for these extracurricular procedures, which can be downright expensive, not to mention exhausting!

For a gentler approach, let's look at some herbal alternatives that have helped others with this trouble. Besides, herbs are more mild and safe as concentrated food sources—there's a good chance that you won't wind up with eight babies at one time if you boost your system with herbs instead of drugs! Having just one baby at a time makes parenting about eight times less hectic!

Ginseng: A Manly Solution

Ginseng (*Korean Panax schin-seng*) (*Siberian Eleutherococcus*) (*Wild American Panax quinquefolium*) is both a male and female remedy for infertility and has been used since ancient times for a host of conditions. The root of the ginseng plant is thick and resembles a manly shape, which could be was how it was first considered to be a manly tonic. Ginseng helps the body to utilize oxygen better, acts as a tonic to the adrenal glands to help them conserve vitamin C, and serves as a tonic to the entire glandular system, thus saving energy.

Herb Lore

Here's my advice to potential parents when it comes to fertility issues. If you and your partner have had troubles for a while, try not to fret because this can negatively affect your goal. I suggest that both of you follow an herbal and nutritional program designed to boost both of your virility and fertility instead of immediately getting tested to see which of you is less fertile. This can only inhibit a man's sense of his self and may make a woman feel guilty. Most of the time, this first approach works before any medical intervention is required.

You might notice a few different types of ginseng: typically, Siberian, Korean, and Wild American ginseng. Which one do you pick, you ask? Well, remember when we talked a little on energetics in the beginning of the book (see Chapter 3, "What to Expect with Herbs")? That will come in handy again here. Wild American ginseng is "cooling" energetically, which makes it especially useful for you guys who tend to run hotter in general. You might want to take this ginseng during the hot months. On the other hand, Korean and Siberian ginseng are similar in their properties and have "warming" energetics, meaning that they have a warming effect on your body. These herbs tend to warm the system slightly, so you will probably want to use them during colder months.

Some say that Wild American ginseng is better suited to women and that Asian ginseng is better for men. It is difficult to say for sure, however, as I have seen each benefit from all three, depending on what effects people are seeking. Use the energetic approach to help you decide, or work with your herbalist.

Ginseng may help boost your fertility, but a combination of herbs to feed your entire reproductive and circulatory system is even better. See the table at the end of this chapter for some more herbs used for the glandular system. Some extra tips include munching on pumpkin seeds, avoiding alcohol and other toxins, switching to boxer shorts, and not exposing yourself to extreme temperatures too often (such as sitting in a hot tub). Sperm needs a balanced temperature to stay active—not too hot and not too cold. Following the tips that relate to impotency can also boost your fertility.

Dong Quai for Wannabe Moms

Dong quai (*Angelica sinensis*) is another Asian herb known for its female-enhancing qualities—in fact, this herb has also been called the ginseng for women. Dong quai seems to have similar effects on the body as estrogen does. You can take this herb to help your skin become soft and supple, help lubricate dry vaginal tissue, stop excess bleeding after giving birth, and promote menstruation when it's late.

Dong quai has warming, moistening (wetting) energetics, and therefore seems to "warm" frigidity. It also can help soothe the nervous system and is used by many women to relax symptoms of premenstrual syndrome.

Sage Advice

Sperm are sensitive little creatures and require just the right environment to keep them thriving. Exposure to excessive heat can lower a man's sperm count. Wearing boxer shorts instead of tighter fitting briefs allows the testicles the proper distance from the body to maintain adequate temperature for lively sperm. So, if you can't stand the heat, get out of the briefs (but not in the kitchen please)!

Sage Advice

A tipped uterus may be why you are not conceiving. Slant board exercises or hanging upside down will help your uterus get to its proper place. Lay back on your slant board with your feet above your head, or hang upside down with inversion boots, and gently pat your lower abdomen vigorously with cupped palms. Do this daily to tone the uterus.

Poison Ivy

Although dong quai has been used successfully by many women to enhance fertility, once you are pregnant you should eliminate the use of dong quai. See the section "Pregnancy and Herbs," in Chapter 4, "Herbs Are Not Just for Hippies Anymore," for herbs you can and can't take during pregnancy.

In nature, seeds are a plant's glandular system. The seed provides everything inside it to blossom into a fully developed, vital plant, given the correct conditions such as water, air, sunshine, and soil. Eating the glandular system of the seeds can help nourish your own reproductive system. Because seeds are usually small, seed butters can make an excellent way to eat seeds—when you're thinking pregnancy, dip your celery stick into some sesame seed butter.

Irritable Bowel Syndrome

Irritable bowel syndrome, colitis, and spastic bowel all share the same symptoms, including recurring abdominal pain with periods of constipation, followed by periods of diarrhea. The spasticity of the bowel is due to abnormal muscular contractions in the colon.

Some possible causes of irritable bowel syndrome include:

➤ Anxiety

➤ Stress

➤ Parasitic infestation

➤ Bacterial or other infection of the bowel

➤ Food allergies

A spastic bowel can be difficult to work with because of the unpredictability of the symptoms. If you are working with constipation, a bowel stimulant such as cascara sagrada will be helpful; however, when you have diarrhea, cascara may make it worse! To be safe, you may want to alternate your use of herbs designed for each symptom until the root cause of your troubles is addressed. See the section "Parasites: Dealing with Uninvited Guests," in Chapter 19, "O, P, and Q: Obvious Painful Questions and Answers," to find some herbal help for this condition.

Irritating Causes

Scientists are finding that our nervous system has direct influence on other systems of the body, such as the immune system, digestion, and the intestines. Thus, dealing with the source of your stress that could be causing your bowel trouble would be helpful in getting rid of this condition. See the section "Anxiety: Panic Not—Herbs to the Rescue," in Chapter 6, "Give Me Another A!" for herbs that will help soothe your nervous system.

Food allergies are also a big culprit when it comes to colitis and irritable bowel. See an allergist or a holistic health provider who can help you determine your allergies. Eliminate wheat and dairy, for starters, since many are allergic to these foods.

More natural help for a spastic bowel:

➤ Magnesium is a mineral that is soothing to the muscles and also the nerves. Taking magnesium will nourish and relax your nerves and also your bowel—this is probably why the anti-diarrhea medication known as Milk of Magnesia® works for the bowel.

➤ Activated charcoal in capsules will help absorb any toxins that might be causing the irritable bowel. I always keep some in my herbal medicine cabinet for poisonings of any kind.

➤ Peppermint oil can aid digestion, and a little dab on the tongue can help ease the problem. Your body could be short of the good intestinal bacteria lactobacillus acidophilus and bifidobacterium (more commonly known as acidophilus and bifidophilus), especially if you have had diarrhea for a while. Supplementing with these bacteria will help bring the bowel into better balance.

Eliminate any food source that seems to trigger symptoms. Make a warm lobelia fomentation and place it over the lower bowel to help settle those spastic contractions.

Slippery Elm: Soothing Solution

If I had irritable bowel syndrome and had only one herb to choose, I would have to choose slippery elm (*Ulmus fulva*). Slippery elm is an herb derived from the inner bark of the elm tree and is a very mucilaginous (literally, slippery) herb. Similar to marshmallow in its effects, these two can be used in place of each other.

Slippery elm, marshmallow, dong quai, and wild yam all offer very soothing and muscle-relaxing effects to the body, which help with colitis by soothing irritated tissues and relaxing muscle contractions. You can add some ginger capsules or tea to support digestive trouble and nausea, and lobelia in small quantities for a relaxing effect.

Insomnia: Waking Up to Herbal Possibilities

So, seen any great infomercials lately? If you have, this could mean that you are watching TV between 2 A.M. and 4 A.M., a sure sign of *insomnia*. And if those infomercials didn't put you to sleep, maybe some of these herbs will do. Who knows—once you find the value of using herbs for your health, you could be the next one to star in an infomercial for your own herbal concoction!

Botanical Bit

Insomnia technically means the inability to fall asleep or to stay asleep for an adequate amount of time. This causes almost chronic tiredness. Although some insomnia is linked to disease, much of it is caused by worry.

How to Get to Sleep at Night

Some Causes of Insomnia	Why/How They Affect You	What to Do
Stress/worry	Stress can keep your mind going and your body tense, causing insomnia.	Fix the problem; if possible, use calming herbs for the nervous system.
Stimulants	Caffeine-containing products, sugar, and vigorous exercise can stimulate the body and keep you up.	Eliminate these things several hours before bedtime.
Parasites	Parasites are usually nocturnal; they wake up and party when you are trying to sleep.	See the section "Parasites: Dealing with Uninvited Guests," in Chapter 19.
Hypoglycemia	When blood sugar drops dramatically, your body will wake you up to warn you to get some food.	Eat a small amount of protein at bedtime (a small handful of nuts).
Thyroid imbalance	The thyroid regulates metabolism, so a problem can throw off your complete cycle.	See the section "Thyroid Problems: Kelp Is on Its Way," in Chapter 21, "T: Terrific Solutions."

Scullcap: Good for a Night Cap

Scullcap (*Scutellaria lateriflora*) stimulates the brain to produce *endorphins* (commonly referred to as "feel-good hormones"), which not only can help you sleep, but also may ease your worry that could be keeping you up. Try a few capsules before bedtime to help you get your zzz's.

Botanical Bit

Endorphins are chemical compounds made by a gland in the brain known as the pituitary gland. Endorphins have pain-relieving properties and are known as the "feel-good hormones." They're also believed to aid in the balance of all the endocrine glands.

Scullcap has been used historically in treatment of convulsions, delirium, emotional trauma, spasms, and restlessness. It also is used as an aphrodisiac (appropriate for this chapter!), so why not offer some to your partner if you both are lying there awake. Skullcap might be beneficial in giving you both something to do with that insomnia!

Scullcap presumably got its name from its appearance—the flower resembles a skull with a hood. Pagan ceremonies have used scullcap as a potion to be exchanged between partners who wished to be together in the afterlife.

Scullcap contains zinc, calcium, magnesium, and potassium. It also contains moderate amounts of vitamins A, C, and E, as well as manganese, silicon, phosphorus, iron, selenium, niacin, and trace amounts of sodium.

More Ways to Catch Your Z's

Melatonin is a controversial hormone used successfully by many to regulate sleep cycles, especially when traveling, and for jet lag. Melatonin is made by your own pineal gland located in the brain and is the hormone believed to be responsible for your sleep/wake cycles, aging, and maybe even your dreams. Usually, supplements are made synthetically or from the pineal gland of a cow. Sunlight suppresses the brain's production of melatonin, but when the sun goes down, melatonin production picks up, and makes you sleepy. Supplementing with this hormone just before bed can help you—especially if you are over 50, when the production of this hormone seems to slow down.

Magnesium and calcium feed the nervous systems, among other things, and may help you get a better night's rest. Because all the minerals in your body need balance, you can use a trace mineral supplement to make sure you are getting everything you need. Other herbs that work synergistically with scullcap include valerian, passion flower, and hops. Sip a nice warm cup of chamomile tea or any combination of these other herbs to help you relax and sleep.

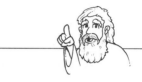

Sage Advice

Why is warm milk such a popular home remedy for insomnia? The amino acid l-tryptophan could be the key ingredient. L-tryptophan acts as a regulator for sleep and mood patterns because it helps the body produce melatonin (the sleep hormone). Warming up milk brings out the tryptophan in the milk and helps you get a good night's sleep.

Herbal Remedies for Common Ailments

Impotence

Best Single Herb: Yohimbe

Best Combinations: Yohimbe; Siberian ginseng, parthenium, saw palmetto, gotu kola, damiana, sarsaparilla, horsetail, garlic, capsicum, chickweed; garlic

Other Helpful Supplements: Niacin; vitamin E; zinc

Possible Causes: Problems with the prostate; thyroid; emotions; or circulatory system

Complementary Help: Exercise; acupuncture; reflexology; counseling

Frigidity

Best Single Herb: Damiana

Best Combinations: (Same combinations as male) Korean or Siberian ginseng; damiana; capsicum; gotu kola

continues

Herbal Remedies for Common Ailments (continued)

Frigidity (continued)

Other Helpful Supplements: Niacin; B-complex; evening primrose oil

Possible Causes: Problems with thyroid, emotions, circulation

Complementary Help: Exercise; counseling; acupuncture; reflexology

Infertility, Male

Best Single Herb: Siberian Ginseng

Best Combinations: Saw palmetto; stinging nettle; Siberian ginseng

Other Helpful Supplements: Zinc; vitamin E with selenium

Possible Causes: Exposure to hot conditions; tight pants; alcohol or other chemical abuse

Complementary Help: Eat pumpkin seeds; switch to boxers

Infertility, Female

Best Single Herb: Dong quai

Best Combinations: Red raspberry, dong quai, ginger, licorice, black cohosh, queen of the meadow, blessed thistle, marshmallow; false unicorn

Other Helpful Supplements: Vitamin E with selenium

Possible Causes: Stress; scar tissue; tipped uterus

Complementary Help: Manage stress; eat raw seeds and seed butters

Irritable Bowel Syndrome (Colitis/Spastic Bowel)

Best Single Herb: Slippery elm

Best Combinations: Slippery elm, marshmallow, dong quai, ginger, wild yam; lobelia

Other Helpful Supplements: Activated charcoal; peppermint oil; bifidophilus or acidophilus; magnesium

Possible Causes: Stress; parasites; food allergies

Complementary Help: Counseling; colonic irrigation; warm fomentations over abdomen

Insomnia

Best Single Herb: Scullcap

Best Combinations: Scullcap; valerian, passion flower, hops

Other Helpful Supplements: Calcium; magnesium; trace minerals; l-tryptophan; melatonin

Possible Causes: Stress; stimulants; diet; parasites; hypoglycemia; thyroid imbalance

Complementary Help: Do not go to bed on full stomach; if hypoglycemic, a *small* amount of protein before bed may help.

The Least You Need to Know

➤ Yohimbe is a powerful herb used as an aid to impotent men, but because of its potency it will usually be found mixed with other herbs.

➤ Damiana can be used to warm women up to the idea of sex.

➤ A few different types of ginseng exist, but most all affect the glandular system, making them useful for both men and women.

➤ Dong quai is known as ginseng for women and may enhance fertility.

➤ A spastic bowel may be soothed with slippery elm bark.

➤ Using the herb scullcap can alleviate insomnia, especially if it is mixed with other nerve toners such as valerian, hops, and passion flower.

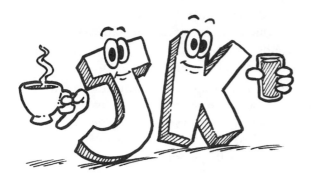

Chapter 15

J and K: For Just the Right Kind of Cure

> **In This Chapter**
>
> ➤ Herbal remedies helpful for jaundice
>
> ➤ Apply herbal applications to injured joints
>
> ➤ Support your kidneys with herbs
>
> ➤ Strengthen the knees with herbs and supplements

"The Lord hath created medicines out of the earth; and he that is wise will not abhor them."
—Ecclesiastics 38:4

So your knees are swollen and you don't know why? Or, you're suffering from or recovering from jaundice and you'd like to use some herbal support? Great, you've come to the right chapter. This chapter will give you tips and herbal remedies to use for joint health, jaundice, kidney function, and specific help for weak knees.

Jaundice: They Call It Mellow Yellow

If you have yellowish skin and eyes, and if it's not Halloween and you're not an alien, you may have jaundice. The yellow color indicates that excess *bilirubin*, a by-product of old blood cells, is floating around your blood stream (as you learned earlier, the skin reflects the condition of the blood).

Three classified types of jaundice exist:

1. **Obstructive jaundice:** Caused by obstruction of the small ducts that allow bile to flow into the intestine. Often, gallstones are a cause of this problem. Symptoms include dark urine, pale feces, and itchy skin.

2. **Hepatocellular jaundice:** Occurs because of a disease of the liver cells, which makes them unable to utilize the bilirubin. (Remember, the liver is a filter.) You may experience hepatocellular jaundice when and if you have hepatitis. (See Chapter 13, "H: Happy Healing with Herbs," for more information on hepatitis.) Symptoms include dark urine, but the feces remains the same in color.

3. **Hemolytic jaundice:** Occurs when a destruction of red cells occurs in the blood, such as in the disease *hemolysis*. With this type of jaundice, the color of the urine and feces remains the same, but the problem usually leads to anemia.

Botanical Bit

Bilirubin is a yellow or orange bile pigment, a colored compound that is basically the waste components of blood that just so happen to color our feces. It's important that your feces be brown (colored with bilirubin)—lack of this pigment could indicate a problem with your liver function.

Hemolytic disease—and thus, jaundice—can happen to a newborn child because of the incompatibility of the mother's blood and her baby's blood. A blood test taken by your doctor early in your pregnancy can detect the possible problem, and it can be handled at that time.

Now that you understand the three types of jaundice a little better, you can see that the first type is caused by problems in or of the gallbladder causing an obstruction of bile flow, the second is related more closely to the liver, and the last is a rare problem associated more closely with the blood. We will primarily discuss how to prevent gallstones that can cause a problem in the first place. Let's take a look.

Accused of Obstruction of Jaundice

Botanical Bit

Hemolysis is the rapid destruction of red blood cells caused by a mismatched blood transfusion, poisoning, infection, or the presence of certain antibodies. It usually leads to anemia.

Find out from your doctor which type of jaundice you have. If it is obstructive jaundice, you probably will want to know if it is a reaction to a drug that may have caused damage to your liver, or if a stone in the bile ducts caused the obstruction. All this information will empower you to take better care of yourself once you recover so that you might never have to suffer the same ailment or related disease in the future.

If you have had jaundice because of gallstones, you can do a gallbladder flush on a quarterly basis to help your body break down stones before they get a chance to lodge somewhere again. See the section "Heartburn: Putting Out the Fire with Marshmallow," in Chapter 13. However, in cases where there is an obstruction to bile flow, NEVER use herbs to try and stimulate the flow. This will only make matters worse.

Also be sure to reduce the amount of fatty foods in your diet, especially fried foods. This will keep cholesterol from clogging up your system. Eat more red beets, which are stimulating to your liver. Also drink fresh carrot juice daily, with a small amount of beet added for a wonderful liver, gallbladder, and bowel tonic drink.

Keeping the liver and bowel cleansed is imperative to your preventative measures. Use herbs as a fiber supplement to keep things moving along if you tend to get constipated. A colonic irrigation program will also help you stay on track. Add vitamin E with selenium to your daily program, as it is a nutrient that aids the circulatory system. Also add vitamin A or beta carotene (which will feed the liver) and a B-complex vitamin (which contains niacin to help keep the circulatory system clean).

Gentian, a Bitter Way to Treat Your Liver

An extremely bitter herb known as gentian (*Gentiana lutea*) has been used to support the liver, stomach, blood, spleen, and entire circulatory system. Gentian reduces liver congestion, promotes bile flow, and stimulates digestion. It is helpful for those in a weakened condition because it helps to strengthen the entire body and stimulates the appetite. Veterinarians have been known to administer gentian to their four-legged patients who have lost their appetite. Gentian is high in iron; the liver is considered an iron organ, and this may be why gentian has been helpful for liver conditions.

A small amount of gentian taken before every meal will assist your body in breaking down fats. Take gentian in a combination of herbs because it is extremely bitter and may also have a strong laxative effect on you. It also has properties that serve as a *cholagogue*, meaning that it stimulates bile secretions. If its laxative effects aren't working for you, make sure you are keeping the bowel clean with other fibers, such as psyllium hulls, or a bowel stimulant, such as cascara sagrada. Gentian is not recommended if you have ulcers.

Other herbs in a combination that will support the liver include: Oregon grape, red beet, dandelion, parsley, horsetail, liverwort, black cohosh, birch, blessed thistle, angelica, chamomile, and golden rod.

Poison Ivy

Gentian is not recommended during pregnancy. Talk to your doctor about using vitamin E, beta carotene, psyllium hulls, and possibly dandelion instead if you are having jaundice problems during pregnancy.

Botanical Bit

An herb with a **cholagogue** property means that the herb will help the body increase its flow of bile. Bile is a substance produced by the liver and stored in the gallbladder. It is used to break down fats during digestion. When bile is released through the bile duct, it also stimulates bowel movement.

Joint Injuries

Joint injuries can happen to anyone due to a fall, playing vigorous sports, break-dancing, bungie-jumping the Brooklyn bridge, climbing the face of Mt. Rushmore, or during other normal activities. Our joints give us mobility, and when they are injured, we can feel very restricted and frustrated. You probably want to heal yourself as quickly as possible when you have an injured joint so that you can get back to those sports again.

But, slow down cowboy or girl—it is important to understand that if joint injuries are a common, recurring problem with you, there could be a deeper underlying problem to address. I know, you hyperactive sports types are now thinking, "Oh great, here we go again—she's getting deep on me." I'll spare you the details this time around: If you just had your first joint injury and would like to help yourself fast-forward through the healing process, take a look at comfrey and the other supplements first. Then we'll get back to the in-depth talk a little later.

Comfrey: Comfy for Them Joints

Comfrey (*Symphytum officinale*) has been used for more than 150 years, both externally and internally, by probably millions of folks; it has been hailed as a miraculous herb for healing bones. Unfortunately, this miraculous herb is banned in many places, but you should understand its value and may want to secure some for yourself before it is gone everywhere. For our purposes, we will discuss the external application of comfrey only. If you cannot get comfrey, I will give you some useful substitutes that have also worked well for many. So make yourself comfy, and we'll talk a little more about this herb.

First, take a look at some of comfrey's values:

➤ It helps the body to promote new cell growth.

➤ It destroys and then prevents amoebic bacteria growth.

➤ It's very rich in trace minerals, calcium, potassium, phosphorus, iron, and vitamins A and C.

➤ It has also been used successfully for burns, wounds, open sores, ulcers, and gangrene, and has an amazing ability to basically weld tissues together.

Poison Ivy

Comfrey has a great reputation amongst herbalists and a bad reputation with the FDA. Because many herbal companies comply with the FDA and do not use it in their formulas, comfrey is hard to find—and even banned in many places. The ban is based on a rat study that showed liver damage after the rat was highly overdosed on the herb. However, most applications of comfrey are used externally anyway!

Because comfrey seems to accelerate tissue repair, soak your injured ankle or wrist into a large bowel or bucket of comfrey decoction to heal injuries quickly. If you have a hip or knee joint injury, for instance, a fomentation or a comfrey poultice would be more appropriate.

For all-over joints (an Evel Knieval type) you can certainly make a tubful and soak in the bath!

Herb Lore

Why is it that something that has been growing out of the ground for hundreds of years and used by many moms to treat their family's injuries has now become banned based on a rat study? How is that possible when at the same time, sweeteners synthesized from petroleum by-products and flavorings made from old tires are being legally added to sodas and many foods daily? When did we get so ignorant that we need the government to take away our thoughtful use of plants as foods and medicines? And what are we thinking when we believe that these manmade chemicals are safe for us just because the FDA approved them? Just a few thoughts to get the brain wheels turning!

Other supplements to consider when comfrey is not available include:

➤ Glucosamine sulfite and chondroitin are supplements that have been used both together and separately to support the joints, with good results.

➤ Calcium with magnesium and vitamin D works as a team to help you absorb the calcium and aid in bone healing.

➤ Uña de gato (cat's claw) or yucca both may help with any inflammation while you recover.

➤ Reducing the inflammation usually will alleviate your pain, but if not, use white willow bark in place of aspirin.

➤ A combination of yarrow (which reduces inner heat associated with injury), mullein, plantain, and rehmannia all have healing properties and support the structural system. If comfrey is not available, a mixture of any of the previously listed herbs will still support your recovery.

Healing Is a Joint Effort

If you are continually getting joint injuries, you may have some other issues going on that could be aggravating your problem. Consider a hair analysis to determine if you could have too much calcium in your body or some sort of great mineral imbalance that needs attention. Yes, too much calcium is possible.

➤ See your joint specialist, and get his or her assessment.

➤ If there is a misalignment in the joints, a chiropractor can help.

➤ If there is some significant deterioration in your cartilage or other joint tissues, you may be having a problem with digestion that could be creating a problem in your structural system. Proper digestion is essential for absorbing the minerals and nutrients needed by our structural system.

Sage Advice

I commonly see people who suffer from arthritis and other structural problems also have problems with overacidity and poor digestion. The only way to get completely well is to support the digestion at the same time you work with the structural system.

Let me explain. Our internal chemistry lab is a very complicated system that requires balance for perfect health. One of these balances is our pH balance between acidity and alkalinity. If the body is too acidic, it can harbor the overgrowth of bacteria, parasites, and fungus—and it even can make a perfect environment for growing cancer. On the other hand, being too alkaline is just as dangerous—and being severely too alkaline means death. Needless to say, balance is important. Diet and physical or emotional stress can throw this pH balance out of kilter.

Pain usually results when the body is too acid, just like in fibromyalgia, arthritis, rheumatism, osteoarthritis, and recurring joint injuries. This is because the body tries to compensate for the overacidity in the body by neutralizing the acid with calcium. Calcium is alkaline and is stored in the bones.

So why are you overly acidic? Here are a few clues:

➤ Your digestion is poor (usually the cause for the overacidity in the first place).

➤ You are not getting enough calcium in your diet.

➤ There is a mineral imbalance in the body (minerals all work together in an intricate balance).

➤ Your absorption of minerals is poor due to mineral imbalance, improper diet, and poor digestion.

➤ You're experiencing high levels of stress.

➤ You're getting lots of physical exercise.

These factors can make it difficult for the body to properly utilize the calcium that you do ingest. In its attempt to compensate and keep you alive, your body takes its alkaline calcium from your largest storehouse of calcium: your bones. This process will eventually weaken your entire structural system, and you will see more injuries and displacements, such as back misalignments, stiff necks, injuries, and aching muscles and joints. I see this happen with the elderly too often; their hips finally give out and they fall, shattering the already weakened bones.

When this calcium-robbing business continues, the body also needs sodium to keep calcium in the blood stream. Guess where it gets the sodium? From your joints! Your joints contain one of the largest stores of sodium in the body. So, now you can see why you would want to support your digestion for the prevention of joint injuries—or any structural problems, for that matter. (See the section "Arthritis: A Flexible Treatment Plan," in Chapter 6, "Give Me Another A!" for some more tips.)

Herbs and supplements that support digestion include:

➤ Papaya

➤ Peppermint

➤ Spearmint

➤ Liquid chlorophyll

➤ Food enzymes with or without hydrochloric acid

➤ Ginger

➤ Catnip

➤ Marshmallow

➤ Pepsin

Kidneys: Never Bean a Problem?

Supporting your digestion and getting the right minerals will take you a long way toward keeping your urinary system healthy, but let's take a look at some herbs that can support that system anyway.

The kidneys are responsible for a lot more than just filtering out waste products. They are also linked to the circulatory system and help keep a mineral balance in the body. They filter out uric acid waste products, so when you eat foods that cause you to be more acidic, you are putting excess stress on the kidneys. Every food we eat is broken down and leaves an acid or alkaline residue. Ideally, our diet should consist of 80 percent alkaline-forming foods and 20 percent acid-forming foods. Here's a table of some foods that are considered acid and alkaline. How well are you doing to stay in balance?

Sage Advice

The right pH balance in the body and supporting digestion are important for structural health. You should also remember that the structural, digestive, and urinary systems all are intimately linked to the health of each other, although our digestion is where most of the problems start.

Acid-Forming Foods	Alkaline-Forming Foods
Beans	Almonds
Berries	Avocados
Bread	Beets
Butter	Cabbage
Cheese	Carrots
Chocolate	Figs
Coffee	Green peas
Crackers	Green peppers
Cream	Lemons
Eggs	Lettuce (leaf lettuce)
Grapefruit	Melons
Lentils	Molasses
Meat	Okra
Milk	Parsley
Nuts (most)	Potatoes
Oils	Raisins
Oranges	Sour cream
Soda	Spinach
Sugar	Squash
Tea	Sweet corn
Wheat	

You can see by the table that most of the acid-forming foods are proteins (meat, cheese, beans, nuts). Therefore, in general, a high-protein diet is not as healthy for your kidneys because they have to filter out the excess acid left over from these foods. For general support for the kidneys, eat more alkaline foods. Also drink liquid chlorophyll daily in your water because it is alkalizing and good for the entire body.

Hydrangea: Like a Rollin' Stone

A kidney stone, a calcification of mineral deposits, is a painful ailment. The pain of having or passing a kidney stone has been described as one of the most painful conditions known to man! The stones can crystallize and cause very sharp, burning pains in the body. They can even be life-threatening if one gets stuck along your urinary tract and inhibits the natural flow of body fluids. Most occurrences of kidney stones happen in the summer time. This is thought to be linked with not drinking enough water to keep the kidneys flowing and stones from forming (during hot weather, the body's need for water increases due to the excess evaporation from the skin).

Fortunately, the herbal kingdom has a stone-solvent herb for us to help break up these little rocks. Hydrangea (*Hydrangea arborescens*) leaves and root have been used for the entire urinary system for bladder infections, kidney infections, gallstones, gout, kidney problems, calculi, and other renal irritations. This herb seems to be able to lessen the pain associated with passing kidney stones and also helps prevent them from forming in the first place. Furthermore, hydrangea is known to help back pain associated with kidney problems and has been used to help enlarged prostate glands.

When peeled, the bark of the hydrangea plant displays seven different colors. Thus, it was nicknamed "seven bark" by our ancestors, who used it as a folk medicine.

A Harvard University study showed that the following program prevented kidney stone formation:

> Vitamin B6
>
> Magnesium
>
> Hydrangea
>
> Pure water
>
> Extra lemon water

Poison Ivy

Some sources say that hydrangea should not be taken in high doses over long periods of time as it can cause chest congestion or dizziness. But you will not need this herb for long. About 12 capsules of hydrangea taken per day along with four marshmallow capsules every four hours will help you pass a stone. Take white willow for extra pain relief.

Parsley: More Than a Plate Decoration

Clean your plate—then eat your parsley! Parsley (*Petroselinum sativum*) is a green, bushy herb commonly served on restaurant plates as a garnish. This is more than just a pretty piece of leaf, though: Parsley is excellent for the urinary system, and it also aids digestion and helps cut garlic breath.

Parsley also serves as a mild aphrodisiac. The word is derived from two Greek words, meaning "rock celery," and it is rich in chlorophyll, to help get rid of excess water retention in the body without depleting potassium, as diuretic drugs can.

Some of the same herbs used for bladder infections are also great used here; these include uva ursi, dandelion, chamomile, cornsilk, and liquid chlorophyll.

Peach Bark: When Your Kidneys Are Not Feeling Peachy

When dealing with a kidney inflammation or infection, peach bark (*Prunus Persica*) is another helpful ingredient used in herbal remedies. The bark and leaves of the peach tree serve as a diuretic and will help flush out toxins from the urinary tract.

Sage Advice

The white part of the watermelon rind contains a high amount of minerals good for the structural and urinary systems. The seeds of the watermelon can be ground and taken as a diuretic.

Peach bark is high in phosphorus, potassium, and magnesium and can be used for problems with the bladder, the uterus, water retention, and the respiratory system (for coughs and bronchitis). If you are fighting a kidney infection, you should also drink lots of water to help your body flush out toxins—add lemon to the water to help purify your system. A spoonful of black strap molasses has proven useful as well.

Down on Your Knees

If you're weak in the knees or are experiencing any type of knee problems, such as inflammation or problems with the knee joint itself, read the previous section on joint injuries; the information on digestion and pH balance may apply to you also.

Other structural problems, such as poor shoes, may be contributing to knee problems. See your podiatrist (foot doctor) to help you. Your chiropractor also can help if you are misaligned. Sometimes the hips can rotate and can eventually affect your knees. If you have a growing boy or girl who is having pain in the knees, he or she may have an overactive thyroid or other gland that is that is resulting in abnormally fast growth and straining the joints. Have your doctor check for any endocrine imbalances.

Herb Lore

Some believe that the knees represent understanding. If you have a continual problem with the knees, then maybe you do not understand your life—an unexplained swollen knee may help you take some time off, slow down, and contemplate the meaning of your life. The knees also share the same energy lines (meridians) with the kidneys. If the kidneys are ill and therefore blocking some of the energy flows through the body, the knees may suffer from the blocked energy. Acupuncture, acupressure, or reflexology can help correct stuck energy.

Plantain Won't Make You Weak in the Knees

If none of the other factors noted for joint injuries seem to fit you, weak knees may indicate a weakness in the kidneys, believe it or not! Supporting your urinary system with herbs such as parsley and uva ursi can be helpful for this problem.

In the meantime, the herb plantain may just be just what the doctor didn't know to order! Plantain (*Plantago major*) is similar to comfrey in its abilities as a healer. It is rich in minerals and vitamins C and K. Plantain also is a mucilaginous herb, which makes it soothing to the tissues and kidneys. You can take this plant externally as well as internally because it is mild and considered safe to use.

Help from the Devil's Claw for Swollen Knees

Devil's claw can be used to help the knees because of its anti-inflammatory properties. This herb is also useful for the kidneys because it helps the body eliminate uric acid. Devil's claw will usually be found in combinations of herbs, especially soothing herbs such as slippery elm, because it can be somewhat irritating to the digestive tract.

Devil's claw has helped many, but it is somewhat slow-acting; it may take you a couple of weeks to feel its positive effects, so be patient.

Carrot juice with goats whey powder added can make an excellent drink for all structural conditions—whey contains many minerals such as sodium, potassium, and other supplements that support the joints. Make and apply a poultice made from soothing herbs such as mullein and plantain to reduce inflammation in the knees or any inflamed areas.

Sage Advice

The skin eliminates uric acid as well as the kidneys. The skin is considered a third kidney and is our largest elimination system. Dry skin brushing is an excellent way to take a load off your kidneys. Brush the body *before* you get in the shower each morning (avoid the face), to eliminate loads of uric acid waste products.

Sage Advice

We have lymph nodes all around our knees and knee caps. If these lymph nodes are swollen, the knee also will appear swollen. A lymphatic drainage massage can help you with this problem.

Herbal Remedies for Common Ailments

Jaundice

Best Single Herb: Dandelion

Best Combinations: Oregon grape; red beet, dandelion, parsley, horsetail, liverwort, black cohosh, birch, blessed thistle, angelica, chamomile, gentian, golden rod; cascara sagrada (for bowels)

Other Helpful Supplements: Vitamin E with selenium; vitamin A or beta carotene; B-complex vitamins

Possible Causes: Gallstones; hepatitis (see Chapter 13)

Complementary Help: Cleanse the bowel; drink carrot juice daily with added red beets for liver stimulation; undergo a gallbladder flush

continues

Herbal Remedies for Common Ailments (continued)

Joint Injury

Best Single Herb: Comfrey

Best Combinations: Comfrey (if available); yarrow, mullein, plantain, rehmannia; yucca or uña de gato/cat's claw (for inflammation); white willow bark (for pain)

Other Helpful Supplements: Calcium/magnesium with vitamin D; trace minerals; food enzymes

Possible Causes: Poor mineral absorption; overuse of joints

Complementary Help: Use a comfrey poultice or fomentation; support digestion

Kidneys, Stones

Best Single Herb: Hydrangea

Best Combinations: Hydrangea; marshmallow

Other Helpful Supplements: Food enzymes; magnesium; vitamin B6

Possible Causes: Overacidity due to poor digestion; mineral imbalance

Complementary Help: Eat a low-protein diet; eliminate sugar and caffeine

Kidneys, Weak

Best Single Herb: Parsley

Best Combinations: Juniper, parsley, uva ursi, dandelion, chamomile; cornsilk; liquid chlorophyll

Other Helpful Supplements: Trace minerals; potassium

Possible Causes: Mineral imbalance; adrenal stress

Complementary Help: Eliminate caffeine and alcohol; eat a low-protein diet; grind up and ingest watermelon seeds; eat white part of watermelon

Kidneys, Infection

Best Single Herb: Peach bark

Best Combinations: Dong quai, golden seal, juniper berry, uva ursi, parsley, ginger, marshmallow; peach bark; parsley; cranberry, buchu root

Other Helpful Supplement: B-complex vitamins

Possible Causes: (see Chapter 7, "B Well," for information on bladder infections)

Complementary Help: Eat a low-protein diet; fast with lemon juice; drink copious amounts of pure water; take black strap molasses

Knees, Weak

Best Single Herb: Plantain

Best Combinations: Yarrow, mullein, plantain, rehmannia; marshmallow fenugreek; parsley; uva ursi; uña de gato; essential fatty acids

Other Helpful Supplements: Food enzymes; glucosamine sulfate; chondroitin

Possible Causes: Weak kidneys; incorrect shoes; structural misalignment; growth problems; overly acidic; insufficient skin elimination

Knees, Weak (continued)

Complementary Help: Support digestion and urinary system; cut back on protein intake; eliminate caffeine; undergo physical therapy; take up dry skin brushing

Knees, Inflammation

Best Single Herb: Yucca

Best Combinations: Yucca; bromelain (pineapple enzyme), hydrangea, yucca, horsetail, celery seed, alfalfa, black cohosh, catnip, yarrow, capsicum, valerian, white willow bark, burdock, slippery elm, sarsaparilla; uña de gato; liquid chlorophyll; essential fatty acids

Other Helpful Supplements: Food enzymes; glucosamine sulfate; chondroitin

Possible Causes: Emotional problems

Complementary Help: Lymphatic drainage massage; acupuncture; reflexology; physical therapy; low-protein diet; daily drink of carrot juice with goat's whey powder added; poultice with mullein, plantain, comfrey

---

The Least You Need to Know

➤ Flush the gallbladder, and support your liver with herbs such as gentian to help prevent jaundice.

➤ Comfrey is banned in many places, but it is an amazing bone-healer when used topically and a wonder herb with proper use internally.

➤ Hydrangea is one of the plant kingdom's best stone solvents.

➤ Support digestion first for any structural or urinary problems.

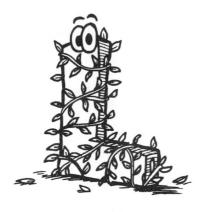

Chapter 16

L: Let Me Heal Naturally

In This Chapter

➤ Gargle with soothing herbs for laryngitis

➤ Herbs that can help ease leg cramps and twitching

➤ Herbs used to fight lupus

➤ Prevent and recover from Lyme disease with herbs

"Why should a man die who has sage in his garden?" —Anonymous, *Regimen Sanitatis, Salernitanum*

Why indeed? Sage is a wonderful herb with properties that help with a subject we will talk about next, laryngitis. Sage is also a word used to describe a wise man or teacher. I think we can learn a lot from our plants as teachers, too, including sage, sagebrush, and all the rest. Other ailments and their herbal solutions covered in this chapter will include leg cramps, lupus, and Lyme's disease. Happy learning and healing!

Laryngitis: Screaming for Attention

Laryngitis is the inflammation and irritation of the larynx, which is commonly referred to as our voice box. This irritation makes the voice sound raspy, which means that the person who has this condition will sound like he's speaking in a whisper. Sometimes it hurts so bad to speak that the person does not speak at all!

Although a little bit of laryngitis may make a woman sound enticingly sexy, this problem is usually caused by some unattractive problems such as allergies, colds, infections, or emotional stress.

Once the ailment has passed, the voice box will usually return to its normal condition on its own. In the meantime, you will need to soothe those vocal cords of yours.

Wisdom of the Sages

The leaves of the sage plant (*Salvia officinalis*) have an affinity for the mucus membranes and, therefore, make an excellent herbal remedy when suffering from laryngitis. Sage also aids the nervous system, making it even more valuable for stress-induced laryngitis. Herbalists and others sometimes get this herb confused with sagebrush, a member of the wormwood or Artemisia family; see Chapter 19, "O, P, and Q: Obvious Painful Questions and Answers," to avoid making the same mistake.

Sage Advice

Make a decoction from sage, slippery elm, and golden seal, cool the mixture slightly, and pour it into a small spray bottle. You can then use the formula as a spray for a sore throat or laryngitis. This mixture of herbs is designed to fight infections, soothe irritated mucus membranes, and dry up excess mucus production.

You can rub the oil of the sage plant around your throat area for some relief, or you can stir up a decoction and use it as a gargle to stop mucus drainage that could be causing your throat irritation.

Taken internally, sage has been helpful for digestion and intestines, and it also tends to "go to the head," making it great for sinus trouble, memory, inflamed gums, mouth sores, and headaches. In addition, sage is high in calcium, potassium, B1, and zinc, and it has drying properties, which is why it is good for laryngitis caused by excess mucus irritation. But be warned: Do not take sage internally if you are breast-feeding—its drying properties can dry up your breast milk! It is also not recommended during pregnancy.

I have put a homemade decoction of sage in a bottle and used it when I was growing my hair long to stimulate my hair growth. You can also use this herb rinse to clear up dandruff problems.

Herbal Lozenges

Of course, sage is not the only herb in the world that has been used successfully for laryngitis and sore throats. Licorice root also is healing for the tissues and can ease the coughing that may be causing your problem. In addition, slippery elm is mucilaginous and soothing to tissues, and golden seal and echinacea will help fight infections. You can use all of these herbs to help you if you have laryngitis.

Sage Advice

Some companies make herbal lozenges from ascorbic acid (vitamin C), zinc, slippery elm, or licorice root. Zinc aids the immune system and seems to work better when slowly ingested, such as when you take it in a slow-dissolving lozenge.

Laryngitis is a condition where you will need to take energetics into account again. Consider the nature of your laryngitis: Is it caused by a wet condition? This would be a mucus condition, such as bronchitis or a head cold, in which mucus draining down the back of your throat is irritating your tissues and causing you to cough.

Or, perhaps your laryngitis is caused by hot, dry, scratchy conditions. If your throat is hot and dry, sage may make it worse because it will only continue to dry your tissues. In this case, use a humidifier and slippery elm or marshmallow to soothe your throat.

What can cause a hot, dry throat condition? Let's take a look at some of the possibilities:

➤ Screaming at your employees, children, spouse, barking dogs next door—or practicing the Tarzan yell

➤ A fever that's drying you out

➤ Summertime allergies

➤ Turning on the dry, hot heat at the start of winter

➤ Singing opera under bright lights

➤ Riding on a motorcycle with your mouth wide open

➤ Sleeping with your mouth open (catching flies)

➤ Eating crackers on a hot day, without water, and reading my book at the same time (which is causing you to inhale the crumbs every time you laugh)

Sage Advice

If you know what has been causing your laryngitis, such as mucus congestion from a cold or bronchitis, see the appropriate herbal remedies listed for each of these ailments in this book so that you can work at the source of your problem. Killing infection and helping your body to recover from your cold will help fast-forward your laryngitis symptoms.

Leg Cramps Cramping Your Style?

Leg cramps can be caused by overexertion of the muscles. Sometimes I will get a cramp in my foot or leg when I am wearing a heeled shoe all day; when I get to bed, my foot or leg will begin to cramp (to get me back I suppose). But some folks who don't wear high heels are still affected by this condition.

Sometimes a cramp or twitch is due to a muscle that has been overworked or stretched improperly. This can happen by any of the following:

➤ Utilizing free weights or exercise equipment incorrectly

➤ Overexertion in any activity

➤ Sitting incorrectly at a desk all day while working

➤ Repetitive movements over long periods of time

➤ Spinal misalignment while doing any activity

Other than overexertion and occasional cramping, ongoing problems with leg cramps or twitches can indicate a mineral imbalance, usually due to a deficiency of at least one mineral. All minerals work to keep each other in balance and need to be in proper quantities to function correctly. For instance, iron is a mineral that is *antagonistic* to calcium, which means that calcium can inhibit or suppress the complete absorption of iron in the body. Therefore, taking a calcium supplement and an iron supplement at different times of the day is best. (That's another reason to rely on herbs to give you the right balance of these minerals.) Leg cramps commonly occur during pregnancy, when the fetus is utilizing many nutrients, so Mom should take more, too.

Poison Ivy

Pay attention to recurring muscle pains, cramps, or spasms because this could be your body's way of warning you that you are overworking your muscles. It could also indicate a mineral imbalance, which can be corrected nutritionally.

Botanical Bit

In the body, some minerals are **antagonistic** to each other, which means that they are not compatible taken together. This also means that one mineral will suppress the absorption of the other.

Do They Call You Thumper?

Leg or other muscle twitches are caused by involuntary spasms. These can happen anywhere in the body, including the hands and shoulders, or under your eyes. My husband thinks that when I say something important and my eye twitches, that means I am thinking more than what I'm saying. Some superstitious folks believe that a twitch in your eye is a sure sign that you're lying—I think it's a sign of mineral imbalance or nervous system depletion.

I once had a client who asked for some help for his twitching leg. His e-mail explained that as soon as he was getting ready to fall asleep each night, his leg would begin twitching uncontrollably! This twitching would aggravate him and keep him awake.

I was amused at his symptom because I couldn't help getting the visual image of a dog shaking its leg when it's tickled. When I realized that this person had a sense of humor, I also couldn't refrain from addressing him as "Thumper." Thumper went along with this name game while he began to take an herbal trace mineral supplement along with an herbal combination that would soothe his nervous system to help him relax.

Thumper says he put some of the liquid supplements in his bowl, lapped 'em right up, and slept like a baby that very first night! He told me that he didn't know anything about herbs and that he might have been "barking up the wrong tree" by consulting me, but so far he has seen results. All kidding aside, since he has taken his herbs, he has not reported any more thumpin'.

Loosening Up with Dulse

I chose the seaweed dulse as the best single herb in this case because we already talked about alfalfa, which is one of the most mineral-rich land plants. Dulse is a sea plant that may be as rich in minerals from the sea as alfalfa is from the soil.

Dulse is very similar to kelp, another sea "weed" used for its rich iodine content. Both of these herbs are also rich in potassium, which works with sodium to keep the acid/alkaline balance in the body, to strengthen the heart and other muscles, and to keep the body healthy. Just a little of this herb goes a long way. It usually comes in a liquid form, and you can add a few drops daily in your water to obtain all that dulse has to offer. Otherwise, an encapsulated combination made from kelp, dulse, watercress, wild cabbage horseradish, and horsetail will supply you with a great array of minerals rich in potassium, among other minerals. Supplementing with extra calcium and magnesium will round out your program and feed your nervous and structural systems to keep you from twitching and cramping.

Sage Advice

Dulse is a rich source of iodine and makes an excellent remedy to feed an underactive thyroid.

Lupus: Jumpin' Through Loops for Herbs

Lupus is a general term used to describe any of several chronic skin diseases. When used alone, it usually refers to tuberculosis (TB) of the skin.

The three types of lupus conditions are:

1. **Lupus erythematosus:** This chronic inflammation of connective tissue affects the skin and internal organs. Symptoms include a red, scaly rash on the face; arthritis; and kidney damage. Considered an *autoimmune disease*, this type of lupus occurs more often in women.

2. **Lupus verrucosus:** This is a tuberculosis infection of the skin, with symptoms of warty lesions on the arms or hands. This happens to people who have had TB before and have become reinfected.

3. **Lupus vulgaris:** This infection of the skin can spread and cause ulcers and severe scarring. Children who have been given a TB inoculation usually suffer this type of lupus caused directly by the injection.

Botanical Bit

An **autoimmune disease** is a disease in which the body attacks itself when the immune system (antibodies) is over-stimulated. Some autoimmune diseases include lupus, pernicious anemia, rheumatic fever, and Hashimoto's disease.

Poison Ivy

Elecampane should not be taken when pregnant or breast-feeding. It is too strong an herb and can make baby "purge" through vomiting or diarrhea.

Elecampane

Elecampane (*Inula heminum*) is one of many herbs I would take if I were suffering from lupus. Add elecampane for its high content of anti-amoebic compounds, compounds that kill or repel bacteria and parasites. If lupus is brought on by a parasitic infection, elecampane is one herb that has a great reputation as a powerful internal cleanser.

In the Middle Ages, elecampane—a yellow herb resembling the daisy and also referred to as wild sunflower—was used as medicine and by veterinarians to treat animals and rid them of parasites. It is helpful in ailments of the respiratory tract and has analgesic (pain-reducing) properties.

The Bigger Picture

Because lupus is a disease of the immune system, it will be helpful to alleviate extra stress in your life while you recover. Stress can suppress your immunity, and this includes the physical stress of digesting solid foods. An herbal supplement can help take the energy out of digestion by supplying the enzymes necessary to break down cooked foods. Calcium, magnesium, and vitamin D supplements may prove useful to feed the structural system, and antioxidants can supply your body with what it needs to help protect your cells from free radical damage.

Of course, you will need to do some investigating to find out what may have triggered your lupus and what may be aggravating the problem. Here are my suggestions:

➤ **Fibromyalgia:** I suggest reading the section "Fibromyalgia: What a Pain!" in Chapter 11, "F: Fantastic Healing Flora," for some other suggestions on helping your body. Fibromyalgia is also a condition in which the body is attacking itself, although not at such an advanced level as is experienced with lupus.

➤ **Parasites/fungus:** Read the sections "Fungus Among Us?" in Chapter 11; and "Parasites: Dealing with Uninvited Guests," in Chapter 19. Many herbalists believe this can be the core issue causing lupus. Do some research on parasites in humans, and ask your doctor to test you for any and all possible parasite infections.

➤ **Dental work:** Speak to your holistic dentist regarding any dental work that you suspect could have an influence on your immune system.

➤ **Breast implants:** Consider problems with a silicone leak if you have breast implants.

➤ **Environmental causes:** Think about exactly when your symptoms started. Try to remember what changed in your environment up to two years before your symptoms started. This will give you clues to seeking an answer. If you suspect environmental allergies, see Chapter 5, "A Is for Ailment," and read *Poisoning Our Children*, by Nancy Sokol Green (The Noble Press, Inc., 1991).

Herb Lore

Lupus means "wolf." It was named this because of the characteristic butterfly-like rash that appears like on the face resembling that of a wolf's markings.

Lyme Disease: Ticking You Off

Lyme disease is caused by spiral bacteria that is carried by ticks. A tick bite spreads the disease, which is characterized by a skin rash, aching muscles and joints, headaches, fever, fatigue, sore throat, and if not treated right away, may lead to arthritis, and sometimes even inflammation of the brain or heart.

Symptoms vary per person, and, unfortunately, many times symptoms appear weeks after the actual tick bite has healed. Usually this disease is treated with antibiotics. If a tick has bitten you, watch your bite for a rash that resembles a bull's eye radiating out from the bite. This bull's eye appears as a red circular spot and can expand in size to 20 inches in diameter. If you see this rash appear, head for the doctors to get it checked.

Sage Advice

Lyme disease is most common during tick season, from April to November. Doesn't leave you with much safe hiking time for harvesting herbs now, does it? Use caution when hiking, and wear long sleeves, pants, and a cap; check yourself and partner occasionally for crawling ticks.

A Brief History of Lyme

Ticks that normally feast on deer are the ticks that carry the bacteria that causes Lyme disease. The condition was named after the town of Old Lyme, Connecticut (nice to name a disease after your town, don't you think?), where Lyme disease was first identified. Some believe the continual encroaching of real estate developments into wildlife habitats is to blame for these new types of diseases. But if you are an outdoor lover, don't fret—you can use herbs as tick repellents to help prevent a bite in the first place (see Chapter 7, "B Well," for more on bites and stings).

Botanical Bit

Adaptogenic herbs are herbs that help the body adapt to stress. These include herbs such as ginseng, suma, astragalus, reishi mushroom, spikenard, and schizandra.

To help fight off infections of any sort, use parthenium, golden seal, yarrow, and a pinch of capsicum as a catalyst. Echinacea and garlic are also well-known infection fighters; take garlic before going out for prevention.

To detoxify after being bit, take four to six capsules of activated charcoal to help stop the spread of poison in the blood. Wash them down with two teaspoons of liquid chlorophyll in a large glass of water. If you are bitten by any questionable bug, take antioxidant vitamins, grape seed or pine bark extract, lots of vitamin C, Oregon grape, and any *adaptogenic* herbs you might have on hand (such as suma), to help your body cope with the stressful side effects of infection.

Suma: Wrestling with Lyme Disease

When you think Suma, do you think sumo wrestling? Well, wipe that vision of a big black thong out of your mind's eye, and let's get back to business! Suma is an adaptogenic herb that can help the body recover from illnesses such as Lyme disease. This herb also has been called Amazon or Brazilian ginseng, and in Spanish it has been referred to as "para todo," which means "for everything."

Suma can help get you back on your feet by helping to regulate sugar balance, acting as an aphrodisiac, and serving an immune stimulant. One herbalist claims that it helps fight the virus responsible for Epstein-Barr, and some recent Japanese research insinuates that suma may inhibit some cancer cells.

Herb Lore

Suma contains a plant component known as germanium, which is concentrated in plants and has an ability to transport heavy metals from the body, helping the body to detoxify and oxygenate. This information is based on studies from Japanese doctor Kazuhiko Asai, who researches organic forms of germanium. Germanium has been used for treating cancer by inhibiting the spread of cancer cells, improve circulation by thinning the blood, and boost the immune system by stimulating the production of interferon.

Herbal Remedies for Common Ailments

Laryngitis

Best Single Herb: Sage (wet conditions); slippery elm (hot/dry conditions)

Best Combinations: Licorice; slippery elm; golden seal, echinacea; sage

Other Helpful Supplements: Zinc; pantothenic acid; citrus bioflavonoids; vitamin A; beta carotene

Possible Causes: Virus or bacterial infection; overuse of voice; dry conditions

Complementary Help: Humidifier; herbal lozenges; sage gargle or tea; sage oil used externally

Legs, Cramps, Twitches

Best Single Herb: Dulse

Best Combinations: Kelp, dulse, watercress, wild cabbage, horseradish, horsetail

Other Helpful Supplements: Magnesium; trace mineral supplement; calcium

Possible Cause: Mineral imbalance

Complementary Help: Stretch daily, exercise lightly

Lupus

Best Single Herb: Elecampane

Best Combinations: Elecampane; black walnut; Essiac tea; suma; red clover; licorice root; alfalfa; uña de gato; grape seed/pine bark extract; barley grass juice powder, wheat grass juice powder, asparagus, astragalus, broccoli, cabbage, ganoderma, parthenium, schizandra, Siberian ginseng, myrrh, pau d'arco; garlic

Other Helpful Supplements: CoQ_{10}; food enzymes; antioxidants, calcium/magnesium with vitamin D

Possible Causes: Candida/parasite infection; environmental poisoning; emotional issues; leak in silicone breast implants; dental work

Complementary Help: Bowel cleansing; dental consultation; juiced barley and wheat grass drunk daily

Lyme Disease

Best Single Herb: Suma

Best Combinations: Liquid chlorophyll; suma, astragalus, Siberian ginseng, ginkgo biloba, gotu kola; Oregon grape; (IGSII) parthenium, golden seal, yarrow, capsicum (infection-fighting); echinacea; garlic

Other Helpful Supplements: Antioxidants; grape seed/pine bark extract; vitamin C; activated charcoal

Possible Causes: Tick and flea bites (check bedding, pets, carpets, and so on)

Complementary Help: Drinking copious amounts of water drinking (with chlorophyll added); prevention

The Least You Need to Know

➤ Sage will help dry up mucus, which can be helpful in treating the cause of some cases of laryngitis.

➤ Dulse is a seaweed similar to kelp that contains a rich source of minerals, especially iodine. Lack of minerals is the cause of most leg cramps.

➤ Elecampane is a powerful anti-parasitic and anti-amoebic remedy that has been useful in an herbal program for lupus.

➤ Suma is an herb that helps your body cope with stress; it can help get you back on your feet when recovering from Lyme disease.

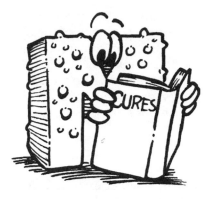

M for More Remedies

*"Anything green that grew out of the mould
Was an excellent herb to our fathers of old."*

—Rudyard Kipling (1865–1936), *Grandmother's Secrets*, Jean Palaiseul

As you've gone through life, you've more than likely experienced measles and mumps in childhood, menstrual problems at puberty, and if you're now pregnant, morning sickness. Guess what you'll be looking forward to soon when junior comes along? Measles, mumps, and if a girl, menstrual troubles! Isn't it funny how life cycles? Well, no worries, this chapter can serve as a reference guide for all of these "M" maladies for you, your children, and their children. We have been taking care of our families for ages with herbs, why stop the cycle now? Read on!

Measles: No Measly Solution

Measles is typically a childhood illness, caused by a contagious virus. The symptoms include a rash that lasts about three to five days, a cough, a fever, and sometimes small red spots with white centers on the inside of the mouth.

This illness usually lasts a short time, but you should take care of yourself for at least a week after you recover to ensure that you avoid further complications from the illness. An inner ear infection or other ailments of the respiratory tract can sometimes follow a measles outbreak. Read the section "Allergies Bee Gone," in Chapter 5, "A is for Ailment," to find some great herbs that will help dry up sinus passages. Also see the section "Colds: A Cure for All Seasons," in Chapter 8, "C's for a Common Cure," for some herbs that will soothe an irritated throat. For some herbs to recover from measles right now, read on.

Were You Vaccinated?

Most of us already have experienced measles in childhood, whether we were vaccinated against it or not. However, exposure to this usually mild infection, through exposure to someone contagious with the measles, will usually ensure lifetime immunity so that you don't have to experience the problem again.

The vaccine against measles is not necessarily 100 percent protection against the virus, nor is it necessarily the reason for the eradication of the disease. Here are some interesting facts:

Sage Advice

If you have been exposed to the measles in any way whatsoever, you should begin taking your herbal remedies right away. You'll boost your immune system and lessen the severity of your symptoms if and when you do catch the disease.

➤ The death rate from measles declined by 95 percent from 1916 to 1958. Note that this occurred years before the introduction of the vaccine.

➤ More than 95 percent of measles cases have a history of vaccination, according to Dr. William Atkinson of the U.S. Center for Disease Control and Prevention.

➤ In Hungary, between December 1988 and May 1989 there were 19,000 cases of measles; 77 percent of these cases were found in people age 17 to 21 who had already received the live measles vaccine.

Whether you were vaccinated against measles or not, you can still utilize the same herbal remedies to help you recover. Let's take a look at an old remedy, boneset.

Boneset, for Bone-Breaking Aches and Pains

The herb boneset (*Eupatorium perfoliatum*) got its name back in the days of the Civil War, when it was used against the flu named breakbone fever. The muscle aches and pains were so severe with this flu that folks believed their bones would break! Boneset helped ease these fever-related pains and earned its name as it did so. It is said that boneset was also used in place of quinine during this time to fight malaria. You can still use boneset to fight the discomfort of the measles and other illness such as the flu.

Boneset works as a diaphoretic (it pushes out fever) and an expectorant (it pushes out mucus); it also resists bacteria and viral infections and helps reduce the muscle pain associated with fevers. Make boneset into a tea or decoction and drink warm to help with fever. The energetic effect seems to change with this herb if taken in a liquid form. For instance, herbalists will tell you to take boneset warm for its diaphoretic effect (making you sweat to break a fever). But if you are chilled and shaking with a fever, boneset is more effective taken as a chilled tea or infusion. Of course, if you take the herb in a pill form or mixed with other herbs, you bypass these specifics.

Other herbs to boost the immune system that are safe for children as well as adults include echinacea and golden seal, safflowers, liquid chlorophyll, marshmallow and fenugreek, slippery elm, and yarrow. Beta carotene and vitamin C both can boost the immune system as well.

Make a fomentation of thyme and apply topically to the rash or use for a sponge bath to help break fever. Garlic and catnip enemas are helpful in fighting infections in little ones and also help reduce mucus in the system. In addition, you can swab Oregon grape onto internal mouth sores to aid in healing.

The essential oil of eucalyptus diffused in a room can help protect others from airborne viruses spread by the coughing, infectious person.

Poison Ivy

Boneset is also an emetic, which means that too much can make you sick. Take only small amounts of this herb at a time, or take it in combination with other herbs historically known to help with colds, flu, and other respiratory ailments.

Menstrual Problems, Balancing on Your Cycle

Menstruation can be viewed as your body's monthly house cleaning. Each month, the body prepares the uterus while the ovaries are busy preparing an egg with the anticipation of attracting the best sperm and creating new life. If no lucky sperm make the grade, the lining of the uterus is shed and the process repeats again.

There are three important stages during this cycle which include:

➤ **Actual menstruation:** This is the three to seven days of your period, when the uterus is shedding its lining. This is when all your hormone levels drop. You can use this time

Sage Advice

If estrogen levels become too high during the follicular phase, women may experience PMS. The liver is responsible for filtering out excess estrogen—consider milk thistle to aid liver functioning. Also avoid fats in the diet, which can raise estrogen levels, avoid sugar, which can affect the blood sugar and make you irritable, and avoid salt, which can make you retain excess water.

as a time of rest, for gentle exercise like walking, and clean eating (less fats and sugar) to help your entire body get the most from this cleansing time.

Botanical Bit

Epimenorrhea is a period that comes in shorter than normal intervals. **Amenorrhea** is an absence of menstruation (other than pregnancy) caused by a host of factors, including glandular abnormalities, diabetes, mental illness, anorexia, stress, and excessive exercise. **Menorrhagia** is abnormally heavy bleeding at menstruation. **Dysmenorrhea** is a painful period that can lead to nausea, vomiting, and fainting.

Poison Ivy

Consider sanitary napkins instead of tampons. Some doctors and holistic practitioners recommend against tampons and believe that blocking the natural flow and release of dead cells may be a factor in endometriosis and other female-related disorders. See Chapter 10, "E: Everywhere an Herb, Herb," and Chapter 19, "O, P, and Q: Obvious Painful Questions and Answers," for herbal help with endometriosis and PMS.

➤ **The follicular phase:** After your period is the time when your body is being prompted by hormones to produce eggs in the ovaries. At this time, estrogen levels begin to build and reach a peak. This is a time when your immune system strengthens in order to rid the body of germs and prepare for new life. (Note that some women become compelled to enthusiastically scrub their homes just before baby is due!) During the last part of this stage, is the time when most women feel their best and strongest (just before ovulation), skin tends to clear, and sexual urges rise. Nature designed this for the female to be better able to attract her mate just at the right time for fertility—isn't that cool?

➤ **The luteal phase:** This is the time when the produced egg leaves the ovary on its journey to the uterus. This is the time when progesterone takes over to prep the lining of the uterus to support a growing fetus. At this time, the immune system drops so that the potential sperm and (hopefully) fertilized egg can do their thing without being attacked by the immune system. If no sperm happens to show, the body goes back to the next phase, menstruation, and the cycle continues.

Menstrual problems are frustrating and include all the symptoms of PMS, irregularity in the cycle, late periods or no periods (*amenorrhea*), periods that come too frequently (*epimenorrhea*), periods that are heavy and may last too long (*menorrhagia*), and painful periods (*dysmenorrhea*).

If you have any of these problems, you should get a check-up and find out what is causing the irregularities or pain. Endometriosis and other abnormal growths, pregnancy, and hormonal imbalances and anorexia can all be factors.

In this section, we will focus on herbs for you ladies who are not pregnant but that need a little herbal help to bring on a late period (amenorrhea).

Pennyroyal for That Womanly Period

Pennyroyal (*Hedeoma pulegioides*), or the more potent version from Europe (*Mentha pulegium*), is an herb that is hard to find. Because of its possible misuse, many manufacturers will not offer it to the consumer. Pennyroyal is an *abortifacient*, which means that it should never be taken while pregnant because it may cause the mother to abort a fetus.

If you are a generally healthy woman, however, pennyroyal can be effective in bringing on a late period. Others have used the herb after giving birth to help the delivery of the placenta (known as the afterbirth). Just a little pennyroyal also may lessen the cramps and bloating associated with menstruation. In this case, a penny goes a long way!

Pennyroyal should also be noted for its use in getting rid of bugs and pests. This herb is one of the most powerful bug repellents and seems to be effective against a wide range of bugs.

Here are some uses of pennyroyal as a bug repellent:

➤ The plant itself has been grown in pots or flower beds surrounding porches to repel mosquitoes. Because of this, it has also been commonly known as mosquito plant.

➤ Used externally, the essential oil repels mosquitoes, fleas, and flies.

➤ The dried herb can be made into a sachet and put in with wool clothing to repel moths.

➤ The dried herb, burned for incense, can also serve as a great repellent.

➤ The plant has been rubbed directly on the skin not only as a bug repellent but also for the relief of poison oak or poison ivy rashes.

Botanical Bit

Abortifacient is an herbal property meaning that an herb may cause miscarriage—therefore, an abortifacient herb is never suggested during pregnancy.

Poison Ivy

Pennyroyal should be taken only in situations where a period is overdue due to stress. Pennyroyal may cause you to abort a fetus or can bring on hemorrhaging if taken when pregnant or if you have a weak uterus. Never take pennyroyal during pregnancy or if you are planning a pregnancy.

Again, remember to avoid any applications of pennyroyal—whether internal or external—if you are pregnant.

Hormonal Helpers

For other female problems, see the associated chapters: Chapter 19 for PMS; Chapter 10 for endometriosis; and Chapter 14, "I: Interesting Illnesses," for infertility. For irregular periods, take vitamin E to help increase fertility and bring more oxygen into the blood; licorice root has helped some of my menopausal clients rid themselves of hot flashes. Licorice root nourishes adrenals, regulates menstruation, and helps the body to release excess water retention. Sip ginger root tea to help promote the menstrual flow once you do get your period. Dong quai has come to the rescue for many women and is used to regulate periods, ease PMS, help menopausal symptoms, nourish female glands, calm nervousness, expel retained placenta after birth, reduce hot flashes, and eliminate anemia.

Sage Advice

Reflexology or acupuncture can release blocked energy, induce relation, and balance the glands. Reflexology has always helped me balance my own cycle, and frequently my female clients will get their period after their reflexology appointments.

Evening primrose oil has also been a saving grace for many women with raging hormones, has been used to help regulate periods, eases PMS symptoms, aids skin and hair health, and boosts the immune system. Try taking up to six evening primrose capsules daily 7 to 10 days before your period is due. Stay consistent. You will need to give your herbal hormonal helpers at least a few months to be able to correctly evaluate if your cycle is becoming regular. Patience and experimentation will be needed unless you are working with a holistic practitioner who can help guide you, of course.

Migraines and Feverfew

Migraines do not need to be explained to you if you have ever had one; these excruciating headaches can incapacitate an individual. When a migraine occurs, blood vessels in the head that were normally constricted open up, and the pressure of the blood in the vessels causes pain. Loss of vision, hallucinations, and loss of motor control (such as speech) can also be inhibited or temporarily lost. You can usually tell when a migraine is developing because you may see a show of colored lights before your eyes, feel spaced out, and may experience sensitivity to bright light at the onset.

Migraines can be triggered by a host of factors, so it is good to learn which factors may be causing yours. A medical doctor told me years ago that a migraine is actually a virus, which is why they tend to come back again and again. I have found migraines to be associated with food allergies and imbalanced hormones. So, finding out what is triggering this virus in the first place will help you know what to do—or what not to do—to avoid them in the first place. Keep a daily diary of your foods, drinks, and whatever goes into your mouth, along with a record of when you experience migraines. This will help you understand what might be your triggering factors. Keeping your immune system strong is always a good idea to suppress a virus, too.

These are some possible causes or triggers of migraine headaches:

➤ Foods, in their order of most common triggers to less frequent include: dairy products, wheat, chocolate, eggs, oranges, tomatoes, corn, coffee. I have also noted yellow cheese, wine, cola, and alcohol to be triggers. (I know, all your favorites, right?)

➤ Poor digestion (due to food intolerance, food allergies, and other allergens or constipation).

➤ Hormonal imbalance (these tend to occur just before a period or during pregnancy).

➤ Liver stress (due to hormonal imbalance, other glandular problems, poor eating habits, or alcohol).

➤ Stress.

➤ Hypoglycemia (see Chapter 13, "H: Happy Healing with Herbs").

➤ Dehydration.

Caffeine can trigger migraines because, with consistent use, this drug tightens the blood vessels. When the caffeine wears off, blood vessels may begin to relax to their normal position, causing pressure in the head—this pressure causes the migraine. Because of caffeine's ability to restrict blood vessels, however, coffee is used therapeutically in hospital emergency rooms to counteract the pain of migraines.

Sage Advice

If you are a daily coffee drinker, slowly eliminate caffeine from your diet so that you can avoid a possible painful migraine.

Read the section "Headaches: It's All in Your Head," in Chapter 13 if you are not sure whether your pain is a migraine or a headache. If you know what is triggering your migraines, you can herbally prevent them from coming on again. The first herb that comes to mind when dealing with migraines should be feverfew (*Tanacetum parthenium*), a pretty little daisy-like flowering herb that has a wonderful reputation with past migraine suffers. Feverfew serves as an anti-inflammatory and an anti-spasmodic, and it even can serve as an insect repellent.

Sage Advice

It is best to use feverfew in a pill form, although it may take consistent use for at least a week for it to work preventatively for you. In rare cases, feverfew taken in a tea can cause mouth sores if used over a long period or in large quantities.

Apply an infusion made from feverfew to the head to help ease headaches, migraines, and fevers—in fact, feverfew got its name from its use for relieving fevers. Most migraines are accompanied by a slight rise in temperature, so feverfew may help in this area also.

Most of my clients have used one concentrated capsule or four to six regular capsules of feverfew daily for migraine prevention—and more if they suspect a migraine coming on. So far, I have heard only success stories when a quality product is used; the feverfew stopped the migraines before they came. The leaves of the feverfew plant are used medicinally to improve circulation, feed the nervous system, and help with tinnitus and dizziness. Feverfew seems to have an affinity for the head and is useful for ailments in this area.

For other causes of migraines, such as liver stress, constipation, food allergies, indigestion, and hormonal imbalances, see the remedies listed under these ailments elsewhere in this book. You also may want to try acupuncture, reflexology, and chiropractic work for relief. Add a daily B-complex vitamin, along with a calcium and magnesium supplement and 400 IUs of vitamin E to feed the circulatory and nervous systems.

Botanical Bit

Anti-abortifacient is an herbal property meaning that an herb may prevent miscarriage during pregnancy.

Morning Sickness: Usurping the Problem Early

Morning sickness occurs due to pregnancy and is usually caused by a toxic system, especially a stressed or over-burdened liver. If you haven't had a chance to do some internal cleansing before you conceived, you will not be able to cleanse now, but remember to do so if you have a chance before the next child. (See Chapter 4's large section dedicated to all phases of pregnancy, too.) In the meantime, let's take a look at some safe herbal remedies during pregnancy.

Red Raspberry: Come to Mama

The leaves of the red raspberry bush (*Rubis idaeus*) are used as a tonic to strengthen the reproductive organs in both men and women. The fruit of the bush is used in jams, jellies, and wines, and you can take red raspberry leaves as a tea or in pill form. This herb is safe for use in pregnancy.

Poison Ivy

Use great caution if you decide to pick red raspberry leaves yourself. Two species, Rubus idaeus and Rubus strigosus, prevent miscarriage, but there are other varieties of red raspberry bushes that are known to promote abortion! Again, please use great caution whenever wildcrafting.

In contrast to pennyroyal, red raspberry serves as an *anti-abortifacient*, meaning that it prevents miscarriage. Red raspberry has been used to regulate hormones, as a tonic for the uterus, and also to tone the uterus after birth. The toning effect may be helpful for the prostate gland in men also. Some women have used red raspberry to correct infertility, aid labor, and ease muscle cramps and afterpains.

Red raspberry also nourishes breast milk and is rich in magnesium, iron, and niacin. It provides vitamin C and manganese, both which may help tone the abdominal wall and make labor less painful. This herb seems to have been made just for women who want to be moms!

Ginger: Not Just Found on Gilligan's Island

Ginger will be highlighted again in the next chapter under nausea and motion sickness because it is one of the best, well-known, and most effective herbal remedies used to combat the problem. In moderate quantities, ginger is also a safe herb used by women with morning sickness. You can buy ginger root in candied form and chew on a small piece if you start to feel sick to your stomach; this has been a godsend to many moms over the years.

If your liver is a problem, or if you tend to be anemic (low red blood count), you can nourish your body with herbs that are rich in iron. Plant forms of iron include red beet, yellow dock, red raspberry, chickweed, burdock, nettle, and mullein. A dab of peppermint oil on your tongue can stop you from feeling sick almost right away, and peppermint tea or peppermint candy has also been used to beat nausea over the years.

Mumps: One Mump or Two?

Mumps is a common childhood viral infection characterized by swelling of the glands in the neck, fever, headache, and sometimes vomiting. The affected person usually feels sick for three to five days but remains infectious until the swelling of the glands has completely gone away.

Sage Advice

Some women use the leaf of the red raspberry topically as a tonic rinse for dark hair. It also can be gargled to help heal mouth sores. To make either of these, use an infusion (tea). In addition, because red raspberry is drying and toning, it makes an effective and safe remedy in a liquid form when given to infants who have diarrhea.

Poison Ivy

Make sure that constipation is not your issue—constipation can not only cause nausea, but it also can give you a headache. See Chapter 4, "Herbs Are Not Just for Hippies Anymore," to find safe herbs useful for constipation during pregnancy and nursing.

If you did not have mumps as a child, catching the illness in adulthood is more serious and needs to be treated immediately. Mumps in adults can cause sterility in men. Some children get the mumps even when they have been vaccinated against it, but you can still help your child with some herbal remedies.

Mullein: Good to the Last Mump

Mullein (*Verbascum thapsus*) is a common herb that's also quite recognizable. This herb grows up to eight feet tall and has stalks that are conical in shape. It has small, yellow flowers that bloom a few at a time and sit close to the stalk. Mullein can be found along most roadsides where it is dry, warm, and open and where the soil has been disturbed. In a pinch, a dried stalk of mullein dipped in pine pitch may be lit and used as a torch.

Native Americans used to smoke the dried leaves of this plant for relief of coughs. The tea also can be drunk, or an infusion can be made and applied to the chest to help break up mucus congestion quickly.

Herb Lore

Native American women used to drink mullein tea to temporarily arrest their menstrual periods. Women who were "on their moon" (as the menstrual bleeding time was referred to), were thought to be closer to the spirit world at that time. The spiritual activity thought to be surrounding the woman at this time was believed to distract from the concentration of the medicine man and others during ceremonies. Therefore, the women could not (and in traditional tribes still cannot) take part in ritualistic ceremonies such as dances, sweat lodges, and other healing ceremonies during this time. Therefore, mullein came in handy since it offered women some control over their periods.

That's all nice and fine, but what can it do for the mumps, you ask? Historically, mullein has been used internally to treat mumps because of its affinity for the glands. You can take it or administer it internally to help with any childhood illness because it is a safe and mild herb. Apply a cooled fomentation of a mixture of mullein, lobelia, and white oak bark externally directly over the swollen lymph glands.

Mullein also has an affinity for the sinuses and can break up congestion. The herb is very soothing to the mucus membranes, which makes it useful for dry, hot, irritated, and hacking coughs. Think of mullein for any type of chest or glandular afflictions.

Speed Mumps

Of course, with any illness due to viral infection, you will want to keep the immune system boosted to help you prevent and recover from the illness. As always, golden seal, echinacea, vitamin C, and garlic are all good remedies taken internally to help fight infections and are all safe for children.

If you have any fomentation left from the previously mentioned remedy, add it to a hot footbath. The heat will bring the blood away from the upper body and down to the feet and may help reduce swelling of those mumps lumps.

Multiple Sclerosis, Multiple Herbs

Multiple sclerosis (MS) is a chronic disease affecting the nervous system. The myelin sheaths that surround and protect the nerves become damaged, which affects the brain and spinal cord and impairs the function of all nerves involved. Unfortunately, I see more and more young people these days suffering from MS, but the good news is that I have also seen folks with MS recover and experience increasingly longer periods without relapse, thanks to herbal remedies and other nutritional supplements.

MS affects different parts of the nerves and brain, so symptoms are scattered and can vary. Symptoms generally include:

➤ An unsteady gait

➤ Shaky hands or legs

➤ Involuntary rapid movement of the eyes

➤ Spasmodic weakness

➤ Affected speech

➤ Blurred vision due to inflammation of the nerves behind the eyes

Now let's talk about some herbs that might help protect you from this disease.

Poison Ivy

Never use a cold footbath when afflicted with the mumps because the blood will be pushed upward. If the glands are swollen around the neck, they are protecting the brain from viral or bacterial infection. You do not want to do anything that forces the infection toward the head. Instead, use cold packs around the neck or swollen areas.

Black Currant Oil

Black currant oil is high in essential fatty acids, such as gamma linoleic acid (GLA). Research has shown that people suffering from degenerative diseases are low in these essential fatty acids, so GLA can help protect the immune system. Evening primrose oil has similar properties to black currant oil, but it contains only half the GLA. Flax seed oil and lecithin are also good sources of essential fatty acids, but they're still not as rich in GLA as black currant oil.

Fatty acids are required to build up the myelin nerve sheaths, and this is why black currant oil can be your best single herb for MS. Essential fatty acids also build hormones, which are required for many biochemical processes and cellular communication.

Black currant oil has helped many and has been used for these conditions:

➤ Allergies

➤ Cancer

➤ Candida

➤ Eczema

➤ Female disorders

➤ Immunity

➤ Mental and nervous system disorders

➤ Multiple sclerosis

➤ Obesity

➤ PMS

➤ Skin ailments (all kinds)

Consider all foods and herbs that feed, support, and build the nervous system if you have MS. Vitamin E aids circulation and serves as an antioxidant, B-complex vitamins feed the brain and nervous system, and lecithin, cell salts, CoQ_{10}, amino acids, and food enzymes have all been helpful supplements. Other helpful herbs besides black currant oil include liquid chlorophyll, black walnut, germanium, skullcap, passion flower, horsetail, and wild yam.

Other MS Considerations

Because the cause of the myelin sheath damage remains unknown, avoid the things that are rumored to be possible causes, even if it is not yet proven scientifically. For instance, several reports on aspartame (more commonly known as Equal or NutriSweet®, a chemical ingredient used to sweeten many sugarless foods and drinks) link the substance to a myriad of symptoms and illnesses including MS, nerve damage, brain lesions, brain tumors, headaches, depression, black-outs, forgetfulness, and other central nervous system disorders. For more information on this and other food additives, read the book *Excitotoxins, The Taste That Kills*, by Dr. Russell Blaylock.

Eliminating all potential toxins going into your body can eliminate the source of what could be causing your problem. Some pesticides are known to be toxic to the nervous system, so search out organic foods whenever possible to keep potentially harmful pesticides out of your system.

Stress-reduction therapies should be incorporated into your life if you suffer from MS. Activities such as swimming, yoga, massage, reflexology, and other bodywork done weekly will help keep your nerves from overreacting and may help slow the damage in the nervous system.

Herb Lore

Aspartame is a chemical substance that contains 10 percent of a toxic substance called methanol. Methanol is an accumulative poison, meaning that it cannot leave the body and will build up to toxic amounts in the system. Maybe the company who produces these products slipped this past the FDA by affirming that the P450 enzymes in the liver can, in fact, break down methanol. But maybe they forgot to mention that the liver breaks down methanol and turns it into formaldehyde! Formaldehyde is another toxic substance used to embalm the dead! *Tip:* Try the sweet herb stevia instead.

Herbal Remedies for Common Ailments

Measles (Rubeola or Rubella)

Best Single Herb: Boneset

Best Combinations: Echinacea, golden seal; boneset; safflowers; liquid chlorophyll; marshmallow, fenugreek; slippery elm; yarrow

Other Helpful Supplements: Beta carotene; vitamin C

Possible Cause: Exposure

Complementary Help: Thyme fomentations; garlic and catnip enema; Oregon grape used externally; eucalyptus diffused in a room

Menstrual Irregularity/Late

Best Single Herb: Pennyroyal

Best Combinations: Black cohosh, squawvine, dong quai, butcher's broom, red raspberry; ginger; licorice root; evening primrose oil

Other Helpful Supplements: Vitamin E

Possible Cause: Stress; glandular imbalance; anorexia

Complementary Help: Reflexology; acupuncture

Migraine Headaches

Best Single Herb: Feverfew

Best Combinations: Feverfew; rose hips, barberry, dandelion, fennel, red beet, horseradish, parsley (supports liver and digestion)

Other Helpful Supplements: B-complex with extra niacin; food enzymes

continues

231

Herbal Remedies for Common Ailments   (continued)

Migraine Headaches (continued)

Possible Cause: Dehydration; poor digestion; food allergies; constipation; spinal misalignment; hormonal imbalance; stressed liver

Complementary Help: Support digestion; cleanse the bowel; seek chiropractic care; undergo acupuncture; drink water; avoid trigger foods (red wine, cheese, caffeine, MSG)

Morning Sickness

Best Single Herb: Red raspberry

Best Combinations: Ginger; peppermint; red raspberry; red beet, yellow dock, red raspberry, chickweed, burdock, nettle, mullein; psyllium hulls (for constipation)

Other Helpful Supplements: B-complex; calcium/magnesium

Possible Causes: Constipation; stressed liver

Complementary Help: Peppermint oil dabbed on tongue

Mumps

Best Single Herb: Mullein

Best Combinations: Mullein; lobelia; white oak bark; echinacea, golden seal; garlic

Other Helpful Supplements: Vitamin C

Possible Cause: Exposure

Complementary Help: Mullein, lobelia, and white oak bark fomentations; hot footbaths

Multiple Sclerosis

Best Single Herb: Black currant oil

Best Combinations: Black currant oil; liquid chlorophyll; black walnut; germanium; skullcap; passion flower; horsetail; wild yam

Other Helpful Supplements: Vitamin E; B-complex; lecithin; cell salts; CoQ_{10}; food enzymes; amino acids

Possible Causes: Stress; malnutrition; environmental toxicity; aspartame

Complementary Help: Undergo stress-reduction therapy; eat organic foods only; read *Fats That Heal, Fats That Kill*, by Udo Erasmus, and *Excitotoxins: The Taste That Kills*, by Dr. Russell Blaylock

The Least You Need to Know

➤ Boneset is an herb traditionally used to aid the body in recovering from colds, flu, measles, and the aches and pains associated with these ailments.

➤ Pennyroyal serves to bring about a late period and also makes a great insect repellent, but it should never be used by anyone when pregnant.

➤ Red raspberry is a plant known for its beneficial effects for pregnant women.

➤ Find out the cause of your migraine, and treat the whole problem; in the meantime, feverfew has been used successfully over the years as a migraine prevention remedy.

➤ Mullein has been used to treat ailments of the respiratory tract and is useful for swollen glands, which makes it a helpful remedy for mumps.

➤ Black currant oil is a rich source of essential fatty acids, which are used to build and protect the nervous system. Black currant oil may be very useful for those suffering with MS.

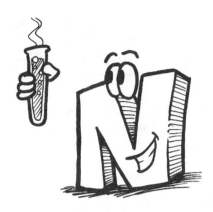

Chapter 18

N: Now You Have a Remedy

In This Chapter

➤ Nourish your nails and nerves with herbs

➤ Herbs that help settle nausea

➤ Combat neuritis with herbs

➤ Herbs you can use for nosebleeds

"We must turn to nature itself, to the observations of the body in health and disease to learn the truth." —Hippocrates (c. 460 B.C.–c. 377 B.C.), Greek physician

It is true that we must observe the body and the nature of nature to understand the ailments we suffer. Some of the first clues that something is going wrong inside can manifest themselves on the outside. These clues can be seen in the condition of our nails, for instance, which is one of the things we will discuss in this chapter. We will also discuss some underlying causes of nosebleeds and some quick herbal remedies to stop them. If that isn't enough, I'll also give you some remedies to combat the inflammation of swollen nerves and the best herb for helping nausea. Now, get ready to read on through the Ns of ailments!

Nail Problems: Nailing Down a Cure

My fingernails are the first to remind me when I haven't been getting enough herbal silicon, calcium, zinc, and other minerals. If I run out of my daily herbal supplements, in less than 10 days my fingernails begin to tear, break, and bend—even though I keep them very short! If healing begins from the inside out, as Hering's Law of Cure states, then I also believe the opposite is true: that illness begins on the inside first, and the outward signs show up last.

The body has the ability to prioritize incoming nutrients. In other words, it will take care of your most critical organs first with the nutrients you feed it. But when the incoming supply runs low, then the less critical things, such as fingernails and hair, suffer. These outward signs are a warning signal that gives you clues to nourish yourself to avoid inner deterioration.

Just like the rest of our structural system, the nails, skin, and hair need minerals for nourishment. One of the main minerals for these parts (considered part of the structural system) is silicon. Silicon is a natural substance found in nature that is extremely tough but flexibly resilient. Think of the seaweed and the herb kelp, which grows in long, rope-like extensions and sways in the sea with the movement of the waves. Kelp is extremely flexible, but the next time some washes up on the beach, try to tear it in half. It's almost like trying to tear a thick telephone book in half! Kelp is rich in silicon, which gives it strength but also flexibility. This is how we want our hair and skin to be. Nails will be firm but should not be brittle; brittle nails will break and fracture frequently under stress. Silicon gives some flexibility to the nails to help them withstand impact.

Botanical Bit

Hering's Law of Cure states, "All healing begins from the head down, the inside out, and in the reverse order as the symptoms have first been acquired."

Botanical Bit

Silica is a compound of silicon and oxygen. It is silicon that gives the hard outer coating to vegetables such as corn, rice, and barley.

Horsetail for Biting Brittle Nails

Horsetail (*Equisetum arvense*) is one of the richest herbs in silicon, and this is why I have chosen it as the best single herb for nail problems. This plant is also known as shavegrass or bottle brush; its spiny projections stick up and out and resemble a brush that could be used to clean bottles, which is where it may have earned this name.

The Latin translation of this herb literally means "horse tail of the fields," and if you have ever felt a horse's tail, you will notice how strong and thick these hairs are. This is an example of how *silica*, a component in silicone, gives hardness to hair.

Horsetail has been used traditionally as an herbal remedy for torn ligaments; arthritis of all types (especially rheumatoid arthritis); inflammations; skin, hair, and nail deficiencies; and bacteria and fungal infections. It also has been used as a diuretic and as a foot bath for stinky or sweaty feet. Horsetail is rich in many minerals and contains trace amounts of gold, which has proven helpful for rheumatism.

Other herbs rich in silicon, calcium, zinc, and other minerals good for the hair, skin, and nails include: rosemary, hyssop, aloe vera, ginkgo biloba, and kelp.

Nail Readings

The nails, skin, and hair are all outward reflections of your inner health, and we can learn to read these signs with practice and study. For instance, some people read faces for signs of health: Who hasn't seen someone who is stressed and over-tired without bags or circles under their eyes? This can also indicate liver or kidney stress. The teeth reflect how nourished we are, as the body can rob calcium from these areas to feed other, more critical body parts.

The nails are no different; they are alive and always growing, and they're quick to show us what might be going on in the body.

Here are some examples:

➤ Dry, brittle nails that break easily could indicate a deficiency in silicon, calcium, and zinc.

➤ Ridges along nails could mean that you have poor digestion or lack hydrochloric acid. Try a food enzyme with hydrochloric acid added for a few weeks, and see if you notice a change. Also consider herbal sources of minerals.

➤ White spots on fingernails may indicate a zinc deficiency. Beware of taking too much zinc, however; about 45–50 mg daily is more than sufficient unless specific conditions apply (such as taking excess calcium). See your doctor or holistic practitioner if you're taking zinc supplements.

➤ Thin, flat, spoon-shaped nails can be a sign of a B-12 deficiency.

➤ A deep blue color to the nails may indicate a lack of oxygen in the tissues due to asthma or emphysema.

➤ Nails that come off or that separate from the fingers may indicate problems with the thyroid.

➤ Thick cuticles can indicate poor digestion of protein. Try food enzymes containing hydrochloric acid, marshmallow and pepsin and eat less protein.

Poison Ivy

Large amounts of horsetail may be toxic, so try to find this great herb mixed with other herbs designed for the structural system. Using this herb over long periods of time can deplete vitamin B1 from the body. This herb may also be somewhat abrasive to the digestive tract and should be taken only occasionally, or in small amounts mixed with other herbs.

Sage Advice

Nutritional sources of zinc include capsicum, spirulina, psyllium, safe, garlic, eyebright, bilberry, and gotu kola. Zinc-rich foods include pumpkin seeds, goat's milk/whey, brewers yeast, and whole grains.

➤ Horizontal ridges across nails can indicate a lack of calcium. However, the nails grow from about a quarter-inch below your nail bed (toward your finger joints). If you bump or damage this nail bed, the impact may make your nail(s) grow out with ridges. I imagine this as the ripple effect, like when you throw a stone into a still pond. The image really makes me think about how we are made up of energy!

➤ A yellowing and thickening of nails can be a deposit of calcium or other minerals that your body is not absorbing or utilizing properly. Work with a holistic practitioner to help with your absorption, and read the section "Got Gas?" in Chapter 12, "G: Great Remedies," for hints on herbs for better digestion. Also check for fungus growth under nails if you see a yellow color. Another possibility is a poor circulatory system that is not fully bringing circulation to the nails.

➤ Nail biting is usually due to a lack of minerals that nourish the nervous system. You may subconsciously be trying to eat your minerals from your fingernails. To end this habit, begin taking some herbal remedies to nourish the rest of your body and see Chapter 6, "Give Me Another A!" for more on anxiety.

Nausea and Motion Sickness: Some Gingerly Advice

I get many phone calls from people asking how to help their car-sick children. I always try to get the parent to nail down a cause first to avoid future problems. My questions to parents of children with car sickness are aimed at finding a root cause and are always the same questions:

➤ Does the child have mucus congestion, or could it be an inner ear infection?

➤ Is the child stressed out?

➤ Is the child eating junk food right before a car trip?

➤ Is the child constipated?

➤ What is the same about each time the child experiences nausea or vomiting during a car ride?

Finding the root cause is important in all ailments and disease, if possible, but my answer for an herbal remedy for motion sickness is almost always the same: Ginger root (*Zingiber officinale*) is tried and true for stopping nausea. Everyone I have spoken with who has had motion sickness and tried ginger root has attested to its effectiveness. In fact, some claim that it is more effective than the drug Dramamine® for motion sickness—better yet, ginger root will not produce the toxic side effects that drugs can.

Peppermint tea is also very soothing to the stomach because it stirs up digestive juices and is an aid to indigestion. A dab of peppermint oil on your tongue when you are nauseous might help. Of course, peppermint is stimulating and will help keep you alert as well; try putting a dab on the very back of your tongue, and then close your mouth and breathe deep for a stimulating mental refresher. See more on peppermint in Chapter 17, "M for More Remedies," in the section on morning sickness.

A reflex point that may help you with nausea is shown in the following figure. Pressing this point has helped many who were nauseous from being on a boat. When I was receiving my first colonic in colon hygiene school, I became nauseous and a kind fellow student and acupuncturist showed me this point. He applied the pressure for me, and my nausea disappeared almost immediately. For some, this method may take longer to be effective.

Here's how to find it:

1. Pronate your hand so that your palm is facing you.
2. With the other hand, place your first two fingers across the base of your wrist. The nausea button is located just below your pointer finger, in the center of the wrist (between the two bones). See the figure showing the spot.
3. Next, take your thumb and press in on the spot. Hold this spot firmly for one minute. Repeat three times.
4. Repeat the procedure on the other wrist.

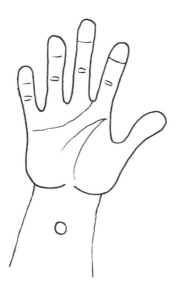

The reflex point for motion sickness is located approximately two finger widths below the wrist joint on both arms.

239

I have also seen this work for folks who have just held one side until their nausea subsided—try it for yourself and see! In the meantime, keep some candied or encapsulated ginger root and a small bottle of peppermint oil with you or in your car's glove compartment. For the best prevention, you can take a couple capsules of ginger root before you leave for a long road trip to keep your stomach settled.

Botanical Bit

Neuritis, or **neuropathy**, is a disease of the peripheral nerves of the body (usually in the toes and fingers) that causes inflammation and can lead to numbness of these areas. **Neuralgia** is nerve pain, usually associated with the swelling of the nerves.

Poison Ivy

Devil's claw may be called a "claw" because of its somewhat abrasive or irritating affect on the digestive tract. You will most likely find this herb in a mixture with other herbs that feed the structural system. If you take devil's claw by itself, try chasing it with an herb that soothes and protects tissues, such as aloe vera.

Neuritis: Numb to the Problem

Neuritis is a disease of the peripheral nerves of the body (usually in the toes and fingers), that causes inflammation and can lead to numbness of these areas. The swelling of the nerves associated with this condition can cause pain (*neuralgia*), skin sensitivity, paralysis, muscular weakness, and slowed reflexes. The term *neuropathy* is also used less specifically to refer to this condition.

Sometimes neuritis can be caused by diabetes, and it is associated with gout and other diseases affecting the proper functioning of the entire structural system (muscles, tendons, bones, joints).

The Devil's Claw Made Me Do It

Devil's claw (*Harpagophytum procumbens*) is an herb that has been used for a host of painful or inflammatory ailments such as arthritis, rheumatism, acne and allergies, kidney and liver problems, and gout because of its anti-inflammatory properties. Because neuritis is an inflammation of the nerves, devil's claw may be useful to you for this condition. It works primarily by helping the body eliminate uric acid (see Chapter 12 for more on gout; see Chapter 15, "J and K: For Just the Right Kind of Cure," for more on devil's claw for inflamed knees).

The root of the devil's claw is taken internally to clean the vascular walls, the blood, and the lymphatic system. It provides iron and magnesium and helps to strengthen the bladder, kidneys, liver, joints, and stomach.

Numb and Number

Stimulating the circulation with herbs will certainly help to prevent the numbness associated with this condition. Capsicum and ginger are both quick to stimulate circulation. Both are very hot and can be toned down a bit to ease digestion when mixed with white willow bark, black cohosh, valerian, and wood betony. If you have diabetes, see Chapter 9, "D Best Herbal Solutions," for more pointers on using herbs.

Consider using the B-complex vitamins to feed the nervous system if you have neuritis. Calcium with magnesium will feed the structural system and may be helpful if you are suffering from nerve pain—especially if the body is over-acidic, calcium may ease this pain. Vitamin E with selenium is a powerful antioxidant and aids the circulatory system; up to 1,200 IU may be useful, but always check with your doctor before taking high doses of vitamins. Too high a dose of vitamin E can cause headaches.

Sage Advice

Reflexology is an excellent therapy that stimulates points on the feet and hands that connect to all other parts of the body. It also helps increase circulation to the extremities and can be instrumental in protecting you from the effects of neuropathy. Diabetics have been aided with the use of reflexology.

Nosebleeds: Herbs That Clot, Herbs That Do Not

Nosebleeds are self-explanatory. They may occur when you have an injury to your nose, of course, or when you are suffering from overly dry conditions or from hay fever or other things that make the tissues inside your nose tear easily.

Nosebleeds that occur regularly can be a problem, so be sure to consider what's causing them. Also please get a check-up by your regular doctor if you suddenly get nosebleeds for no apparent reason; you could have a physical problem in the nasal cavity or brain.

Here's a look at some possible causes of nosebleeds once a medical problem is ruled out:

➤ You could have weak blood capillaries that are easily broken. Blood capillaries should be strengthened to ensure a healthy circulatory system. We'll talk later about some herbs that can do that.

➤ Hot herbs, such as ginger or horseradish, taken over a long period of time can heat up and dry out sensitive mucous tissues, causing the nose to bleed from dryness. Consider the herbs you are on if you have been taking them a long time, and stop any herbs you suspect may be causing the problem.

➤ Environmental toxins, such as pesticides sprayed over farms in the area, could be contributing to your nosebleeds.

➤ Pest-control services nearby or around your own home or office area could be irritating your nose.

➤ You could be exposed to harsh cleaning supplies.

➤ You could be overexposed to chlorine, perhaps if you work in or around a heavily chlorinated pool.

241

➤ You could be exposed to industrial chemicals.

➤ Lawn fertilizers could be irritating your nose.

All these things can become hazardous if you are constantly or continually exposed to them. Some people are much more sensitive than others, and everyone has an individual tolerance to these environmental pollutants; however, if you are having nosebleeds and the doctors cannot find any physical causes, consider taking a look at what is in your environment. Personally, I am very sensitive to smells, especially to unnatural chemicals. Of course, consider the source *after* you stop that bleeding!

Herb Lore

While living briefly near Clearwater, Florida, I suddenly came down with almost daily nosebleeds! I did not know what the problem was because I had not changed anything in my lifestyle. Then I discovered that during the time I was there, the government was spraying a toxic pesticide called malathion throughout a nearby town to kill off the spread of a tiny fruit fly. Although the pesticide was sprayed nearly 20 miles away, my nose bled daily until two weeks after the spraying had stopped!

Bugleweed for When Your Nose Hits the Grindstone

Bugleweed (*Lycopus virginicus*) is an herb historically used for the respiratory and nervous systems. It has strong astringent properties and may help stop bleeding because it contracts tissues. Taken internally, bugleweed has been used to tone the heart muscle, aid heart palpitations, tone an overgrowth of the thyroid, calm anxiety, and ease coughing.

If you use this herb as a tea, it is recommended that you use the fresh herb. This may be because the herb is a member of the mint family, and the fresh herb may make it more tasty. The fresh herb can also be applied externally for bleeding cuts or noses. Bugleweed is not recommended for use during pregnancy.

Sage Advice

Bugleweed is an herb you can remember for nosebleeds because a "bugle" is a type of a horn. Some refer to the nose as a honker, a horn, or even a bugle!

Nosy About Herbs

Herbs that strengthen the blood capillaries include an extract from grape seeds and pine bark and are known as *proanthocyananidins* (commonly referred to as Pycnogenol®, the trade name for the proanthocyananidin bioflavonols from the pine bark). These substances have a powerful effect on strengthening blood capillaries. When capillaries are easily broken, you can bruise very easily because any light bang or smack can break these delicate blood vessels. Strengthening the blood capillaries, then, can help prevent easy bruising.

Citrus bioflavonoids work in a similar way to grape seed and pine bark. These can be found as extras with vitamin C tablets and can sometimes be purchased as a single supplement. Some herb companies may add extra vegetable citrus bioflavonoids along with the grape seed or pine bark extracts.

Calcium serves as the tissue and bone knitter in the body, and can help bleeding wounds mend. An herbal or vitamin source of calcium should be considered if you are having regular nosebleeds.

Liquid chlorophyll is the blood of the plant, and its makeup is similar to our hemoglobin (red blood cells); see the section "Bad Breath (Halitosis): A Refreshing Remedy," in Chapter 7, "B Well," for more on chlorophyll. I have had many herbalists tell me that they keep extra liquid chlorophyll around in a pantry to stop bleeding in emergencies. Taken internally, liquid chlorophyll can build up the red blood count and help filter out air pollution from the air we breathe. This is especially helpful internally if you believe external pollution is to blame for your nosebleeds. Chlorophyll may help protect you on the inside as well.

Poison Ivy

If you bruise easily, also get checked for anemia. This could also be an indication of possible liver problems or kidney dysfunction.

Here are some external uses for herbs that can be used to stop a nosebleed in its tracks:

➤ Extract of capsicum, soaked on a cotton ball and placed in the nose. This herbal remedy will probably sting, but the hot herb serves to kind of sear the flesh wound and will usually stop bleeding on contact.

➤ A cotton ball soaked in liquid chlorophyll and placed in the nose. This remedy will not sting, but it may take a moment to work. Apply pressure, and be sure to stand over a sink to catch any dripping chlorophyll. Like human blood, this green pigment of plant blood will permanently stain clothing and carpets.

➤ Golden seal powder has been used to help stop bleeding, too. Wet your finger, dip it in some of this herb powder, and place it in the nostril that is bleeding.

Overall, it is important to get your nose to stop bleeding first with any of these remedies. Later, in Chapter 26, "An Herbal First Aid Kit," we will go over some more of these herbs so you can be prepared anytime for these unexpected nuisances. In the meantime, keep your nose clean, and let's get on with the next set of remedies!

Herbal Remedies for Common Ailments

Nails, Biting, Brittle

Best Single Herb: Horsetail

Best Combinations: Horsetail, rosemary, hyssop, aloe vera, ginkgo biloba; kelp

Other Helpful Supplements: Zinc; vitamin E; food enzymes with hydrochloric acid; vitamin C; calcium/magnesium with vitamin D

Possible Causes: Weak digestion; thyroid problems; malnutrition

Complementary Help: Support digestion

Nausea/Motion Sickness

Best Single Herb: Ginger

Best Combinations: Ginger; peppermint; chamomile

Other Helpful Supplements: B-complex vitamins; magnesium; activated charcoal

Possible Causes: Inner ear infection; motion sickness; constipation; liver stress; stress/nerves; morning sickness; hormonal imbalance

Complementary Help: Peppermint oil on tongue (keep with you or in your vehicle); candied ginger; peppermint tea

Neuritis (Neuropathy)

Best Single Herb: Devil's claw

Best Combinations: White willow bark, black cohosh, capsicum, valerian, ginger, hops, wood betony, devil's claw

Other Helpful Supplements: B-complex vitamins; calcium/magnesium; vitamin E with selenium

Possible Causes: Diabetes; poor circulation

Complementary Help: Reflexology

Nosebleeds

Best Single Herb: Bugleweed

Best Combinations: Bugleweed; golden seal; capsicum; liquid chlorophyll; grape seed/pine bark extract

Other Helpful Supplements: Vitamin C with citrus bioflavonoids; calcium

Possible Causes: Weak blood capillaries; environmental toxins/poisoning

Complementary Help: Golden seal "snuff"; liquid chlorophyll cotton ball packs; capsicum applied topically

The Least You Need to Know

➤ Nails can give clues about conditions of the body. Horsetail is rich in silicone and minerals and will nourish hair, skin, and nails.

➤ Ginger is one of the best herbal remedies for nausea and is safe for children and pregnant women.

➤ Devil's claw has been used to combat arthritis, gout, and rheumatism because of its anti-inflammatory properties, which may also make it useful for fighting neuritis.

➤ Bugleweed is an astringent herb used to tone internal organs; it makes a good remedy for nosebleeds.

Part 4
Yuckies from O to Z

This section concludes the last portion of the alphabet with herbal remedies for common and not-so-common ailments from osteoporosis and PMS, to herbal help for smokers who want to quit. Also included is a supplemental plan for weight loss.

By the time you are through, you should have an herbal solution for almost anything you suffer from—and, to top it off, you will have been properly introduced to the pros and cons of more than 100 herbs! Not bad for a complete herbal idiot, hmmm?

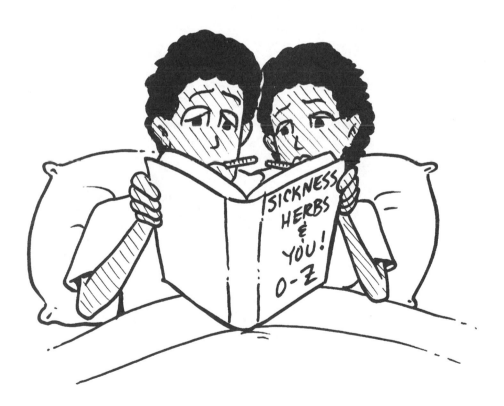

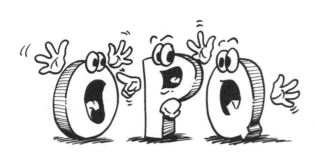

Chapter 19

O, P, and Q: Obvious Painful Questions and Answers

In This Chapter

➤ The nourishing properties of nettle

➤ Nourish the pancreas with cedar berries

➤ Rid yourself of parasites

➤ Fight pneumonia with herbs

➤ An effective herb for prostate trouble

"I hate to tell you that sickness is sometimes a blessing. Sickness has moved more people into the health field than anything else. As soon as you get tired of being tired and sick of being sick, you will seek Nature's real health. It is not pleasant to go through sickness, but it is a necessary earthy experience." —Bernard Jensen, D.C., Ph.D., N.D., *Food Healing For Man* (Bernard Jensen Publisher, 1983).

I agree with Dr. Jensen. Sometimes it seems that we have to go through many ailments and struggle to find out a cure—and then we wind up sharing this with the world! So let's take a look at some more ailments so you might cure yourself and share what you know with others. Get ready to look at osteoporosis, parasites, pneumonia, and inflammation of the pancreas and prostate—and, of course, the herbs that can help you through each of these.

Osteoporosis: A Hole Cure

Osteoporosis is a loss of bony tissue and condition in which the bones become porous, making them brittle and easily broken or fractured. It is estimated that one in three women in the United States will suffer from this in their lifetime. (And since you purchased this book, these statistics won't need to apply to you now will they?)

Prevention is the key for fighting osteoporosis, and it's not too late to start now.

Many factors cause osteoporosis, including:

➤ Infections

➤ Injuries

➤ Osteoporosis of an adjacent bone

➤ Cushing's disease

➤ Long-term steroid therapy

➤ Calcium and other mineral deficiency

➤ Lack of estrogen (as in menopause or a hysterectomy)

Osteoporosis is commonly found in women. Regular exercise will build bone strength and is one of the best preventative therapies against osteoporosis.

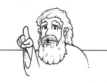

Sage Advice

World-renowned holistic practitioner Dr. Paavo Airola says that honey increases calcium retention in the structural system. Raw honey is best because the enzymes are intact. Add a little to your herb tea daily, or take some on a slice of whole-wheat bread with peanut butter. Any way you do it, honey can help your bones—so eat your honey, honey!

Nettle for the Holey

Nettle (*Urtica dioica*) also earned another well-deserved common name, stinging nettle. This plant's nasty stinging hairs under its leaves will give you blisters and burning if you are unfortunate to touch it. Some people have stung themselves on purpose, however, claiming that if you suffer from arthritis, the sting of the nettle will offer an immediate cure. I wouldn't recommend this because I'm not into sadomasochism, but for those of you who get stung unwittingly, the remedy for the sting is in the juice of the plant. If you don't want to be anywhere near it, try some yellow dock or plantain on your rash; this is also an effective antidote.

Singing properties aside, nettle is a wonderfully useful herb. It is salty to the taste, and if you remember what that means from Chapter 3, "What to Expect with Herbs," when we talked about energetics, you might remember that the salty taste indicates a high amount of minerals, making it a *nutritive*. Nettle is rich in iron, calcium, phosphorus, magnesium, zinc, and vitamins A, Bs, C, D, and K.

Botanical Bit

Nutritive is an herbal property meaning that the plant has plenty of food value and may be used as a nourishing food.

You can use nettle for osteoporosis to feed your body necessary minerals from nature. Nettle is also known by many moms as a great enhancer of breast milk. Likewise, if you are a farmer or have chickens, try feeding nettle to your chickens to help them produce more eggs. This herb has been used to treat infertility in females and has come in handy as a remedy for arthritis, gout, kidney inflammation, rickets, and jaundice. I could go on and on about the uses of this herb, but for now, we will get onto some other herbs and supplements that can help you with osteoporosis.

Other Herbs to Fill in the Gaps

Many times, those suffering with osteoporosis are already taking calcium supplements, but the calcium needs to be absorbed to be properly utilized. If digestion is insufficient to break down and absorb calcium, the minerals won't help in the rebuilding of bone tissue. (See more on this in the section "Arthritis: A Flexible Treatment Plan," in Chapter 6, "Give Me Another A!"; then take a look at Chapter 12, "G: Great Remedies," for tips on digesting better.)

Consider supplementing with a natural form of calcium (herbs), such as the combination listed in the table in the end of this chapter, since herbs will ensure you that you are getting a wide range of minerals. Otherwise, make sure your vitamin calcium supplement includes vitamin D. This vitamin is synthesized by our body when we get sunshine and helps us utilize calcium.

Some controversy arises over whether drinking distilled water leeches out minerals from the body. I suggest drinking distilled water only if you are on a short cleansing diet. Drink purified water, such as reverse osmosis water, instead. Wouldn't it be nice if they had "reverse osteoporosis" water? (See Chapter 1, "What Are Herbs and Why Should I Use Them?" for an explanation of reverse osmosis water.)

Juicing and ingesting vegetables daily will help you get easily absorbed minerals in your diet. Eat carrots for calcium and celery for sodium. Add powdered goat's whey to this mixture for extra minerals. Also eat a more wholesome diet with more alkaline foods in case you are over-acidic (acid can be eating away at the holes in your bones). See Chapter 15, "J and K: For Just the Right Kind of Cure," for more on acid and alkaline foods.

Sage Advice

You only need about 15 minutes per week in the sunshine for your skin to capture the vitamin D that you need, but some of us don't get out much! Make sure you are getting your minimum sunshine intake—it's good for you and your bones.

Pancreas Trouble: A Cedar Berry Cure

The pancreas is an organ that serves many functions. It is a pinkish, semi-oblong-shaped organ about six to eight inches in length. It is located on your left side midway between your diaphragm and waist. The pancreas sits a little behind and a little below the stomach.

Pancreatitis is an inflammation of the pancreas that is frequently diagnosed as idiosyncratic pancreatitis by physicians. This term cracks me up because it is such a long, technical-sounding term that, when interpreted simply means, "The pancreas is swollen, and we don't know why!" As far as I'm concerned, you could use this term for other things, such as "idiosyncratic shop-a-holic," meaning, "I'm addicted to shopping, and I don't know why!"

Seriously, if you have a swollen pancreas, consult your physician to find out why, if possible. Alcohol may cause the pancreas to inflame, as can a virus, malnutrition, and any injury to the body near the pancreas. If you have a swollen pancreas, the root cause could be because of inadequate digestion, low blood sugar (hypoglycemia), or high blood sugar (diabetes). (See the corresponding chapters for more on these ailments.)

Take herbs that are helpful in toning the body tissues, such as cedar berries (*Juniperus virginiana*). The berries of this plant, which take about two to three years to ripen, are the medicinal parts of this herb. Cedar berries have been used to aid inflammations of all types, including gout, ureteritis, arthritis, and hemorrhoids. Some claim that cedar berries also help combat the side effects experienced after immunizations.

Poison Ivy

Although good for contracting inflamed tissues, cedar berries should be avoided if you have inflammations due to kidney or bladder infections, or if you are pregnant.

You can apply the essential oil of the cedar berries as a topical application to help dandruff and achy joints or as an insect repellent. The oil acts as an astringent, so its topical applications can help shrink cold sores, hemorrhoids, and acne.

See the table at the end of this chapter for an excellent combination that includes cedar berries and 13 other herbs used to nourish the pancreas and soothe inflammation.

Parasites: Dealing with Uninvited Guests

Parasites are organisms that live off a host (you) that do not contribute to the welfare of that host. Basically life-suckers, parasites are linked to a myriad of illnesses, and parasite infestation can be very damaging to the system. Several different types of parasites exist, from microscopic organisms to large intestinal tapeworms. Because most of you will be terribly grossed out by this topic, I'll spare you the gruesome details. However, I think that everyone should be aware that more of us than you might think have parasites.

In this section, I'll also make you aware of some of the signs of infestation, and I'll give you some preventative measures to take. Then we can get on with the herbal remedies.

Parasites can be transferred through contact with the following contaminated items:

➤ Animals

➤ Feces

➤ Meat

➤ Soil

➤ Vegetables

➤ Water

Parasites can enter our body via the mouth or through the skin.

How can you tell if you might have a parasitic infection? Here are some things to look for:

➤ Sudden, unexplained illness

➤ Dramatic weight loss or weight gain

➤ Diarrhea, intestinal distress

➤ Vomiting, nausea

➤ Grinding teeth, especially at night

➤ Sugar cravings

➤ Abdominal bloating

➤ Lowered immunity

➤ Insomnia

➤ General body aches, pains, weakness

➤ Liver problems, anemia, cirrhosis

These ailments can be caused by a host of things (no pun intended!) but are common among my clients who suffer from parasite infections.

When utilizing herbs to kill off a parasite infection, get some guidance from your holistic practitioner and herbalist because the process can sometimes take more than a month—and sometimes several months—to complete.

Try this regimen that my clients have followed with success:

1. Take your parasite-killing herbs (examples are given in the table at the end of this chapter) for 10 days, and avoid eating sugar, meat, cheese, and bread.

Sage Advice

Think of bugs and parasites as nature's undertakers—they invade only when conditions are ripe. Keep the body clean, digestion strong, and tissues oxygenated so parasites cannot take a foothold.

Poison Ivy

Avoid sugar when dealing with a parasite infection. Sugar is a favorite food of parasites, and you will need to starve the party to get rid of them for good.

2. Replace these foods with lots of rice, steamed vegetables, tofu, beans, salads, and other wholesome foods.

3. Then, continue on your clean diet and discontinue the parasite-killing herbs for 10 days. (You can continue on your food enzyme supplement with hydrochloric acid for protection.)

4. After this 10-day rest period, resume taking your herbs for another 10 days. This will ensure that you have killed off any eggs that may have hatched from the first batch of the nasties.

Don't be discouraged if you have to go through this process for another month or so—it will depend on how strong of a foothold the buggers have on you. You can also increase your garlic intake to speed up the process.

Wormwood, Would You?

In case you're out in the bushes identifying different herbs, let's clear up a common problem in identifying or labeling sage. There is the herb sage, and then there is the herb sagebrush. Sagebrush is commonly referred to as just sage, for short, but sage and sagebrush actually come from two separate families. Sagebrush is part of the Artemisia family (also referred to as the wormwood family). We're going to talk about the wormwood or Artemisia family here for its usefulness in fighting parasites. This family contains three different herbs, and all are quite different.

Let's get this wormwood, sage, sagebrush thing straight:

Wormwood is a common name for the herb *Artemisia absinthium, Artemisia frigida,* or *Artemisia tilesii.* This is the herb we will discuss for its effects on ridding the body of parasites.

Mugwort is the common name for the herb *Artemisia vulgaris.* This herb is also used to fight parasite infections and can be used together with wormwood for enhanced effect.

Sagebrush is the common name for the herb *Artemisia tridentata* and is the common, bush-like herb you see in the mountains, deserts, and plains of North America. We'll talk a little more about this common plant here, too, because it's one of my favorites. This herb has been used for respiratory ailments and many other conditions of the body. See the following photo of sagebrush taken early in the spring to help identify this herb.

Sage does not belong in the Artemisia family at all—its Latin name is *Salvia officinalis,* and it's used for sinuses, the bladder, mucus membranes, sore throats, and nerves. For more on the uses of sage, see the section "Laryngitis: Screaming for Attention," in Chapter 16, "L: Let Me Heal Naturally."

Growing up in Colorado (and now living in Idaho), I have been surrounded by sage-brush (*Artemisia tridentata*) almost everywhere outdoors. I love its bittersweet smell and have harvested it for use as incense. The plant burns easily, and with an incense holder and a piece of self-igniting charcoal, you can burn the fresh herb for quite a while. Use sagebrush for a psychic cleansing for your environment and self. When moving into a new home that was previously occupied or buying a previously owned vehicle, a smoky sagebrush cleansing will help purify others energies and makes the space feel cleaner.

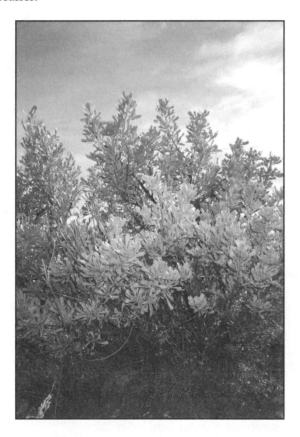

Artcmisia tridentata, *commonly known as sagebrush and sometimes called sage.*

The sagebrush is the silver-green, somewhat fuzzy plant you see in the Western high deserts and plains of North America. Next time you watch a cowboy Western movie, notice the sagebrush that is always growing abundantly in the dusty, rocky ground. Pick some for its wonderful smell, and remember its differences from the other herb: sage.

Now back to the other Artemisia family members that specifically have been used as *verimfuge*s (parasite killers) and *anthelmintics* (parasite expellers).

255

Herb Lore

Having the opportunity to be involved with a tribe of Lakota Sioux Native Americans helped me see what a useful and revered herb sagebrush is. Women added a pinch of it to soups and stews; fresh sprigs were added to the flames of the sweat lodge fire; and the medicine man always cleansed the energy of each person who entered the healing ceremonies with the smoke of burning sagebrush. Sometimes when flesh offerings were given, the medicine man would pick some sprigs and immediately dress the wounds with the leaves; the application stopped bleeding immediately.

Wormwood is a plant that may have received its name because pests are repelled by it. You can take wormwood internally but only in small doses; this herb can kill and send unwanted parasites from your body, and it may work specifically well for roundworms and thread worms. You will usually find wormwood mixed with other herbs in combinations because too much of this herb can be toxic to the system. Parasites aren't the only pests that dislike this herb—mice also are repelled by it. In fact, it is said that writers and authors in the days of old used to add the juice of the wormwood plant to their ink to protect mice from chewing on their papers! (Isn't it funny how times have changed? Now authors couldn't survive without a mouse!)

Botanical Bit

A **verimfuge** is a term used for an herb that has properties that push parasites from the body. This term has been used interchangeably with *anthelmintic, parasiticide,* and *antiparasitic*. An **anthelmintic** is a term used for an herb that has properties that kill parasites. This term has been used interchangeably with *verimfuge, parasiticide,* and *antiparasitic*.

You can also use dried wormwood to make sachets for protecting your closets and sweater drawers from moths. Try wormwood as a tea or decoction, and apply it externally for use as a topical insect repellent and to combat lice, scabies, and itchy skin.

In folklore, the dried herb of the wormwood plant was used to protect a person from spells given by the evil eye. So, it seems, wormwood has been used for a long time to rid unwanted things from our body and from our environment.

Other Herbs to Evict Unwanted Tenants

Many herbs can be used safely in combination or separately to fight parasitic infections and to protect you from them in the first place. For protection, take a food enzyme

256

supplement with hydrochloric acid before every meal, especially when eating out or traveling. (See Chapter 11, "F: Fantastic Healing Flora," for more on food poisoning and how to avoid it.) Food poisoning is usually caused by bacterial infections, but parasites can be contracted the same way—either way, hydrochloric acid should kill them both!

Here's a list of well-known herbs that kill and rid the body of parasites:

➤ Wormwood

➤ Elecampane (see more in Chapter 16)

➤ Mugwort

➤ Spearmint (see more in Chapter 23, "V, W, X, Y, Z, and Other Technical Words")

➤ Turmeric (a spice used in cooking—especially in Indian curries)

➤ Ginger (see more in Chapter 17, "M for More Remedies"; and Chapter 18, "N: Now You Have a Remedy")

➤ Garlic (see more in Chapter 7, "B Well")

➤ Clove (see more in Chapter 21, "T: Terrific Solutions"; and Chapter 26, "An Herbal First Aid Kit")

➤ Cascara sagrada (see more in Chapter 8, "C's for a Common Cure")

➤ Black Walnut (see more in Chapter 11)

Any combinations of these herbs can serve as an internal fumigation for your parasites! Not all of these are safe for use if pregnant or nursing, so see the contraindications listed back in Chapter 4, "Herbs Are Not Just for Hippies Anymore," before utilizing these herbs.

Sage Advice

If you and your physician cannot pinpoint the exact cause of your ailments, consider a parasite infection.

Premenstrual Syndrome (PMS)

Premenstrual syndrome encompasses a variety of symptoms, which is why it is referred to as a syndrome. Symptoms of PMS include irritability, moodiness, nausea, bloating, cramping, facial break-outs, swollen abdomen or breasts, and tension. These symptoms are usually caused by an overproduction of estrogen and a lack of progesterone production, which is caused by unknown reasons. (We have to keep those men guessing don't we?) Actually, since the liver has the job of filtering excess estrogens from the blood, a couple capsules of milk thistle added to your daily herb program can help. Milk thistle cleanses and boosts a sluggish liver and can help keep your hormones balanced.

Several herbs listed in this book can help you during any of these symptoms. For instance, see Chapter 5, "A Is for Ailment," for acne; Chapter 18 for nausea; and

Chapter 17 for menstrual troubles. Here we will address an herb used to help tame the wild feelings and tension that accompany PMS symptoms.

Wild Yam to Tame a Wild Woman

Wild yam (*Dioscorea villosa*) is another one of God's gifts to women. This herb has been misunderstood by some; it can be confused with the potato-like vegetable tuber, sometimes called sweet potatoes or candied yams that are served at many holiday dinners. Wild yam is different from these vegetables; although the herb is a root, too, it is derived from a tropical vine found in Mexico.

The Japanese discovered that they could derive steroid components from the wild Mexican yam species and process them many times to create steroid drugs. Drugs derived from the wild yam include oral birth control pills and corticosteroids. (However, if you really don't want to get pregnant ladies, don't rely on wild yam as a viable birth control!)

A component in wild yam called diosgenin is a hormone-like substance that acts like progesterone in the body. *Progesterone* is a female hormone that helps keep estrogen in check. When progesterone and estrogen are in the right balance in the body, women do not experience PMS symptoms.

Botanical Bit

Progesterone is a hormone made in the ovaries that helps keep estrogen levels in balance within the body to create harmony. If progesterone levels drop for some reason (menopause, PMS, and other unknown causes), there is nothing to keep estrogen in balance. The result is experienced as the cranky symptoms of estrogen overload—otherwise known as PMS.

This is why supplementing with wild yam during your usual PMS time can be helpful. This herb taken 10 days to two weeks before menstruation can ease PMS symptoms by assisting a hormonal balance. Wild yam is also used to relax muscle tissue, which can help ease menstrual cramps. Consider supplementing with wild yam if you have any spasmodic conditions in the muscles because this herb may be able to ease the pain associated with tension and cramping. Two capsules taken three times daily have been helpful for many, but dosage is always an individual thing.

A PMS Plan

Evening primrose oil contains hormone-like substances and has also been helpful as a supplement for PMS suffers. My recommendation is that you try wild yam or evening primrose oil separately. If one doesn't seem to work for you, try the other. How many tablets or capsules you take will depend on your body and will differ for everyone. If you are not working with an herbalist or practitioner who can guide you, read the label on the bottle and start there.

Cleansing the bowel can help take away that bloated feeling you get when PMS-ing. Also, B-complex tablets will help your body rid itself of excess water and should be considered as a daily supplement; you can increase your intake during PMS times.

Here are some helpful tips in keeping you more steady during your cycle:

➤ Supplement with wild yam or evening primrose oil capsules 10 days before your scheduled period, or try the combination listed in the table at the end of the chapter.

➤ Avoid excess salt in the diet, which can cause water retention and lead to bloating and irritability.

➤ Take extra B-complex vitamins to help get rid of excess water.

➤ Avoid fatty foods such as dairy products. These can actually have a change on your own hormones, so eat more vegetables, fruits, and grains.

➤ Try reflexology. This therapy has been studied extensively for its effectiveness on PMS symptoms.

Also keep your blood sugar in check; fluctuating blood sugar levels (see Chapter 13, "H: Happy Healing with Herbs," on hypoglycemia) caused by sugar consumption and a weak liver (see the same chapter under hepatitis for more on the liver) can cause a person to be irritable with or without PMS.

Pneumonia: Clearing Up Quick with Horseradish

Pneumonia is an inflammation of the lung(s) causing chest pain, difficulty breathing, and coughing. The air sacs in the lungs can become filled with pus, which hardens the lungs. Bacteria generally causes this illness, which means that your lungs can be more prone to pneumonia if you are exposed to air pollution on a constant basis.

Horseradish (*Armoracia rusticana*) makes an excellent herb to use for any ailments of the respiratory tract. Horseradish is extremely hot—if you don't believe me, taste a spoonful of the condiment. You won't get it far from your nose before you can tell what a pungent herb this is.

Because of its strong, pungent odor, horseradish is used in small quantities and will usually be found mixed with other herbs used for the respiratory system, including fenugreek and mullein. Horseradish has also been helpful for bronchitis, catarrh, coughs, flu, and hay fever.

Of course, anything that aids your other eliminatory systems, such as bowel cleansing, will aid your respiratory system as well. An old home remedy for pneumonia (the same home remedy for earaches) includes the use of a baked onion on the chest. See Chapter 10, "E: Everywhere an Herb, Herb," for this home remedy and for more details on using onion.

Poison Ivy

Horseradish should not be used directly on the skin, as its volatile, essential oils can cause a burn. It should be taken internally in small doses only; in large quantities, this herb can make you vomit. Also, people with an underactive thyroid should not use horseradish.

Prostate Trouble: The Pressure Is On

Prostate trouble usually comes in the form of an enlarged prostate gland, which is the small, donut-shaped gland surrounding the neck of the bladder in males. *Prostatitis* is an inflammation of the prostate gland due to a bacteria infection. Either can cause difficulty with urination and may interrupt sexual function.

How can you tell if you could have prostate trouble? Here's a list of the most common symptoms:

➤ A need to urinate often, especially in the middle of the night

➤ A weak or interrupted urinary stream

➤ A feeling that you cannot empty your bladder completely

➤ A feeling of delay or hesitation when you start to urinate

➤ A feeling that you must urinate right away

➤ Continuing pain in the lower back, pelvis, or upper thighs

He Saw Palmetto and Was Cured

If you tell almost anyone who knows anything about herbs these days (even a complete idiot) that you have prostate trouble, you won't be surprised to hear about the herb saw palmetto (*Serenoa serrulata*). Saw palmetto berries are used as a tonic to all the glands in the body and also prove helpful as a diuretic. These berries have been used not only for prostate problems, but also for respiratory ailments, diabetes, nerve problems, and digestive trouble.

In addition, this herb helps those who wish to put on weight, and it has been observed that animals that munch on these berries in the wild get plump!

Besides being helpful for the prostate gland, saw palmetto is also used for asthma, bladder health, chronic bronchitis, head colds, gonorrhea, impotence, kidney disease, lung congestion, neuralgia, and sterility.

Women use this herb for breast problems, frigidity, hot flashes, gonorrhea, reproductive organs, sexual stimulation, and urinary problems.

> **Sage Advice**
>
> Saw palmetto is also a well-known aphrodisiac—added to damiana, it makes a powerful remedy to help both men and women get back that loving feeling.

Herbs for Prostate Health

Although saw palmetto has been one of the best-known herbs for men suffering from prostate conditions, a few more can prove useful as well. Because zinc is a mineral that is carried in the prostate, this gland may need some more for replenishment. An herbal source of zinc is pumpkin seeds—or, you can eat raw pumpkin seeds, but you'll have to eat a lot of them and chew them well to get enough zinc to help correct your problem.

Nettle is another excellent male tonic (listed earlier in this chapter) because it has astringent-like effects on the tissues. It not only can help tighten swollen or inflamed tissues, but it also provides lots of minerals to nourish your body. Siberian ginseng is another overall body tonic, and grape seed and/or pine bark extract are powerful antioxidants for the prostate and other tissues of the body.

If you are suffering from an enlarged prostate, cut back on your coffee intake, get some exercise, and do some bowel cleansing. These can all enhance your herbal program and get you back into shape.

Herbal Remedies for Common Ailments

Osteoporosis

Best Single Herb: Nettle

Best Combinations: Alfalfa, marshmallow, plantain, horsetail, oatstraw, wheat grass, hops; liquid chlorophyll; sarsaparilla (for hormonal balance); wild yam

Other Helpful Supplements: Food enzymes with hydrochloric acid (especially a protein digestive aid); Omega-3 oils; and vitamin D

Possible Causes: Improper digestion; mineral imbalance; calcium deficiency

Complementary Help: Eat raw honey; don't drink distilled water; avoid meat, carbonated beverages, citrus fruits, and coffee; juice carrots and celery, eat powdered goat's whey (add to juices), nuts, seeds, and fresh fish (salmon)

Pancreatitis

Best Single Herb: Cedar berries

Best Combinations: Golden seal, juniper berry, uva ursi, cedar berries, mullein, yarrow, garlic, slippery elm, capsicum, dandelion, marshmallow, nettle, white oak, licorice

Other Helpful Supplements: Calcium/magnesium; B-complex vitamins

Possible Causes: Virus; injury; malnutrition; alcoholism; scar tissue

Complementary Help: Support digestion (see Chapter 9, "D Best Herbal Solutions," for diabetes; see Chapter 13 for hypoglycemia)

Parasites

Best Single Herb: Wormwood

Best Combinations: Elecampane, mugwort (*Artemisia vulgaris*), spearmint, turmeric, ginger, garlic, clove, wormwood (*Artemisia absinthium*); cascara sagrada; black walnut

Other Helpful Supplements: Acidophilus; food enzymes with hydrochloric acid

Possible Causes: Poor stomach acid; problems with the drinking water; transfer from food or pets

Complementary Help: Wash fruits and vegetables thoroughly; cleanse the bowel; avoid sugar

continues

261

Herbal Remedies for Common Ailments   (continued)

Premenstrual Syndrome (PMS)

Best Single Herb: Wild yam

Best Combinations: Wild yam; evening primrose oil; red raspberry, dong quai, ginger, licorice, black cohosh, queen of the meadow, blessed thistle, marshmallow

Other Helpful Supplements: B-complex vitamins; calcium/magnesium with vitamin D

Possible Causes: Constipation; water retention; hypoglycemia; stressed liver

Complementary Help: Avoid fatty foods; reflexology; acupuncture; cleansing the bowel

Pneumonia

Best Single Herb: Horseradish

Best Combinations: Boneset, fennel, fenugreek, horseradish, mullein; lobelia (for coughing); garlic (for infection)

Other Helpful Supplements: Beta carotene or vitamin A; zinc; vitamin E with selenium

Possible Causes: Overexposure to respiratory pollutants or irritants (chemicals, dusts, fumes); smoking

Complementary Help: Cleanse the bowel; diffuse essential oil of oregano or eucalyptus oil; place a baked onion on the chest

Prostate Trouble

Best Single Herb: Saw palmetto

Best Combinations: Saw palmetto; nettles; Siberian ginseng; pumpkin seeds; grape seed or pine bark extract

Other Helpful Supplements: Zinc; vitamin E with selenium

Possible Causes: Constipation; lack of exercise; caffeine abuse

Complementary Help: Bowel cleansing

The Least You Need to Know

➤ Nettle is an herb rich in minerals and can be useful in the prevention of osteoporosis.

➤ Cedar berries are used to help counteract inflammation in the body.

➤ Parasites can be killed and naturally removed by the body using herbs of the Artemisia family, garlic, black walnut, cloves, and elecampane.

➤ Wild yam works to ease PMS symptoms by helping keep estrogen levels in check.

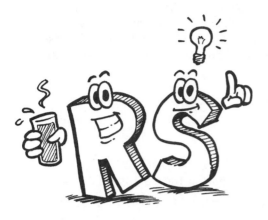

Chapter 20

R and S: For Remarkable Recoveries and Super Solutions

In This Chapter

➤ What to do for radiation poisoning

➤ Why calendula can be useful for shingles

➤ Thyme's potency to aid recovery from sinusitis

➤ Why lobelia might help you stop smoking

➤ One of the best herbs used to ease stress

"In nature there are neither rewards nor punishments—there are consequences." —Robert G. Ingersoll (1833–1899), American lawyer and agnostic. *Lectures & Essays,* "Some Reasons Why"

Nature is neutral. She has her laws. If they are obeyed, then the consequence is good health. If ignored, the consequence is ill health. Fortunately, Mother Nature also provides solutions to help get us back on track when we have ignored her laws of healthy living. Herbs are part of that solution. This chapter will address some habits that disobey nature's laws, such as smoking, stressful lifestyles, and exposure to radiation, all of which can have harmful consequences. Now let's see what we can do about these things and other ailments.

Radiation Poisoning

Fortunately, radiation poisoning or sickness is not such a common problem. This sickness is usually associated with radiation treatments for cancer or some other type of deliberate exposure to radiation on a continual basis. Symptoms of this fatal sickness usually include diarrhea, nausea or vomiting, and noted changes in blood chemistry.

Radiation is a general term meaning "to radiate," which in physics is the term for the emission and movement of waves through space. This section is intended to help you detox your body from the general radiation many of us are exposed to daily. These herbal remedies can also help you before you can get medical treatment if you experience a serious exposure to radiation.

These are some examples of being exposed to radiation:

➤ Having diagnostic X-rays taken at the dentist, doctor, or chiropractor offices; at hospitals; and elsewhere

➤ Working in any of these offices, whether you take the X-rays or not

➤ Undergoing radiation treatments for cancer

➤ Repeatedly or continually exposing yourself to microwave ovens, such as when working in a restaurant or a food store

➤ Living near a nuclear testing site where there is a danger of nuclear fall-out

➤ Living or working next to or near power plants

➤ Consistently exposing yourself to irradiated foods (foods such as meats that have been blasted with rays for preservation purposes) or crops exposed to fall-out or other radioactive pollutants

➤ Excessive airplane travel

Poison Ivy

Do not try to treat yourself with herbs or home remedies if you have radiation poisoning—you could die. If you are suffering from serious exposure to radiation, seek competent medical help, and use the suggestions here until you can get to a doctor.

If you have some daily exposure to any of these forms of radiation, you can use herbs and supplements for daily protection. You should also consider detoxing each month or every other week, just for prevention's sake. If nothing else, it can make you feel refreshed and clean, and it may just help you prevent long-term damage.

Algin: You're Soaking in It

Algin is a component in the seaweed herb kelp (see Chapter 21, "T: Terrific Solutions," for more on kelp), which makes algin very "kelpful." You can take kelp if you cannot find the supplement algin, but because algin is the concentrated substance found in kelp, this herb has been proven useful in radiation exposure; you will need to take more kelp than you would an extracted algin supplement.

Botanical Bit

Strontium 90 is a radioactive substance harmful to the body. It can accumulate in food substances high in calcium; when you ingest the food, the calcium that is used by your bones will carry the pollutant to the bones, where it will damage your bone marrow. The algin found in brown kelp can help block this absorption.

Algin is very effective in eliminating the body of toxic materials such as radioactive *Strontium 90*, mercury, barium, tin, cadmium, and excess zinc. The algin is a non-digestible fiber and protects the body from absorbing these poisons by attracting and then grabbing hold of the toxic materials, and then excreting them from the body via the bowel and urinary tract. There are no dangers in taking this kelp extract, either, which makes it an excellent daily supplement for those who are continually exposed to forms of radiation.

If you have been exposed to radiation of any kind, soak in a bathtub with algin and/or Epson salt added to the bath water. I would also take four capsules of algin every four hours or so if this was the only supplement I was taking. Other supplements can help speed up or enhance the effects of the algin by working synergistically—let's take a look at a few more.

Other X-Rated Cures

Exposure to anything toxic will increase the amount of free radicals in your body. The best way to protect your body from the effects of free radical damage is to supplement with antioxidant vitamins and herbs.

Some of the main vitamins, herbs, and minerals used for their antioxidant-boosting abilities include:

➤ Vitamin C (try to find one with extra citrus bioflavonoids)

➤ Vitamin E (with selenium, a trace mineral that enhances the vitamin)

➤ Beta carotene (or vitamin A—your body will synthesize vitamin A from beta carotene in the liver, and beta carotene is safer to take in larger doses)

➤ Zinc (not too much—25 to 50 mg daily only, unless prescribed by your doctor)

➤ Red clover (contains much of the antioxidant properties found in vitamin E)

➤ Grape seed extract or pine bark extract, found together or separately (more potent than vitamin C or E as an antioxidant)

Sage Advice

Your thyroid gland is specifically vulnerable to radiation, and protection of the thyroid is critical when dealing with radiation. See Chapter 21 for more on the functions of your thyroid and to learn one of the favorite herbs used by those with thyroid problems.

Utilizing liquid chlorophyll in your daily water intake and taking a liquid aloe vera will also protect your cells from the effects of radiation exposure.

Shingles: Better on Your Roof

Shingles is an ailment that usually strikes middle-age women and men, but it is especially common and can be more harmful in those with weak immune systems and the elderly. This ailment is recognized as a severely itchy or painful red rash that appears across the trunk of the body and sometimes on the face. Most of the time this rash lasts about three weeks until the blistered scabs heal. However, in some with particularly weak immune systems, the problem may linger for months and can lead to nerve pain that can continue for years.

Shingles is related to the chicken pox and herpes virus (all of the same family). It is thought that the chicken pox virus lurks in the body inactive for decades; when we experience a crisis or other major stress in mid-life that causes the immune system to become vulnerable, the virus then resurfaces as shingles. Therefore, when working with shingles, you will need to take into consideration herbs that nourish your nervous system (see the section "S-T-R-E-S-S: That's the Way We Spell Success," later in this chapter; also see the section "Anxiety: Panic Not—Herbs to the Rescue," in Chapter 6, "Give Me Another A!"). You will want to boost your immune system with herbs to help fight off the virus and to help you recover.

Calendula: Scratching the Itch

Calendula (*Calendula officinalis*) is an excellent herb to help you with your painful rash because it has properties that make it work as an anti-inflammatory, anti-fungal, antiseptic, anti-spasmodic, a sedative, and an astringent. Sounds like it can ease that itch, doesn't it?

Make a poultice or fomentation from the flowers of the calendula plant and apply it directly to your rash to help with inflammation and itching. Although I have never had shingles, I have used calendula topically for other skin ailments to prevent infection with success. An old saying states something to the effect of, wherever calendula is, no puss will form. Calendula then, may help prevent your shingle blisters from becoming infected.

When taken internally in small doses, calendula works as a sedative and thus may help ease the stress and tension that brought out your shingles in the first place. You will usually find calendula flowers in topical applications at the health food stores. This herb also may be an ingredient in some herbal combinations, or as a homeopathic ingredient, or you might find the flowers in bulk. I would follow this lead and use calendula topically or in a homeopathic form. Then consider some of the herbs we'll discuss next for internal use.

Sage Advice

A vitamin E oil capsule that's punctured and applied topically to a rash or any other skin wound during the healing process has proven useful in preventing scarring.

Nervous System Support

White willow bark has been used for pain—remember, this was the herb that aspirin was derived from. A good mixture of eight herbs that can help the pain associated with shingles is listed in the table at the end of this chapter. B-complex vitamins also will feed the nervous system, and the amino acid l-lysine has been reported to help suppress the herpes virus and makes it of value in fighting a shingles outbreak.

Take a calcium and magnesium supplement to help your muscles relax and to accelerate tissue healing once your rash begins to clear. Acidophilus supplementation or eating extra yogurt with live acidophilus cultures will help you absorb your nutrients better and will aid in boosting your immune system, too. See more tips for fighting herpes in the section "Cold Sore No More (Herpes Simplex)," in Chapter 8, "C's for a Common Cure."

Sinusitis: Sniffing Out a Cure

Sinusitis is the inflammation of the sinus passages. Symptoms include headache, clogged nose, inability to breathe through the nose, pressure in the sinuses, a runny or dripping nose, and post nasal drip, causing an irritated throat.

Sinusitis is usually caused by an allergy, which causes the sinuses to react by sneezing and producing mucus. The allergy can then lead to a localized infection, causing more irritation to the sinus passages that can then be called sinusitis. Make sure you boost your immune system when dealing with sinusitis, and be sure to read the section "Allergies Bee Gone," in Chapter 5, "A Is for Ailment," for more. Until then, you can use a little thyme to clear your head. Let's talk about the best use of thyme next.

Thyme for a Solution

Thyme (pronounced *time*) (*Thymus vulgaris*) is an excellent herb that has been used in a variety of herbal combinations for boosting the immune system. This herb has been especially helpful in ailments of the respiratory system (sinuses, lungs, and bronchials). Thyme is used as a spice in soups, stews, chili, and other foods and helps you digest fats. This herb is not recommended in high doses for pregnant women, but having some as a spice in your food should be safe for you. A little bit is also an excellent and safe remedy for children with colds and the flu.

I have seen fenugreek and thyme stop a runny nose within 20 minutes after ingestion, so thyme's anti-bacterial and antiseptic properties might be just the thing your body needs to kill off your sinus infection. Don't be surprised, however, if you experience a temporary increase in mucus leaving your sinus cavities or lungs; thyme is an expectorant and will help your body rid itself of excess mucus through the lungs. Thyme may also be useful for combating shingles because it helps boost the immune system.

Poison Ivy

Thyme should not be taken in large doses if you are pregnant. Also, it is better to acquire your thyme from a reputable manufacturer because picking your own can be dangerous—the different species of thyme can vary in potency by 10,000 times.

Herb Lore

Thyme is interesting in that its effects will change depending on how much you take. For example, taking tiny amounts of the herb will create a sedating effect and can relax you and help you get the rest you need when you are sick. However, larger doses act as a stimulant and may make you feel more energetic to pull you through the day. Thyme has also been used for bronchitis, colds, colic, digestion, fevers, gas, hysteria, infections, menstrual cramps, nightmares, skin conditions, toothaches, and whooping cough.

Sinus Up for More Herbs

Other herbs useful to the respiratory system and sinuses include golden seal, yerba santa, and ephedra. See the table at the end of this chapter for a good combination of herbs and some vitamins that will aid your recovery.

Sage Advice

Reflexology points to help break up sinus congestion and relieve pain associated with sinusitis include all fingers and toes. You can place reflexology clips temporarily on your fingers or toes to stimulate these reflexes, or use your fingers and squeeze these areas for relief. Consult *The Complete Idiot's Guide to Reflexology* (Alpha Books, 1999), for more on this topic.

When suffering from a sinus infection, stop eating or drinking products that create more mucus in your body. Eliminate wheat, dairy, and sugar while fighting your infection, and avoid any foods that cause mucus for you. Also, bowel cleansing can help eliminate respiratory congestion—see the section "Constipation: All Dressed Up and Nowhere to Go," in Chapter 8 for a great cleansing drink.

Smoking—Quitting

When I first pleaded with my grandmother to stop smoking, she exclaimed, "But I thought you enjoyed my cooking!" So much for getting what you ask for. Although eating burnt food is not particularly pleasant, puffing on a cigarette is more detrimental to your health and to the health of those around you.

Most of us ex-smokers or never-been-smokers know what the hazards of smoking are already, so those of you can skip this part. If you are a smoker, however, here are some reasons to quit—just in case you weren't aware. Smoking:

➤ Increases the risk of lung, throat, tongue, and mouth cancers

➤ Increases the risk of arteriosclerosis and other heart and circulatory diseases

➤ Exposes you to about 2,000 chemicals for every puff you take

➤ Discolors your fingers, teeth, and skin

➤ Deadens skin tone, color, and elasticity

➤ Makes you stink, even when you are not smoking

➤ Increases risk for respiratory infections such as bronchitis, pneumonia, and emphysema

➤ Decreases oxygen supply in the blood and to the brain and can cloud thinking

➤ Wrinkles the skin around the lips, causing you to appear older

➤ Decreases the general health of those around you

As you can see, there are plenty of reasons why you might want to kick the habit. First, let's talk about a few reasons you might be smoking. Then we'll talk about some herbs that might give you the physical support to help you through your withdrawal.

Slaying the Fire-Breathing Dragon

Of course, the first step toward breaking the smoking habit is the desire to quit! Nothing can force you to quit if you don't *want* to quit. However, a dramatic positive addition to your life—such as cleansing the body with herbs and incorporating a wholesome diet, vigorous exercise, or fasting—can make the thought of a cigarette unpleasing and even repulsive to you.

To illustrate, here's a story of a client who claimed to be upset with me. She said that the herbal program we designed for her made her feel much better. She claimed to no longer be constipated. Her skin was clear, and her energy had picked up dramatically. She had even lost those few extra pounds that she had not been able to lose for years. I couldn't understand why she was upset with all these positive things that she had earned.

Then she told me that she had to give up smoking because of the herbs. She used to be an occasional smoker, but after she started her program, she became nauseous after smoking half of a cigarette. Finally, she couldn't smoke a few puffs without becoming ill. She said she was "forced" to give up the cigarettes completely and that she did not know what to do with her hands during social situations because she was so used to holding a cigarette!

The reasons people smoke vary—some started out of peer pressure, as young adults and the habit is ingrained. Others feed their need to be loved and nourished through the physical mechanics of smoking cigarettes, and still others say they "need" cigarettes to feel relaxed. Well, if you're ready to quit smoking cigarettes or to give up chewing tobacco, a wonder herb can help you break the habit and recover from the side effects—not to mention serve as a much less toxic way to feed the nervous system. Let's talk about this herb next.

Poison Ivy

Lobelia is not recommended for people in weak conditions, people who are prone to fainting, or people who have blood pressure problems. Lobelia is considered poisonous by the FDA, so be cautious and use it with discretion so that we can keep this valuable herb to help ourselves when we need it.

Sage Advice

The herb lobelia is an emetic, which means that it can make you vomit, so go lightly when ingesting it. Remember these common names for lobelia to remind you to not take too much: pukeweed, gagroot, and vomitwort.

Lobelia: Put That in Your Pipe and Smoke It

Lobelia (*Lobelia inflata* or *Lobelia siphilitica*) (pronounced *low-beel-ya*) is an herb tried and true for helping many smokers quit. The species Lobelia inflata is the herb you will most likely see spelled out on herb bottles, as it has less of the emetic (vomit-inducing) quality than the other relative, Lobelia siphilitica. We have already discussed some of lobelia's usefulness for asthma in Chapter 6 and as an emetic for food poisoning in Chapter 11, "F: Fantastic Healing Flora." However, this herb really is tops when it comes to quitting and recovering from cigarette smoking and tobacco chewing. This is probably because lobelia contains the active ingredient lobeline, which is almost identical to nicotine and has similar effects on the nervous system. However, lobelia has none of the toxic side effects that cigarettes have on the body.

If you continue to smoke while taking lobelia, the smoking could make you feel ill while on this herb. Lobelia is a strong herb and is not meant for daily use over long periods of time; it is more useful to relieve acute conditions over a fairly short period of time. Try one capsule a day, or one capsule twice a day, to help you quit. If this is not helping, increase by one capsule, and see how you do.

After you quit, lobelia can be used for a couple of weeks to help your lungs eliminate excess tar and mucus, to calm the nerves, and to help your body rejuvenate.

S-T-R-E-S-S: That's the Way We Spell Success

Who hasn't heard of stress these days? It seems to enter our vocabulary daily. One definition of stress is mental or emotional pressure. This is stress you can't see, but your body still knows it's there. Unfortunately, stress is not always caused by negative things, such as work-related stress, or bad-relationship stress, or car-trouble-induced stress. In fact, some of the top related stresses are good things.

Read over these examples of some positive things that cause a great deal of stress in our lives, if you have more than two or three of these things going on at once, you could benefit from extra stress-reducing herbs and supplements:

➤ Weddings

➤ A new marriage

➤ Travel

➤ A move to a new home—even when it is your dream home!

➤ A promotion at work

➤ A new baby

➤ High goals you set for yourself and then work toward

➤ Starting your own business, and being successful

➤ Retirement preparations

Needless to say, the universe has a way of keeping in balance, and along with the positive things that come your way, you can be sure you'll experience negative side effects from stress to make up for it. Stress is linked to a host of related ailments and can make your immune system more vulnerable to other illness. If you are overburdened with good or bad things in your life that are causing you stress, take some time to sip the herbal tea.

Chamomile for Soothing the Right Nerve

Chamomile (*Matricaria recutita*) is one of the safest and most effective herbs to use to gently calm your nerves and ease stress. It has been used successfully to calm intestinal cramps; ease colic, indigestion, stress, and ulcers; and ease restlessness. What's more, this herb is safe enough to be shared by pregnant and nursing moms and babies.

Herb Lore

Recently, a nursing mom asked me about what she could do for her colicky baby. I told her about the soothing effects of chamomile, and she sipped a couple cups of tea before breast-feeding her baby that evening. The next day she told me that she hadn't slept so well in weeks—and her baby woke up only once during the night!

Chamomile flowers are used as a hair rinse for blond hair to help keep the hair's color. This herb, also called wild pineapple or ground apple, grows low to the ground and gives off a wonderful smell—similar to pineapple—when picked fresh. I find it interesting that wild chamomile grows in areas such as driveways and where people walk constantly—I have always found it under my feet, literally. I have a theory, based on

Poison Ivy

Although chamomile is considered a very safe herb, a small percentage of folks may be allergic to it. The people who have a severe sensitivity to ragweed seem to be the most vulnerable.

Sage Advice

Kava kava has been used as a staple herb in the Pacific Islands for more than 3,000 years to ease anxiety. Kavalactones, the active ingredient in this herb, serve to relax muscles and sedate the nerves without the toxic side effects that tranquilizers can have. Several studies have shown that kava actually increases mental mood and alertness, while creating a euphoric-type state.

the doctrine of signatures, that chamomile grows in areas where it receives much abuse or stress, and that is what makes it such a good herbal remedy for this condition!

Researchers have found that a plant's medicinal parts are actually part of the plant's own immune system. When a plant is attacked, such as when its leaves are plucked or when it's trampled on, the medicinal qualities actually get stronger. So, maybe the chamomile that is trampled on will serve as a more potent stress-relieving remedy than a chamomile that is pampered. I don't know for sure, but, as always, there are many thoughts to ponder while sipping that nice, relaxing cup of chamomile tea. Ahhh!

More De-Stressing Solutions

Plenty of remedies in the herbal kingdom can help ease your mind and body. Passion flower and hops are also favorites. (See more on hops in Chapter 6 in the section "Anxiety: Panic Not—Herbs to the Rescue.") The B-complex vitamins are always helpful as well because your body utilizes more of these B vitamins when under stress.

Add some adaptogen herbs that help your body adapt to stress if you are feeling worn-out due to lifestyle. Suma, astragalus, ginseng, and gotu kola are all excellent herbal tonics that can help pull you back together after a stressful period or keep you going through the rough times. Avoid taking these herbs just before bed, however, because they can keep you awake.

Other great therapies that are helpful to many with stress include massage, aromatherapy, reflexology, meditation, and exercise.

Herbal Remedies for Common Ailments

Radiation

Best Single Herb: Algin

Best Combinations: Algin or kelp; bee pollen; aloe vera; liquid chlorophyll

Other Helpful Supplements: All antioxidants; CoQ_{10}; amino acids

Possible Causes: Radiated foods; repeated X-ray exposure; continual microwave exposure; nuclear fall-out

Complementary Help: Epson salt bath

Shingles

Best Single Herb: Calendula

Best Combinations: White willow bark, black cohosh, capsicum, valerian, ginger, hops, wood betony, devil's claw; elecampane; licorice root; uña de gato

Other Helpful Supplements: B-complex vitamins; acidophilus; l-lysine or all essential amino acids; calcium/magnesium with vitamin D; vitamins A and D; zinc; trace minerals

Possible Causes: Stress; anxiety; low immune system

Complementary Help: Calendula fomentation; vitamin E oil applied externally when healing to prevent scarring; stress reduction (See Chapter 8 for more on cold sores, as shingles belongs to the same herpes family.)

Sinusitis

Best Single Herb: Thyme

Best Combinations: Fenugreek, thyme; burdock, golden seal, parsley, althea, ephedra, capsicum, horehound, yerba santa; bee pollen; bayberry

Other Helpful Supplements: Vitamin A or beta carotene; vitamin C; pantothenic acid

Possible Causes: Old catarrh; lowered immune system; body trying to cleanse old bacteria

Complementary Help: Cleanse bowel; take golden seal "snuff"; avoid dairy and sugar (see Chapter 5 for more on allergies); use self-help with reflexology, squeeze the toes and fingers firmly

Smoking, Quitting

Best Single Herb: Lobelia

Best Combinations: Lobelia, St. John's wort; black cohosh, capsicum, valerian, passion flower, scullcap, hops, wood betony; liquid chlorophyll

Other Helpful Supplements: All antioxidants

Possible Causes: Nervousness; not feeling nourished or loved emotionally; addiction

Complementary Help: Vigorous exercise; herbal cleansing or fasting to clear all toxins from body and eradicate cravings

Stress

Best Single Herb: Chamomile

Best Combinations: Chamomile, passion flower, hops, fennel, marshmallow, feverfew; suma, astragalus, Siberian ginseng, ginkgo biloba, gotu kola

Other Helpful Supplements: B-complex vitamins

Possible Causes: Lifestyle

Complementary Help: Massage; reflexology; stress management; chamomile eye pillow; chamomile tea

The Least You Need to Know

➤ Algin can be used to rid the body of toxic chemicals.

➤ Calendula is used as an anti-inflammatory herb and may help ease the pain associated with shingles when applied topically.

➤ Thyme is a powerful and useful herb used for many respiratory ailments.

➤ Lobelia can help break the smoking habit.

➤ Chamomile is a safe and effective herb used to calm the nervous system.

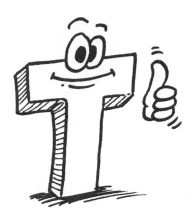

Chapter 21

T: Terrific Solutions

> ## In This Chapter
>
> ➤ Herbs used topically to deaden tooth pain
>
> ➤ An herbal poultice to ease tendonitis
>
> ➤ Help ringing in the ears with herbs
>
> ➤ An herb that stimulates the thyroid
>
> ➤ An essential oil to help tonsillitis

"I watched what method Nature might take, with intention of subduing the symptom by treading in her footsteps." —Thomas Sydenham (1624–1689) *Medical Observations*

Nature has an intelligence that we can learn from. When we are ill, our bodies react in certain ways. A careful observer can recognize how the body works to cure us and then utilize herbs that assist the body in that process.

This next chapter will teach you about how to take care of some common problems beginning with the letter T. Ironically, most of the things we'll discuss are from the neck up and include the teeth, the thyroid, the tonsils, and ringing in the ears! Let's get on with it so you can get some herbal "T" for your problems.

A Toothful Solution

Having problems with your teeth is no fun. First and foremost, of course, you need to have proper hygiene habits, such as brushing after meals and flossing at least once per day. Second, regular dental check-ups and cleanings will help you keep your oral health in top condition.

Some people are afraid to go to the dentist, but it is better to go more frequently—especially if you are worried—because the sooner your dentist can catch a problem, the easier it will be to fix for both of you. Letting cavities, cracks, and receding gum lines go unattended can only lead to more serious problems requiring much more time in the dental chair. A cavity now could require a crown or even a root canal farther down the line. So be sure that you stay on top of your oral health, and then use these herbal remedies for your internal environment and help you in emergencies when you can't get to your dentist right away.

Numbing Tooth Pain with Cloves

Clove (*Eugenia caryophyllata*) is a very powerful aromatic herb that has been used for thousands of years as a pain-killer. The dried flower buds have been used to numb pain, to kill bacteria and parasites, and to help expel mucus. Topically, clove oil is the best application to numb the pain of a toothache. Rub a small amount around the tooth that is bothering you as a topical analgesic, and call your dentist to have the underlying problem corrected.

If you have a child who is teething, a drop of diluted clove oil can be applied to your finger and rubbed onto your baby's gums. Use only a small amount of this oil, and dilute it first with olive oil (1 part clove oil to about 20 parts olive oil). Do not give clove oil to babies internally, however—cloves are extremely powerful and need to be used with caution, especially the concentrated essential oil. Too much can be toxic for adults, and it is too strong for babies internally. It can give children nausea or headaches. See Chapter 26, "An Herbal First Aid Kit," for more on the uses of the essential oil of cloves. Birch or peppermint oil placed on gums in this same manner can be used as a substitute for clove oil for teething babies or toothaches.

Sage Advice

Ask your hygienist to show you how to brush correctly—believe it or not, there are right and wrong ways of brushing. You can even damage your gums by using the wrong type of brush! Don't be embarrassed to ask for clarity; your hygienist will be happy to instruct you on the proper ways to brush and floss.

Poison Ivy

Use caution when using clove oil on yourself—and especially with babies. This concentrated oil is extremely powerful and could make you very sick when used in excess.

More to Chew On

Because your teeth are bones and are considered part of your overall structural system, herbs and supplements that will support your overall structural system can also strengthen and nourish your teeth. For instance, a calcium and magnesium supplement that includes vitamin D is one of the best minerals you can feed your bones. Vitamin C with extra citrus bioflavonoids will also help you absorb calcium and nourish the tissues that surround your teeth. Alfalfa is another excellent herb that is rich in organic minerals, and liquid chlorophyll (the blood of the alfalfa plant) will help you keep calcium in the body, where it belongs!

If you are having lots of dental caries (cavities) despite your great oral hygiene, then consider your nutrition. To help you with a tooth infection, try garlic. When you have a tooth abscess, the infection can be spread throughout your blood stream and can cause you to feel ill. The garlic will help fight off the bad bacteria and will keep your immune system fighting. But, for your dentist's sake, take an enterically coated garlic tablet instead of chewing the raw cloves!

For tooth pain, until you can get to your dentist, try this combination: white willow bark, valerian, wild lettuce, and capsicum. These are great for relaxing you (pain usually causes tension) and curbing the pain associated with toothaches. For infections of the gums, brush with black walnut powder, or use some myrrh to pack around gums. Herbs used historically to prevent tooth decay include:

Sage Advice

Soda pop creates an acid environment and can wreak havoc on your dental health. Sugary gum and hard candies create an environment for decay to begin. Dried fruit such as raisins and fruit rolls are sticky and can be just as bad for the teeth. Try sugarless snacks instead, and brush and floss after meals.

➤ Wild bergamot (*Monarda fistulosa*) contains the active ingredient (thymol) used in the mouthwash Listerine®, known to kill bacteria in the mouth. This herb also contains geraniol, known as a decay-prevention compound.

➤ Stevia (*Stevia rebaudiana*) is a controversial herb that can be used as a sugar replacement. It is said to be 100 times sweeter than table sugar, so only a pinch is needed to sweeten foods or drinks. Using this herb instead of sugar could help you prevent sugar-induced tooth decay.

➤ Chaparral (*Larrea divaricata*) can be made into a mouthwash and used to prevent tooth decay. This herb contains antiseptic properties and has been used for toothaches in folk medicine for centuries.

➤ Myrrh also contains antiseptic properties and can be used as a mouthwash or dental pack. For more on myrrh, see the section "Gingivitis to Your Party?" in Chapter 12, "G: Great Remedies."

See Chapter 12 for more on herbs for oral health.

Tendonitis

Tendonitis is the inflammation of the tendons, which are the cords of collagen fibers that attach a muscle to a bone. Tendons assist in concentrating the pull of the muscle on a small area of bone. This swelling is usually associated with one specific area due to repeated injuries or overuse of a specific limb. This can happen in sports or work, or in some other type of overactivity or injury.

Usually tendonitis will not require medical treatment because the inflammation will subside with rest. However, when needed, medical treatment usually involves corti-sone shots applied directly to the inflamed area, or administration of other anti-inflammatory drugs. See the section "Fibromyalgia: What a Pain!" in Chapter 11, "F: Fantastic Healing Flora"; the section "Down on Your Knees" in Chapter 15, "J and K: For Just the Right Kind of Cure"; and the section "Arthritis: A Flexible Treatment Plan" in Chapter 6, "Give Me Another A!" for more on herbs that have been used for anti-inflammatory purposes.

Poison Ivy

If you lift free weights as part of a workout routine, tendonitis could cause you a problem. Be sure to work with a competent physical fitness instructor, and get a good tendon warm-up before you begin lifting. These tendons are easily damaged if they're not stretched before lifting a heavier amount of weight.

A Tendency to Ease Pain with Lemongrass

Lemongrass (*Cymbopogon citratus*) is a grassy-looking herb that gives off a fresh, lemony scent. You will find this herb most commonly for sale as an essential oil or as an ingredient in other mixtures of herbs. Lemongrass has been used to kill viruses and bacteria, as well as being used as a digestive tonic and a diuretic. Externally, it has been used to reduce muscle soreness, backaches, and rheumatism pain, and as an insect repellent.

Herb Lore

Lemongrass is an herb native to Southeast Asia and is commonly used in a mixture of spices in Vietnamese and Thai dishes. Use the essential oil of lemongrass to rub directly onto your affected areas. It not only can ease your pain, but will relax you and give you that lemon-fresh scent!

For tendonitis, lemongrass is best used as a topical application. Here are a couple ways you can use this sedative-type herb topically:

➤ Make a poultice and apply it directly to the inflamed area.

➤ Add some dried lemongrass (you can place the herb in a nylon stocking or a coffee filter tied with string to avoid a messy tub) or the essential oil of lemongrass to the bath water. This can be used for overall tendon, muscle, or other structural system-related soreness.

➤ Add the essential oil of lemongrass to your favorite massage lotion and massage it into the inflamed area.

Reducing Inflammation

Licorice root helps the body produce cortisone and is a much safer alternative to try before getting cortisone injections. Uña de gato (cat's claw) has also been useful for its anti-inflammatory properties.

We just talked about the use of cloves as an effective pain-killer for teething and toothaches, but diluted clove oil or birch oil can also be applied to an area with tendonitis to help ease pain. Comfrey leaf poultice is also an effective therapy used with success by many for any type of structural or joint injury, inflammation, and pain. Many herbalists have nicknamed comfrey as the "bone mender" because of its wonderful healing properties. See Chapter 15 for more on comfrey.

Sage Advice

Other supplements such as glucosamine and chondroitin work by building the cross linking of cartilage between joints and can be helpful for many with joint, tendon, and other structural system-related problems.

Tinnitus (Ringing in Ears)

For most of us, a high-pitched temporary ringing in the ears goes unnoticed shortly after it passes, and an occasional ringing in the ears is really nothing to be concerned over. However, many folks have a ringing, whooshing, buzzing, or some other constant sound in one or both ears on a consistent basis. This constant ringing in the ears is called tinnitus, and its causes can be linked to several different conditions.

Possible causes of ringing in the ears can include:

➤ Head trauma that caused damage to the ear drum

➤ Excess wax and debris in the ears (see the section "Earaches," in Chapter 10, "E: Everywhere an Herb, Herb," to find a natural way to have the ears cleaned)

➤ High blood pressure (see the section "Blood Pressure: Easier to Deal with Than Peer Pressure," in Chapter 7, "B Well")

➤ Ear infections caused by fungus (see the section "Fungus Among Us?" in Chapter 11)

➤ Excessive exposure to medications, smoking, or noise

➤ Temporal mandibular joint problems (the joint where the two jaw bones meet); this can sometimes be corrected by a chiropractor

➤ Lack of blood supply to the head area (decreased circulation)

Herb Lore

To try to help you keep your sense of humor while you find the root cause of your problem, I've devised the following questionnaire. How can you tell if you have a problem with tinnitus? (1) Your favorite winter song chorus goes something like this: "Sleigh bells ring, are ya listenin'? In your head, bells are whistlin'." (2) Earrings have a whole new meaning. (3) Every new name you hear rings a bell. (4) You sheepishly ask people, "Is that noise in my head bothering you?"

Discern what your probable cause for your condition is, look up the corresponding chapters related to your base cause, and then work to clear that problem. If you don't have any discernable underlying causes, try some of the remedies here.

Gotu Kola: The Real Un-Cola

Gotu kola (*Centella asiatica*) is another one of my favorite herbs that's similar to ginkgo biloba in its uses as a brain tonic. These two herbs make a powerful team when taken together. Gotu kola is an herb that, like ginkgo biloba (see the section "Alzheimer's Disease: Don't Forget to Take Your Herbs," in Chapter 5, "A Is for Ailment," for more on ginkgo), has an affinity for the brain. This means that it is attracted to and nourishes the brain and nervous system.

Gotu kola has been used as an anti-aging regenerative herb because it is thought to stimulate collagen, increase blood circulation, and help detoxify the body of chemicals. You will see some sodas with a gotu kola or ginseng base in many health food stores, and this is a common sight in Asia.

It is said that gotu kola helps to integrate both hemispheres of the brain—how's that for whole thinking! Gotu kola has been used by those suffering from a nervous breakdown and to help balance and tone the entire glandular system. The old saying about gotu kola sums it up nicely in a catchy phrase that goes something like this: "Gotu kola every day will keep old age away!"

Gotu kola is a favorite food of one of my favorite animals, the wild elephant. The herb is known for its benefits toward longevity and as a brain food. Could munching on this herb be the reason for the long life of an elephant—and the reason why an elephant never forgets?

Poison Ivy

Although gotu kola is a wonderful brain food, too much of a good thing is not necessarily better! In large quantities, gotu kola can give you a headache (too much blood flowing to the brain) or can make you feel itchy, dizzy, or faint.

Other uses for gotu kola include: mental fatigue, nervous breakdowns, fatigue, memory, high blood pressure, concentration, thyroid stimulant, and boosting vitality.

Help for Ringing in the New Ear

Make sure you're getting the right amount of minerals in your diet. If you are unsure, a safe way to get your daily minerals is by supplementing with alfalfa tablets. We all need calcium and magnesium. Vitamin D helps you absorb the calcium. Magnesium should be about two times more than the calcium intake; this mineral helps regulate your blood pressure, which is sometimes an underlying cause of ear ringing. For more on vitamins and minerals, read *The Complete Idiot's Guide to Vitamins and Minerals*.

The B-complex vitamins are nutrients important to brain and circulatory system function, and these should be considered when you have ringing in the ears. Foods rich in the B vitamins include wheat germ, bananas, avocados, most nuts and legumes, and beef liver.

Thyroid Problems: Kelp Is on Its Way

The thyroid gland is a butterfly-shaped gland located in the throat area that straddles your windpipe. This gland is responsible for many functions, including the regulation of your metabolism. Your metabolism is your body's rate of speed, and it regulates your hair, skin, nail, and other body tissue growth, as well as governing weight and fat distribution. In addition, your metabolism is intricately linked to your hormone production balance. Therefore, if the thyroid is not working well, you can have a host of problems.

For help with an underactive thyroid, I strongly recommend kelp. Kelp (*Fucus vesiculosis*) is a seaweed plant that contains a substance called algin (for more on algin, see Chapter 20, "R and S: For Remarkable Recoveries and Super Solutions"). The algin in kelp has been extracted and used to pull radioactive substances and other harmful toxins from the body; the thyroid is particularly sensitive to radioactivity.

Sage Advice

After being faced with taking the synthetic thyroid hormone known as Synthroid®, my clients who have had poor thyroid activity have tried a combination of kelp, Irish moss, parsley, hops, and capsicum instead. This literally changed their thyroid's hormone production, and they have not needed the synthetic drug.

Sage Advice

Kelp is a sea plant and benefits the oceans by soaking in water and filtering it. Much like a clam, its role is to help clean the water. So, when you take kelp to feed your thyroid, you want to make sure it is harvested from non-toxic waters. Make sure that the herb company you buy from has a strict quality control department to screen out potentially toxic kelp.

As a salt water plant, kelp contains a rich amount of iodine (did you ever hear of iodized salt?). The thyroid contains a small amount of iodine, and the natural iodine in kelp can nourish your thyroid gland and help it to function properly. The symptoms of thyroid imbalance vary, so see your doctor to get your thyroid tested before supplementing with herbs. Too much kelp could over-stimulate the thyroid, especially if your thyroid is functioning properly.

Botanical Bit

Chelated minerals are minerals that are bound to proteins for better absorption in the body. A target chelated mineral is one that is bound to a specific amino acid geared toward a particular body organ when it is ingested.

Kelp has been recorded to have anti-bacterial, antioxidant, anti-tumor, diuretic, and expectorant qualities. It also has been used in the baths of those who are trying to rid their body of cellulite. I like to purchase kelp in bulk and fill up the salt shaker with it instead of table salt. As a nutritive herb, kelp is very salty to taste; when my visitors ask for salt, they are getting this nourishing herb instead (and they don't seem to notice the difference!).

Irish moss, dulse, and watercress are all other plants that contain many of the same nutrients and properties of kelp, and these can be just as nourishing to your thyroid.

Here are some other things you can do to protect your thyroid:

➤ Eat an iodine-rich salad at least a couple times per week, including raw asparagus tips, cabbage, avocado, leaf lettuce (not head lettuce), green onions, sweet green peppers, and whipped and goat cheese. Add salmon for more iodine, if you are a fish eater.

➤ Keep your hormones balanced. All the endocrine glands work together to maintain balance, so have your other glands checked for any problems.

➤ Limit radiation exposure. (See the section "Radiation Poisoning," in Chapter 20, for more.)

➤ Limit drinking distilled water, which can leech minerals from your body.

➤ Find a *chelated* mineral supplement (sometimes referred to as target minerals) targeted for your thyroid.

Tonsillitis: Tea Tree for Two, and Two for Tea Tree

Our tonsils are located on either side of the back part of the throat and are part of our lymphatic system. The tonsils were once thought of as useless, but now we know that they have the job of filtering out possible invaders before they can cause damage to the body, making them an important part of our immune system.

Most of us have suffered with *tonsillitis* at one time or another, usually in childhood during the time when we caught colds and flu. Some of you have even had your tonsils removed because of recurring tonsillitis!

The streptococcal infection (commonly called strep throat) is the common bacterial infection associated with tonsillitis, and it can cause small white pus pockets on the tonsils. Your doctor can give you a throat culture to determine whether you have strep throat. Usually antibiotics are prescribed for treatment.

Symptoms of tonsillitis include inflammation, heat, sore throat, trouble swallowing, and fever. If you have tonsillitis due to strep throat, try some of the remedies listed under colds (see Chapter 8, "C's for a Common Cure") and the flu (see Chapter 11) to boost your immune system and help you recover. Another good combination of herbs used to fight infections is included in the table at the end of this chapter.

In the meantime, let's talk about an herbal remedy that will help you alleviate the pain and local infection that may be causing your tonsils to swell. The essential oil of tea tree, referred to as tea tree oil or melaleuca (*Melaleuca alternifolia*), can be used topically to help kill infections and numb the pain of a sore throat.

The essential oil has been used topically as an antibacterial, anti-fungal, antiseptic, and anti-viral remedy. It has also been used to fight the staphylococcus infection when used as a throat spray.

Do not use tea tree oil internally without supervision, however. This herb is very powerful and is not recommended for internal use, although some have used a drop of tea tree oil in warm water as a healing douche to treat Candida (yeast infections) and cystitis or other urinary tract infections. Some have placed a drop or two into hot water and breathed in the vapors to help kill lung and sinus infections. But mostly, tea tree oil is used topically.

Here's a recipe for a tea tree oil throat spray:

Botanical Bit

Tonsillitis is the inflammation of the tonsils, usually due to infection.

Poison Ivy

Tea tree oil should be used for top-ical applications only, unless instructed otherwise by a competent health practitioner. Even then, it should be used only in small amounts. When taken in larger amounts, this herb can make you sick to your stomach or give you a headache.

1 glass bottle with spray pump

1 cup of water or liquid chlorophyll

1 capsicum capsule

1 slippery elm capsule

4 drops of tea tree oil

2 drops of lemon oil

Heat water, empty capsicum and slippery elm capsules into water, and stir. Let cool slightly (so the essential oils do not evaporate when added to the solution). Add the oils, stir, and pour into the spray bottle. Spray on the back of throat as needed for pain.

You can also dip a Q-tip® directly into a bottle of tea tree oil and swab it onto your tonsils. Or, you can gargle with the mixture instead.

I like to take slippery elm internally anytime I have a sore throat to soothe my irritated tissues. Cleansing the bowel will help rid the body of any toxins that are lingering and irritating the immune system. And, of course, vitamins C and A are both antioxidants that will help you fight any free radical damage caused by your infection.

Herbal Remedies for Common Ailments

Teeth, Teething, Toothaches

Best Single Herb: Cloves

Best Combinations: White willow bark, valerian, wild lettuce, capsicum; garlic (for infection); black walnut extract (brush)

Other Helpful Supplements: Vitamin C; calcium/magnesium with vitamin D

Possible Causes: Blood sugar imbalance; poor oral hygiene

Complementary Help: Visit the dentist; check your blood sugar; floss

Tendonitis

Best Single Herb: Lemongrass

Best Combinations: Lemongrass (used externally); licorice root; uña de gato

Other Helpful Supplements: Glucosamine sulfite; chondroitin; magnesium

Possible Causes: Overuse or misuse of body

Complementary Help: External application of essential oil of birch; tofu or comfrey leaf poultice; treatment for inflammation (see Chapter 14, "I: Interesting Illnesses") and arthritis (see Chapter 6)

Tinnitus

Best Single Herb: Gotu kola

Best Combinations: Ginkgo biloba, gotu kola; blessed thistle; Korean ginseng

Other Helpful Supplements: Calcium/magnesium with vitamin D; B-complex vitamins

Possible Causes: High blood pressure; hearing loss; injury

Complementary Help: Ear coning; acupuncture; reflexology; treatments for high blood pressure (see Chapter 7) or cholesterol (see Chapter 8)

Thyroid Problems

Best Single Herb: Kelp

Best Combinations: Kelp, Irish moss, parsley, hops, capsicum; dulse; watercress

Other Helpful Supplements: Chelated minerals; zinc; manganese

Possible Causes: Radiation damage; glandular imbalance

Complementary Help: Do thyroid exercises; balance the hormones; eat iodine-rich salads; limit distilled water intake

Tonsillitis

Best Single Herb: Tea tree

Best Combinations: Parthenium, golden seal, yarrow, capsicum; mullein; lobelia; white oak bark; tea tree

Other Helpful Supplements: Vitamins C and A

Possible Causes: Viral infection; toxins in body

Complementary Help: Cleanse the bowel; gargle with any of the following diluted mixes: tea tree oil, sea salt, lemon oil, capsicum, slippery elm

---

The Least You Need to Know

➤ The oil of cloves can serve as a topical analgesic for toothaches or teething babies.

➤ Lemongrass, used externally in a bath or as a poultice, can ease the pain of tendonitis.

➤ Gotu kola is a brain tonic-type herb similar to ginkgo biloba in its properties; it can be useful in small amounts to help get rid of ringing in the ears.

➤ Kelp is rich in iodine and is a nutritious food for your thyroid.

➤ Tea tree oil may be used topically to help fight an infection causing tonsillitis and can help relieve the pain of a sore throat.

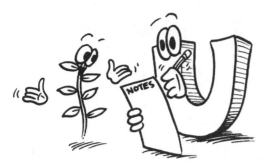

Chapter 22

U: Understanding the Power of Herbs

In This Chapter

➤ Herbs that help with ulcers

➤ Put on weight using a nutrient-rich herb

➤ Tame urinary problems with herbs

➤ Support the uterus before and after childbirth with herbs

"A single untried popular remedy often throws the scientific doctor into hysterics."
—Chinese proverb

Now we will talk about a few ailments and body parts that start with the letter U, including ulcers, problems of being underweight, urinary problems, and trouble affecting the uterus. Now, let me show "U" how to use some great herbs to support your healing.

Ulcers Eating Away at You?

Ulcers can occur in two places: inside the body in the alimentary canal (digestive tract), as in duodenal ulcers, or gastric or peptic ulcers; or on the outside skin, as in diabetic ulcers due to improper circulation, bed sores due to pressure, and mouth ulcers (canker sores). Some ulcers found in the alimentary canal can be linked to an overgrowth of bacteria known as Heliocobactor pylori, commonly referred to as H. pylori. To effectively treat your ulcer, you will need to work with the specific cause of the ulcer. If it is aggravated by stress, refer to Chapter 6, "Give Me Another A!" and Chapter 20, "R and S: For Remarkable Recoveries and Super Solutions," for more help with anxiety and stress. If you have ulcers due to diabetes, read about diabetes in Chapter 9, "D Best Herbal Solutions," for more. Here we'll talk about some herbs that offer pain relief by soothing the tissues and I'll give you the scoop on the best herb to kill the H-pylori bacteria, but first, let's get rid of that pain with some luck of the Irish.

Botanical Bit

An **emollient**, or **demulcent**, is used to describe an herb that has properties that soothe and soften tissue. Some examples of emollients and demulcents include aloe vera, marshmallow, slippery elm, plantain, and kelp.

Irish Moss: Gift from the Sea

Irish moss (*Chondrus crispus*) is an herb found in the sea that was used as a food by the Irish during famine times. This herb serves as an *emollient*, or *demulcent*, meaning that it soothes and softens tissue. This makes it useful for the inflammation and irritation that accompanies ulcerated tissues. Irish moss can be used to reduce duodenal and peptic ulcers and reduce the gastric secretions (acid) that aggravate these conditions. If you are using this herb to soothe your pain, be sure not to forget about treating the bottom-line cause of your ulcer. Just because the pain has been eliminated doesn't mean the causative factors are gone.

Irish moss is also used as a food binder or thickener in puddings and ice cream. Sometimes you will see carrageenan listed on the ingredient label on these foods. This is another name for Irish moss. Topically, Irish moss has been used to treat wrinkles and is a common ingredient in many natural body, face, and hand creams and lotions.

Poison Ivy

Because Irish moss has some blood-thinning qualities, it should not be taken at the same time as blood-thinning medications; it could enhance the effect of the drug.

Because Irish moss grows in the sea, it is rich in iodine. In fact, you may see this herb added to combinations of herbs designed to balance or nourish the thyroid, or it may be used in weight-loss products to help boost the metabolism by feeding the thyroid iodine.

Irish moss has also been used to soothe tissues in the respiratory tract. This herb contains protein and is a nourishing food.

Soothing Ulcer Irritations

For ulcers caused by irritation due to H. pylori, some herbs have been shown to inhibit the growth of bacteria and are instrumental in fixing the cause of the problem. These herbs include pau d'arco, cloves, and inula racemosa (a species of the herb elecampane). Licorice root also helps soothe digestive tract inflammation and ulcer pain. Look for deglycyrrhizinated licorice extract (DGLE) specifically created to work against H-pylori infection, while counteracting discomfort.

Golden seal is an herb used by diabetics to help lower blood sugar and is also an excellent remedy for ulcers. Add some capsicum and myrrh, and you have a pain-killing, antibiotic-type effect. Aloe vera is another soothing, healing herb that is rich in calcium and that helps mend ulcerated tissues and soothe inflammation surrounding ulcers.

Mouth ulcers, known as canker sores, can be very painful. A drop of peppermint oil on your finger applied directly to the sore can help numb the pain. Treat yourself internally for canker sores as you would for any other ulcers of the alimentary canal. The body is usually in an overacid condition when you get a canker sore, so steer clear of acid-producing foods and eat more alkaline foods (see Chapter 15, "J and K: For Just the Right Kind of Cure," for a list of acid and alkaline foods). Chlorophyll is an excellent way to alkalize your system. You can also use liquid chlorophyll as a mouthwash to speed the healing process.

Author and researcher F. Batmanghelidj, M.D., believes that when we become dehydrated, we are prone to ulcers of all types, and so do I; here's why. The stomach creates hydrochloric acid to aid in the digestion of foods. Because of the special lining in the stomach designed to handle this acid, the stomach is the only place in the body that it can exist without causing severe tissue damage. When the stomach is finished churning a meal, the food is passed into the duodenum for further processing. In order to protect the duodenum and rest of the digestive tract from being burnt with this acid, the pancreas must create and secrete a bicarbonate solution into the duodenum as the food (and acid) is being passed along. The pancreas requires lots of water for this function. Of course, if the pancreas does not have the supplies it needs (plenty of water), damaging acids will pass into the duodenum and cause ulcers. See how simple natural healing is? All your body really needs is the right materials to help it do its job.

In addition, avoid these instigators that can aggravate ulcers:

➤ Stress

➤ Cigarette smoking

➤ Coffee, cola, chocolate, and other caffeine-containing foods

➤ Alcohol

Sage Advice

If you suffer from duodenal ulcers, you'll have to give up the gum-chewing habit. The chewing action tricks the body into thinking that there is food entering the stomach, causing the secretion of gastric juices, but in reality you have no food in the stomach to soak up this excess acid. This can only aggravate and add to your problem.

Poison Ivy

Antacids suppress stomach acid production and therefore inhibit proper digestion and can cause more serious problems later. Don't treat your ulcer by suppressing the pain—find the cause, and utilize herbs. Drugs like Tagamet® and Zantac® not only stop your stomach from doing what it is supposed to do but also inhibit bone formation and can lead to liver problems and candida.

Support your digestive process when you have an ulcer by taking food enzymes without HCl before each meal. Usually two tablets or capsules are sufficient. Omega-3 oils have been used successfully to help with alimentary canal ulcers, and calcium is a tissue-knitter and also is alkaline in nature, which will tame some of that acid problem. Take extra beta carotene, too. Beta carotene will be converted into vitamin A in the liver, and it helps heal skin tissues and mucus membranes. You can skip the beta carotene supplement if you drink at least eight ounces of fresh carrot juice daily, which contains calcium and is also a source for vitamin A. Add a tablespoon of whole-leaf aloe vera juice to each glass of water, and drink at least one quart of water daily. This remedy alone has helped many heal their ulcers completely, sometimes within weeks.

Are You Underweight or Under Control?

Being underweight can be as frustrating for a person as being overweight is for the obese. In the United States, at least, we seem to have an obsession with being thin; yet, most of the country is overweight! So, if you have a problem with being too skinny, let's take a look at some of the possibilities first; then I'll give you some tips on eating, and we'll talk about herbs and other supplements that can help you bulk up to your body's capacity. If you have the more common problem of wanting to lose fat, see Chapter 23, "V, W, X, Y, Z, and Other Technical Words," for more (or less).

People are underweight for different reasons, some based on an inadequate self-perception. In other words, you could be healthy and at the ideal weight for your body, but you feel inadequate for some reason. Of course, herbs cannot change your perceptions of yourself. If you are seriously ill, you will probably not be eating much and may become severely underweight. You also may have an overactive thyroid, poor absorption, or other fixable problems. Find out from your physician if you are clinically underweight, and find out how much your body can reasonably handle without stressing your structural system. Then set some reasonable goals for yourself. You will want to build muscle when gaining weight, not unhealthy fat.

Herbs cannot do everything for everyone, so let's take a look at what herbs can and can't do for weight management.

Herbs and Weight Management

Herbs and a Diet of Concentrated Foods Can...	But Herbs Cannot...
Help with general bulk building, such as building extra muscle	Change your body type
Help balance hormones or metabolism	Change genetic malfunction
Relax nerves	Force you to incorporate stress-free living
Enhance digestion and absorption of nutrients	Cure bulimia
Stimulate appetite	Cure anorexia

Herbs alone cannot cure the things listed in the "cannot" category, but they can aid in the recovery from some of these things. Mental disturbances such as anorexia and bulimia must be addressed by a mental health professional, and then a weight-producing herbal/supplemental/food program can be put into place effectively if it's still needed. If you are underweight due to a severe illness, you can use these nutritious, weight-building herbs to build your strength back up as you are recovering. Make sure to check for parasite infection if you suddenly drop weight. As always, find the core of your problem first, and then work with the herbs that will help with your core issue. Only then can true healing and balancing take place. Now let's take a look at some herbs and supplements that, in general, can help beef you up.

Herb Lore

The supplement is known as 5-hydroxy-tryptophan and is a metabolized form of the amino l-tryptophan. It could serve as a solution for anorexia, depression, and other mental illnesses. The body uses this supplement to make the hormone serotonin, a neurotransmitter that plays a role in mood, appetite, and sleep. Make sure your supplement contains B6 and zinc since these nutrients make the substance more available to your cells. *Caution:* This supplement should not be taken by pregnant or nursing women or if you are on medications, nor should it be taken if you are also taking a product that contains ma huang (ephedra).

Spirulina: A Weighty Solution

Spirulina, an algae otherwise called food plankton, is particularly rich in protein. This herb is grown in and collected from lakes, and it contains all eight essential amino acids. Spirulina also is an excellent supplement for strict vegetarians to take as a source of B12, a vitamin that is normally found only in red meat.

The rich chlorophyll content in spirulina also helps build the blood and nourishes the body with minerals such as potassium, magnesium, selenium, zinc, iron, phosphorus, calcium, and manganese.

Anyone with blood sugar imbalances (diabetics or hypoglycemics) can especially benefit from the positive qualities in spirulina. It is a rich source of protein and therefore has an ability to balance fluctuating blood sugar levels. If you are pregnant and/or nursing, spirulina can serve as a rich source

Poison Ivy

An absence of vitamin B12 in the diet can lead to pernicious anemia (low blood count). Strict vegetarians can receive B12 through the use of spirulina supplementation.

291

of natural vitamins for you. Spirulina's chlorophyll content can help keep you from becoming anemic during pregnancy, and it can enrich breast milk while nursing. Not only can this herb make you feel more energetic and give you more stamina, but it also can help relieve stress and provide a sense of euphoria at the same time.

This protein-rich food can help you build muscle as well. Take four capsules two to three times a day for weight-building; you can also add it to your daily weight-building smoothie. To steady blood sugar, take a capsule or two between meals.

Here's a recipe that might help you add some pounds. Add the following to your blender, and mix:

8 ounces soy milk

1 frozen banana

4 capsules spirulina (emptied into mixture)

$^1/_2$ handful of any of the following: cashews, sunflower seeds, sesame seeds, flax seed

A tablespoon or two of organic yogurt, with live acidophilus cultures

Flavor with any of the following if needed: a splash of fruit juice, a few drops of vanilla, or a teaspoon or two of carob powder with a pinch of stevia for sweetening.

Sage Advice

The Sunspire company makes chocolate candies called Sundrops®, which are just like M&M's® without the refined sugar, chemical dies, or wax; ask your local health food store to carry them for you.

Drink this concoction daily for enhanced weight production.

He Ain't Heavy—but He's Trying

If you are a parent of a growing boy who desires to build his weight, please don't allow him to pig out on junk food, candy bars, and sugary snacks. This only has detrimental effects on their overall health, blood sugar, and hormone balance. Junk food can also trigger adolescent acne and can encourage obesity and poor dietary habits that are hard to break.

Instead, leave out bowls of dried fruit pieces and nuts for snacking. Some juice-sweetened organic chocolate candies thrown in the mixture is okay, too.

Dried fruits and raw nuts and seeds are concentrated foods that will help put on healthy bulk. Make sure that you (or your children) are drinking lots of extra water if you are eating dehydrated fruits.

Consider an amino acid supplement to help you put on extra pounds. The B-complex vitamins may stimulate your appetite if you take them before instead of after meals. Other herbs that are full of nutrients and that can help you gain healthful weight are listed in the next table. These include saw palmetto, bee pollen, marshmallow, alfalfa, and chamomile.

Herb Lore

Farmers who raise pigs for slaughter cleverly discovered that baked potatoes will help you put on weight. The farmers used to feed their pigs raw potatoes, but they somehow realized that by cooking the potatoes first, the pigs fattened up faster. Now many pigs receive cooked potatoes only!

Urinary Problems: Urine for a Treat

We have already addressed problems with the urinary tract during our discussions about bladder infections in Chapter 7, "B Well," and kidney problems in Chapter 15. But for general malice wrought on the urinary tract, such as incontinence, infections of the urinary tract, and water retention, I'd like to introduce you to a popular herb that you will probably see more and more of for its positive effects on the urinary system. The herb is called uva ursi.

Uva Ursi Is Good for U

Uva ursi (*Arctostaphylos uva-ursi*) is also called bearberry. The Greek translation of *uva* is "grape," and *ursi* means "of the bear"—put together, this plant can also be referred to as bearberry, although I cannot verify whether bears eat the berries from the uva ursi plant. I plan to question the next one I run into!

For human consumption, the berries can be cooked or made into a cider. When chewed raw, they are bland but will stimulate the flow of saliva in your mouth and help you quench your thirst—in fact, uva ursi has been used as a survival herb.

It was only a decade earlier, when I consulted with an herbalist who put me on capsules of uva ursi for a bladder infection, that I found its medicinal uses for the urinary system.

Poison Ivy

Uva ursi contracts the tissues in the genito-urinary region, so you should not take this herb if you are pregnant because it may limit blood flow to the uterus. Too much of this herb and frequent doses can irritate the stomach. Use uva ursi as you would an antibiotic—not for more than 10 days in a row.

Uva ursi acts as an antiseptic, astringent, diuretic, and vasoconstrictor (that is, it reduces blood flow). It can be helpful in cases of severe diarrhea to slow things down, and it has been used as a mouthwash for thrush and as a douche for urinary trouble and infection. Uva ursi should be used as a medicine, for temporary use as needed. For urinary tract infections take two capsules twice daily, not more than 10 days in a row. Or you can make a tea (add chamomile for a better taste) and take ¹/₂ cup two times a day. Uva ursi is best taken for wet conditions such as water-retentive type ailments. Don't take it if you are dehydrated.

Herb Lore

If you live in the West, you have probably seen uva ursi growing. This is a green, leafed plant with small red berries and small, oval, shiny leaves that grow low to the ground and spread wide. I first discovered this plant on my parent's mountain property in Colorado, where a distant, elderly neighbor of ours (who was also a mountain man and a teacher of nature) identified it as kinnik-kinnik. He told me that the Native Americans used to smoke a mixture of kinnik-kinnik and tobacco, and that they would use it as a cleansing smoke in their sweat lodges.

Sage Advice

Kegel exercises were designed especially to help women prone to bladder prolapses or anyone with incontinence (trouble holding back urine). To perform Kegels, tighten your lower pelvis muscles as if you were restricting urine flow. Contractions should be held for six to 10 seconds, followed by relaxing the muscles completely. This should be done four or five times in a row, three to four times a day.

And Don't Forget ...

When there is infection in the body, a bowel cleansing is always helpful to eliminate excess toxins from circulating throughout the body. Do a dry-skin brush daily to take a load off your kidneys; read Chapters 7 and 15 for more on kidney and bladder health.

For overall nutrition for the urinary tract, see the combination of herbs listed in the table at the end of this chapter. This table contains nutrients that will act as an antiseptic for the urinary tract. Use this combination to strengthen the urinary system, and then maintain your health with proper nutrition and your daily herbal program. (I'll give you a daily program later in the book.) Also incorporate Kegel exercises to strengthen the pelvic floor muscles, and sip cornsilk and/or parsley tea each night for urinary nourishment.

Uterine Problems

When there's a problem with the uterus, it may be due to a weakness or a prolapsus. A prolapsed uterus is a uterus that has either tipped backward because of other sagging organs putting pressure directly on it, because of a lack of tissue integrity of the uterus, causing it to sag.

To help a tipped uterus, consider the colon. If the lower bowel is heavy with waste materials due to constipation, the bowel can sag under this weight and can drop down on top of the uterus, causing discomfort, problems conceiving, or painful periods.

Try cleansing the bowel if you have trouble with your uterus. Any organ that is lying underneath a constipated, toxic-laden, heavy colon can only create an unhealthy environment for that organ. The position can cause constricted blood flow and may encourage adhesions or other growths to occur. Read Chapter 3, "What to Expect with Herbs," for more on cleansing with herbs.

Other things that can help a prolapsed transverse colon or a prolapsed uterus are slant board exercises. All you need for a slant board exercise is an exercise incline bench or some other type of board that you can raise one end of and lie on safely with your feet higher than your head. These exercises are designed to bring back tone to a prolapsed colon, but the uterus will be affected also.

1. Lie on your back with your head at the low end of the board.
2. Gently and rapidly tap the area below your belly button with your cupped hand for a few minutes.
3. You can also find a tennis ball or similar ball and roll it around the same area.

Gravitational force will help pull the bowel and uterus back into place, and the tapping and rolling motions will bring blood supply to the area and may help give tone back to the muscles. This exercise is also helpful if you experience tiredness, a groggy head, or forgetfulness.

Motherwort for the Weak Uterus

Motherwort (*Leonurus cardiaca*) is an herb used for its antispasmodic, astringent, diuretic, and nervine properties. This herb is considered a tonic made for female problems because it has been used to ease the pain associated with menstruation, to

Poison Ivy

Be careful getting up from this position! If you are not used to it, you can become dizzy because of the extra blood and oxygen flow to the brain.

Poison Ivy

Because of its laxative effects, motherwort should not be used during pregnancy, but it may be used to help ease pain during childbirth.

295

relieve pain during childbirth, and to ease frigidity. Motherwort has some laxative effects as well. The Japanese celebrate motherwort at a festival called Kikousouki, where they add the flowers of the plant to their food and eat them.

Although this herb can be used to ease pain during labor, it should not be taken during pregnancy.

Red raspberry is an herb that can help support the uterus during pregnancy. A tea containing red raspberry, witch hazel, and motherwort or bayberry can be made into a douche and used to help contract and tone the uterus.

Squawvine Support

Sage Advice

Magnesium acts as a muscle-relaxant and can help in labor pain. Aroma-therapists also have diffused tangerine into the birthing room to calm and relax nerves and to soothe the soul.

Squawvine (*Mitchella repens*) is used to help support the tone of the uterus while pregnant, as well as during and after childbirth. Native American women have taken squawvine as a tea during pregnancy to aid delivery and to help nourish breast milk.

Unlike motherwort, which should be used only during labor, squawvine is a uterine tonic that is safe to use during pregnancy. This herb can be combined with black cohosh, dong quai, butcher's broom, and red raspberry and taken five weeks before your scheduled delivery date to help make labor easier. My clients who have used this combination have always had great testimonials about the effects of this combination, even when giving birth to a first child (which can be a more difficult delivery, for some).

Squawvine also has been used as a diuretic and has been helpful in eliminating stones from the kidneys and the bladder. Pregnancy and breastfeeding can make the nipples sore, and a squawvine fomentation has helped ease this tenderness for many women.

Herbal Remedies for Common Ailments

Ulcers

Best Single Herb: Irish moss

Best Combinations: Golden seal, capsicum, myrrh; aloe vera; Irish moss; liquid chlorophyll

Other Helpful Supplements: Food enzymes (without hydrochloric acid); Omega-3 oils; calcium; vitamin A

Possible Causes: H. pylori bacteria overgrowth; dehydration; stress; hiatal hernia; over-acidic body condition

Complementary Help: Drink lots of water; practice stress management; avoid caffeine, cigarettes, and alcohol; drink carrot juice and eat alkaline foods

Underweight

Best Single Herb: Spirulina

Best Combinations: Spirulina; saw palmetto; chamomile; alfalfa; marshmallow; bee pollen

Other Helpful Supplements: B-complex vitamins; amino acids

Possible Causes: Overactive thyroid; nervous tension; parasites

Complementary Help: Dried fruit; nuts and seeds; baked potatoes

Urinary Problems

Best Single Herb: Uva ursi

Best Combinations: Uva ursi, hydrangea, parsley, dandelion, schizandra, Siberian ginseng, lemon, dong quai, cornsilk, horsetail, hops (for strengthening)

Other Helpful Supplements: B-complex vitamins

Possible Causes: Infection; constipation

Complementary Help: Dry-skin brushing; Kegel exercises; bowel cleansing; treatments for bladder problems (see Chapter 7) or kidney problems (see Chapter 15)

Uterus, Weak/Prolapsed

Best Single Herb: Motherwort

Best Combinations: Motherwort; red raspberry

Other Helpful Supplements: B-complex vitamins

Possible Causes: Constipation; prolapsed transverse colon

Complementary Help: Slant board exercises; bowel cleansing; bayberry or witch hazel tea or decoction used as douche

Uterus Support During Childbirth

Best Single Herb: Squawvine

Best Combinations: Squawvine; black cohosh, squawvine, dong quai, butcher's broom, red raspberry (five weeks or less before scheduled child delivery only)

Other Helpful Supplements: Magnesium

Possible Causes: Not applicable

Complementary Help: Tangerine oil to relax during delivery

The Least You Need to Know

➤ Irish moss is seaweed used for ulcers because of its soothing effect on tissues.

➤ Spirulina is a nutritious herb containing amino acids that can be helpful for those who want to gain weight.

➤ Uva ursi is a strong tonic for the urinary system and can be used temporarily to help fight off urinary system troubles.

➤ Motherwort should not be used during pregnancy, but the herb can help alleviate labor pains when taken just before or during labor.

➤ Squawvine is an herb historically used by Native American women during pregnancy to help tone the uterus and aid in delivery.

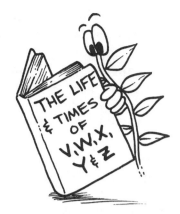

V, W, X, Y, Z, and Other Technical Words

In This Chapter

➤ Use herbs topically on your varicose veins

➤ Herbs used for vertigo

➤ Correct vomiting with settling herbs

➤ Get rid of warts with herbal remedies

➤ Avoid excess water retention with help from nature

➤ Herbs that help with weight loss

Think of this horror scenario: You are feeling overweight and have excess water retention, and because of this pressure on your body, you suffer from varicose veins. To top it off, you have not been able to get rid of the warts on your hands. You are so sick of yourself that it makes you vomit, which makes you dizzy (vertigo)! Wow! I hope this doesn't sound like you—but if it does, then this entire chapter is dedicated to you specifically!

We'll cover all these ailments and give you a game plan to deal with them. So, be happy—you really don't have such problems all at once, and let's learn how you can help yourself with the ones you do have!

Varicose Veins: Veinity Will Get You Nowhere

Varicose veins are bluish, bulging veins that usually appear as twisted ropes just under the surface of the skin. Symptoms include aches or heaviness in the limbs and swelling of the legs and ankles. These veins seem more prominent if you have been standing for long periods of time. Although rare, you may have a deep varicose vein that is painful, but it may not show up at the surface of your skin. Varicose veins can become serious if left untreated.

Many times you will see varicose veins surrounded by broken blood capillaries, known as spider-burst veins. These small broken blood vessels can resemble intricate road maps on a fair-skinned person. Many times these broken blood vessels show up around the ankles, in the lower legs, and elsewhere in the feet, although they can occur anywhere in the body.

Possible causes of varicose veins are listed in the table at the end of this chapter, but to expand a little here, I should mention that varicose veins and broken blood vessels can indicate the inadequate nourishment of your entire circulatory system. Consider taking herbs to strengthen your blood capillaries to prevent further damage.

Varicose veins are usually caused by pressure on the veins. Have your cholesterol checked; if fat is clogging up your veins, this can put pressure on these weakened vessels and cause problems (see the section "High Cholesterol: Cutting Through the Fat," in Chapter 8, "C's for a Common Cure").

Sitting with your legs crossed will create pressure and can increase your problem as well. Constipation adds internal pressure to the body and organs and can cause varicose veins and hemorrhoids, so bowel cleansing is always in order if you suffer from these problems.

Sage Advice

Remember the liver must be cleansed if you have high cholesterol since the liver is responsible for emulsifying fats. Milk thistle helps cleanse and support a sluggish liver and will help it do its job better.

Sage Advice

Try this cool trick: Label an ice cube tray and fill a few of the squares with distilled witch hazel. After the liquid is frozen, put the frozen cubes in a freezer bag—and again label it clearly! You don't want to add it to your drinks! When someone has a bump, cold sore, or other painful swelling, the witch hazel ice cube can be applied.

Witch Hazel Has Broken Blood Vessels?

Witch hazel (*Hamamelis virginiana*) is an herb that was listed as an official drug in the United States, and it is still used by many as a safe remedy for many applications. This herb has been used as an anti-bacterial, anti-inflammatory, astringent, hemostatic (controls bleeding), syptic sedative, and tonic. The bark, twigs, and leaves of the witch hazel plant are used for these purposes. I suggest using this herb topically, but some have used the herb to make a tea; they drink two cups per day to help strengthen blood vessels. Topically, use as a decoction and apply with cheese cloth, with the legs raised.

Distilled witch hazel is commonly found alongside hydrogen peroxide and rubbing alcohol at your local pharmacy; this herb should be used only externally.

Witch hazel contains flavonoids, natural substances found in plants that are powerful antioxidants that can strengthen blood vessels. Grape seed and pine bark extract also contain these powerful nutrients. You can soak a cotton ball in the distilled witch hazel from your pharmacy and apply it directly to small affected areas; otherwise, pour some into a shallow dish, soak a piece of cheesecloth in the solution, and then apply the rag to the affected area. If you use it room temperature or cooler, this will heighten the effect. This is especially helpful for the pain associated with varicose veins.

Herb Lore

It is said that witch hazel got its name from the early days when dowsing, or "witching," for water was popular. Frequently, branches from the witch hazel plant were used for this divining practice, thus it received its witchy name!

If your varicose veins are in your feet, use a cool footbath with witch hazel added to ease your soreness and inflammation. Witch hazel has such strong astringent-like qualities that it is used as an active ingredient in over-the-counter hemorrhoid medications such as Preparation H® and Tucks®. This is probably the reason why Preparation H® cream has been used by some famous Hollywood beauties as their secret anti-wrinkle cream remedy!

Witch hazel can be applied to all areas of inflammation on the skin, or areas that you wish to tighten temporarily. This includes varicose veins, hemorrhoids, pimples, cold sores, wrinkles, and bruises.

More Witch Doctor Potions

Witch hazel applied to a protruding varicose vein might help the swelling subside, but you will always need to consider what caused your problem in the first place. If you have clogged veins or arteries due to high cholesterol, consider adding butcher's broom to your diet. (See the section "Hemorrhoids: A Swell Solution," in Chapter 13, "H: Happy Healing with Herbs," for more on butcher's broom.) Another great herb to try is horse chestnut. Horse chestnut and butcher's broom together make an excellent combination to fight varicose veins internally. White oak bark or bilberry capsules can be taken internally to help reduce swelling (both are strong astringent herbs), and rose hips, rich in vitamin C and bioflavonoids, will nourish and help strengthen your circulatory system.

Exercise is an important factor in preventing varicose veins, hemorrhoids, and broken blood vessels. Also see your chiropractor for adjustments to ensure that your blood flow is not being restricted, and try the slant board exercises discussed in the previous chapter to help take the pressure off the lower body.

Vertigo: Helping a Dizzy Blonde

Occasionally having a dizzy spell—such as when you are bent over for a long period of time and then quickly stand, or when you are too hot, tired, or hungry and then get dizzy—is not the same as vertigo. Vertigo is the incapacitating sensation that the world is spinning or tilted, and usually leads to vomiting.

Some possible causes of vertigo include:

➤ Inner ear problem, damage, or infection (an infection could be caused by excess debris, ear wax, mucus in the ear—get an ear coning or other type of ear cleansing)

➤ Injury or problem in the brain stem

Poison Ivy

To rule out any serious problems linked to vertigo, see your doctor for an examination—and make sure that someone else drives you!

Recurring dizziness can be caused by other underlying problems, such as:

➤ Poor circulation to the head, or blood pressure that's too high or low

➤ Spinal misalignment

➤ Anemia

➤ Excess wax or debris in the ear

➤ Lack of oxygen to the inner ear tissues

➤ Hypoglycemia

➤ Vitamin B deficiency

➤ Stress

If your dizziness is due to an inner ear infection or poor circulation, give the following herbs a try.

Wood Betony for Grounding

Wood betony (*Betonica officinalis*) is not that common of an herb, but you will probably see it in combination with other herbs. This herb has historically been used as a pain-killer, an antiseptic, an astringent, a brain tonic, a nerve calmer, and a circulatory stimulant. Therefore, wood betony may be helpful in not only killing the bacteria or virus causing your ear infection, but also nourishing the brain and relaxing the central nervous system.

Too much wood betony can make you sick to your stomach. Herbalists are very careful about making anyone feel ill, although in some cases you may need to feel worse before you feel better with natural healing!

Poison Ivy

Large doses of wood betony may cause you to vomit. This herb should not be used during pregnancy; however, in very small doses it is safe for children.

Wood betony is a good herb for most problems of the head and for cleaning the blood via the liver. It has been used for bronchitis, colds, coughs, dizziness, headaches, jaundice, menstrual cramps, nerve disorders, and externally on wounds, ulcers, and splinters (to help pull out a splinter, bruise the leaves and apply to the area). In the wild, animals are said to seek wood betony when they are wounded. It aids the immune system, relaxes muscles, opens blood vessels, and a European study found it to reduce high blood pressure.

Adults can take one to two capsules daily for vertigo, or as recommended on the bottle.

Other Herbs for the Ride

Other herbs useful in aiding the circulatory system include a combination of ginkgo biloba and hawthorn berry. If you are having circulatory problems, look up my suggestions for herbs for blood pressure in Chapter 7, "B Well," and under cholesterol in Chapter 8. Also see the table at the end of this chapter for some other supplements helpful for the circulatory system that may help heal the root cause of your dizziness.

Ear coning is my favorite remedy for cleaning out the ears. You can read more on ear coning in Chapter 10, "E: Everywhere an Herb, Herb," or in my other book, *The Complete Idiot's Guide to Reflexology*. Otherwise, ask your holistic practitioner to help you. Ear coning might help draw out excess debris that can be causing a recurring infection.

Herb Lore

One of my clients had recurring vertigo due to inner ear infections. I coned her ears and was amazed at the amount of debris that was pulled from them! We did another, and another—up to five in three weeks, until the cones came out clear. She obviously had stored large amounts of mucus in her system, and this was probably the cause of the reoccurring infections. She has not had any problems since, but she maintains her ear conings quarterly for prevention.

Vomiting: Regurgitating an Old Remedy

I'm sure you really won't need me to explain what vomiting is—at some time or another, we all have been inflicted with this reaction! Vomiting is a reaction of the stomach, usually triggered to protect you from something that is deemed harmful to the body.

For example, when you catch a flu bug or swallow something poisonous, your body's immediate reaction is to regurgitate the substance. Thank goodness for this mechanism—it protects you from absorbing poisons that reach the stomach. On the other hand, sometimes vomiting can be dangerous, especially when a person is in a weakened condition or if the person is tiny, like an infant or a young child. A couple of great herbal remedies can help stop this problem and settle the stomach—so let's take a look.

Herb Lore

The stomach carries worry, so the vomiting mechanism can be triggered by anxiety and resistance to what we are experiencing. Think about the "butterflies" in your stomach you get before you are about to do something important. Naturally, you are worried—and, naturally, the stomach reacts. Because herbs work on more than just the physical level, they can also help ease your worry and stop you from getting sick.

Sage Advice

If you make a spearmint tea or infusion, do not boil the herb. Boiling it will cause the essential oils to evaporate, and the oils are the most medicinal part of this plant. See how to make an infusion or tea in Chapter 1 under "Tea for Two? Different Applications of Herbs."

Spearmint to Calm the Stomach

Spearmint (*Mentha viridus*) is a favorite anti-vomiting remedy herb. This good-tasting herb from the mint family is a popular plant used to flavor candies, gum, foods, and liquid chlorophyll. Its leaves have been used as a remedy to rid the intestines of gas and to rid the body of excess water. Spearmint can aid circulation and bring stimulation to the body and mental processes.

Spearmint is a great anti-spasmodic and is also especially soothing to the stomach, which makes its properties ideal for countering the effects of vomiting. This is especially true when someone is suffering from "dry heaves," meaning that the stomach is empty, but the regurgitation process is still active (ugh!). A sip of spearmint, or a dab of spearmint essential oil on the tongue can ease the spastic stomach. You also can rub some of the essential oil of spearmint directly onto your skin over your stomach or rub a little near your temples to relax you. Keep in mind that because spearmint belongs to the mint family, it is very strong—and the essential oil is even stronger. If you have sensitive skin, make sure to dilute the oil before applying it directly to your body.

Other Things to Try

A great combination to help stop vomiting and ease nausea is listed in the table at the end of this chapter. The mixture contains ginger as the first ingredient, which is well-known for its anti-nausea effect. If you're having trouble swallowing a pill, make a tea from the powdered herbs of this combination, and add a drop of the spearmint or leaf of spearmint last, for flavor. Sip the warm tea slowly, to calm your stomach.

When the vomiting is serious, due to poisoning or swallowing something contaminated, take a few tablespoons of hydrated bentonite to absorb and protect the body from the poison. This mixture is liquefied clay and has no nutritive value, but it is used for emergency poisonings or for detoxifying cleanses.

Warts: A Bumpy Road to Recovery

Warts are actually caused by a virus. They can occur anywhere on the body, but they're most commonly found on the hands. On the soles of the feet, warts are called plantar warts (denoting the plantar aspect of the foot).

Consult your podiatrist about plantar warts, although you might want to try some of these herbal remedies first before you have them burned away. Treat the source of the problem internally with herbs. Having them removed medically is only treating the temporary symptom and not addressing the core issue. I have seen many different external remedies work for ridding my clients of warts, and unfortunately, they are all different! I will give you some to try for yourself, and I will be grateful if you send me your letters on what works for you! (Maybe it could be the subject of my next book, *The Complete Idiot's Guide to Wart Remedies!?* Well, I wouldn't go that far, but it is an interesting subject!)

Poison Ivy

Genital warts are transmitted by sexual contact and may have to be frozen or surgically removed by your physician. See your doctor for genital warts because these are contagious and you may need to be treated medically.

Let's look at some herbs that may help you get rid of the source of your warts.

Reishi Mushroom

The Reishi mushroom (*Ganoderma lucidum*) has also been referred to as the lucky fungus. This mushroom has become quite popular in the United States in recent years, but it has a long history as a sacred herb in the Orient. Reishi is used by Taoist monks, who believe that it enhances the receptivity of the spirit. In China, the herb is said to bring immortality.

This herb is used to help normalize blood pressure, reduce cholesterol, relax the muscles, numb pain, kill bacteria, reduce swellings, rejuvenate the body and tissues, tone the heart, stimulate the body and help it adapt to stress, boost the immune system, and aid in the fight against cancer, especially tumors. Nice to have this fungus among us, eh?

As you can see, Reishi is used for more than just warts, and you should see some beneficial side effects with the use of this mushroom. This herb is generally considered safe, but if you use it regularly and also use medications, use caution—the herb may inhibit the absorption of some drugs. Reishi contains polysaccharides, which are thought to help the immune system eat up free radical cells. This has made this mushroom popular in use with herbal and nutritional cancer-prevention programs. All these positive properties of this valuable fungus make Reishi a safe and effective herb for boosting the immune system and helping the body rid itself of warts. To help you get rid of your warts and boost your overall vitality and health, take six to 10 capsules of Reishi spread out through the day. This remedy can be taken in very large quantities with no toxic side effects. If you are fighting a serious illness, you can double or triple this amount. Work with a professional who can get you on a holistic program to help you if you are ill.

More Folk Remedies

So many herbal remedies exist to rid yourself of warts that I cannot list them all here, but I will give you some of my favorites that have been effective:

➤ Take four pau d'arco capsules twice daily, and take a pau d'arco tea, lotion, infusion, or poultice externally for six weeks.

➤ Break the stem of a fresh, blooming dandelion before noon and before dark. Apply the white liquid to the wart directly. Do this twice each day for 10 days, and the wart will fall off.

➤ Apply tea tree oil to the wart two to four times each day until the wart dissolves.

➤ Puncture a vitamin E capsule, and apply it to the wart daily. Cover the area with a bandage. (This has helped some within two weeks!)

➤ Apply castor oil each evening and each morning until the wart leaves.

➤ Take one teaspoon of colloidal silver twice daily internally, and add a dab to the wart twice per day for 10 days. (Do not take silver for more than 10 days at a time.)

➤ Soak gauze with apple cider vinegar, and apply to the wart overnight. The next morning, the wart will be gone.

I don't know why some of these remedies work for some and not for others, but they are safe—and at least one of them should work for you!

Internally, vitamins A and D help boost the immune system and feed the skin, and these vitamins have helped many get rid of their warts. This is probably because vitamin A in particular has been shown to be low in those suffering from viral infections. Because these vitamins are stored in our body, be sure that you are not taking large doses for too long. Recommended Daily Allowances (RDA) for adults taking vitamin A are 4,000 to 5,000 IU (international units). If you are not working with an herbalist or nutritionist, you might consider taking beta carotene instead. Your liver can convert beta carotene to vitamin A for you when your body needs it.

Sage Advice

You can get your vitamin D from the sunshine; otherwise, an average adult can take between 200 IU and 600 IU daily.

Water Retention Prevention (Edema)

Retaining excess water in your body is uncomfortable. This problem seems to be more common in women than men. When you are holding excess water, you will notice your rings feel tight on your fingers, your abdomen may feel or look bloated, your ankles are swollen, and your face looks puffy. Ironically, these can be signs of dehydration. When your body is not receiving enough water, it protects you by holding onto excess water around your cells, causing your puffiness. So, the No. 1 remedy to stimulate the release of excess water is to drink more water! See Chapter 1, "What Are Herbs and Why Should I Use Them?" for how much you need.

Here are some causes of general water retention:

➤ Not drinking enough water.

➤ Eating too many spices, including spicy foods, sodium (salty) foods, MSG, potato chips, cheese, restaurant food, prepared foods, and sodas. Sodium makes you retain water, but does not hydrate the cells.

➤ Static lymph flow, from traveling, sitting for long periods of time in cars, or traveling in planes.

➤ Hormones: PMS, for instance, can cause a temporary change in your water balance.

➤ Constipation: The body retains water to protect you from the toxins floating around in the blood stream.

Edema is the technical term for water retention, but it is also used to refer to a more serious problem resulting from underlying disease or allergic reaction.

Some causes of edema (also referred to as dropsy) include:

Poison Ivy

Other known side effects of diuretics include ringing in the ears, dizziness, rashes, itching, sensitivity to sunlight, diarrhea or constipation, muscle cramps (potassium is found in muscles, too), fever with sore throat, blurred vision, loss of appetite, increases in blood sugar, gout, numbness in hands or feet, and headaches. Report these symptoms to your prescribing physician immediately.

➤ Kidney failure

➤ Heart failure

➤ Cirrhosis of the liver

➤ Acute nephritis

➤ Starvation

➤ Allergic reaction

➤ Steroid drug reaction

If you have any of these serious problems, you will need emergency care right away.

In cases of edema, your medical treatments will usually include the administration of synthetic diuretics to stimulate the kidneys to release the excess water. These diuretics deplete the body of potassium. Because potassium is a mineral found in the heart, the side effects of diuretics may be detrimental to the heart.

Let's take a look at some herbs that can stimulate the kidneys to release excess water from the body without any toxic side effects.

Juniper Berries: Please Release Me, Let Me Go

Juniper berries (*Juniperus communis*) is a favorite herb remedy for those suffering from occasional water retention. Along with drinking plenty of pure water, juniper berries act as nature's diuretic.

Many different types of junipers exist; following is a photo of one growing in front of my home. This photo was taken early in the spring, so no berries have shown up yet. But when they do, they are bluish-gray in color.

Four to six capsules a day should prove more than adequate for the average adult to get rid of excess water. Use juniper berries as a temporary remedy. You can use juniper daily up to six weeks without any problems, but this is a very strong herb, so stop taking it if you begin to have symptoms such as:

➤ Pain in the kidneys (the kidneys are located about mid-back, one on either side of the spine)

➤ Intestinal irritation or diarrhea

➤ Elevated blood pressure

➤ Rapid heartbeat

Fortunately, if you overdose on herbs, the symptoms subside shortly after you discontinue taking them. With drugs, the results can be fatal.

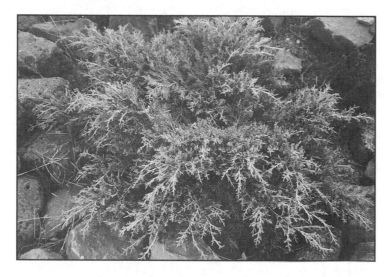

Juniper bush showing no berries yet.

Juniper berries are used for more than just water retention. Here are some other great past uses—some of which are still used today:

➤ Chewing the berries before meals can help stimulate hydrochloric acid production in the stomach, which will aid your digestion.

➤ The berries may help clean out tar residues left in the lungs after you quit smoking.

➤ Native Americans used juniper as a form of birth control.

➤ The essential oil has been an effective bug repellent.

➤ Berries can be roasted and used as a coffee substitute.

➤ Juniper can bring on an overdue period.

➤ Juniper can help rid the body of parasites.

➤ Juniper can help in reducing inflammation associated with arthritis.

Poison Ivy

Juniper berries are effective and strong and should not be taken by pregnant women or small children. Although they possess antiseptic properties helpful against infection, juniper berries should not be taken if you have a kidney infection, nor should you take them daily for more than six weeks.

Juniper also has been burned in Native American sweat lodges for purification, and the berries are used in the making of the alcohol gin.

Dam, It Worked!—In the Flow with Herbs

Juniper berries sure are popular as a natural diuretic, but some other herbs serve just as well as herbal diuretics, including these:

Sage Advice

The B-complex vitamins will help you release excess water retention. If you have kidney problems, try a low-protein (low-acid) diet to take the burden off your kidneys. (See Chapter 15 for more on eating right for kidney health.)

➤ Uva ursi (see Chapter 22, "U: Understanding the Power of Herbs")

➤ Parsley (see Chapter 15, "J and K: For Just the Right Kind of Cure")

➤ Cornsilk

➤ Buchu

➤ Cranberries (see Chapter 7)

A popular combination of herbs used to support the kidneys and serve as a natural diuretic is listed in the table at the end of the chapter.

If you are constipated, your body will hold excess water; read Chapter 8 for some effective herbal laxatives.

Weight Loss: A Wide Range of Possibilities

The weight-loss challenge is a heavy one indeed. There are some basics on keeping trim and lean, such as exercise and a healthy diet filled with lots of vegetables and fruits, but some fantastic herbs can aid you in losing those excess pounds, too.

First let me tell you that, before herbs, I was overweight. Despite exercising five days a week in my aerobic class, drinking $3/4$ of a gallon of water daily, and following a vegetarian diet, I was still overweight. This is what led me to my herbalist and iridologist. She put me on a program not specifically geared toward losing weight, but to get at some of my core problems.

Once these imbalances were nourished with the herbal program, an extra 35 pounds just melted off, never to return! The herbs have also heightened my senses and have literally taken away the cravings for bad things I used to crave.

Now let's talk about a few core reasons you can't seem to get rid of your excess baggage.

Besides pure overindulgence in foods and a total lack of exercise, excess weight can be caused by other factors that you need to address for an overall approach to losing and maintaining your ideal weight. Look at the following table to get an idea of some reasons you could be feeling pudgy.

Some Reasons for Excess Weight

Cause	Reason(s)	Herbal Solution(s)
Glandular imbalance	A. Your thyroid can be under-active, causing your metabolism to slow down. B. The pituitary regulates fat distribution and may be out of balance. C. Hormones that are out of balance may cause excess weight.	A. Kelp B. Alfalfa and gotu kola C. Evening primrose oil (See Chapter 21, "T: Terrific Solutions," for more on the thyroid.)
Constipation	You will retain excess water and look heavier, which may also make you feel heavier and therefore crave heavier foods.	Cascara sagrada and psyllium hulls (See Chapter 8 for more on constipation.)
Poor digestion	A. When the pancreas is insufficient, your blood sugar can fluctuate wildly, causing you to crave sugar and carbohydrates. B. When your absorption is insufficient, your body is not being nourished properly and your appetite button gets triggered more than necessary, causing you to overeat.	A. Cedar berries and/or golden seal (for high blood sugar); licorice root (for low blood sugar). Chromium will help balance blood sugar. (See the section "Diabetes: How Sweet It Isn't," in Chapter 9; and the section "Hypoglycemia: A Sweet Solution," in Chapter 13.) B. Marshmallow and pepsin, or food enzymes with hydrochloric acid, will help break down proteins and undigested proteins left in the colon; take papaya or pineapple before meals. Acidophilus supplements can aid absorption of nutrients.
Poor food combining	When you eat foods that inhibit the digestion of the other foods (such as starches and proteins at the same meal), the result is poor digestion, which leads to excess weight.	No herbs will make up completely for poor food combining, but pineapple and/or papaya and pepper-mint will help. (See Chapter 12 for food-combining tips.)

Herb Lore

Herbs help you reach your ideal weight because of their ability to fill in your nutritional voids; cleanse excess mucus, feces, cholesterol, and toxins from the body; release excess water retention; balance the glands that regulate fat storage and metabolism; aid your digestion; elevate your taste buds for wholesome foods; and give you the extra energy you need to exercise! When you get on an herbal program designed for your particular needs, your body will eventually regulate itself to your ideal weight. Aren't you happy we have herbs?

Chickweed for the Hungry

Chickweed (*Stellaria media*) is one of my favorite ingredients for general weight loss. This is the one herb that I always think of first when asked by passersby what herb they can take to help them lose weight. Take one to two capsules of chickweed between each meal to help you lose weight. Chickweed contains a rich amount of lecithin, a fat emulsifier, which makes chickweed a cholesterol remedy also. I like it for its appetite-suppressant effect. This herb also serves as a mild laxative and is rich in vitamin C, calcium, and phosphorus, so it will nourish you as you lose weight.

Chickweed is a favorite of at least 30 species of birds, so maybe this is where the saying comes from—if you want to lose weight, you should eat like a bird!

Sage Advice

Two great combinations to use to cleanse and curb the appetite are found in the table at the end of the chapter. The second combination, a mix of brindall berries, gymnema, marshmallow, and psyllium, will help your body resist absorbing so much sugar and will help with sugar cravings.

L-carnitine also is listed in the table in the end of this chapter because this amino acid is instrumental in encouraging fat metabolism. Other herbs, of course, can help boost metabolism and thermogenesis (including Chinese ephedra, but it is not suited for everyone; read more about this herb in Chapter 6, "Give Me Another A!").

Garcinia cambogia is a fruit that is a part of many weight-loss remedies because it has been shown to help burn up excess calories in the body, suppress the appetite, inhibit the conversion of excess carbohydrates to fat, and increase the body's stores of energy fuel.

Pineapple or papaya has helped many lose weight as well. The enzymes help digestion, and these fruits can be eaten before any meal. Improving digestion is also very helpful in weight loss.

A Lighter Solution

You may notice that everyone is shaped a little differently. You may also notice that there are groups of similar shapes in certain people—long ones, tall ones, short ones, big ones. Some systems can classify your body into a particular type, and then you can adhere to your type's best supplements and diet. I like to use glandular body typing.

Here's a brief look at each type; seek out a holistic health practitioner who can help you find your type and get you on a diet that suits you best. Each practitioner you seek may have a different method, such as blood types, constitutional typing, metabolic typing, and so on. But, just for fun, take a look at the categories here to see if you can pinpoint your type.

Sage Advice

A simple remedy you can use is to take four capsules of psyllium hulls 20 minutes before each meal, along with one full glass of water. The psyllium will expand in your digestive tract and make you feel full, so you will eat less.

Glandular Body Types

Glandular Type	Where Fat Is Gained Predominately	Best Herb
Pituitary	Gains fat evenly all over body	Slippery elm
Adrenal	Gains fat mostly in upper body; small on bottom; thin legs; large on top and in bust and back area	Peppermint
Gonadal	Gains weight on bottom; pear shape; thinner on top; larger butt, hips, and thighs	Dandelion
Thyroid	Tall and mostly thin, but gains weight around middle (like wearing an inflated rubber tire tube around waist), prone to "beer" belly	Bayberry
Thymus	Mixture between adrenal and thyroid; balanced body; depends on which type is most resembled—use herbs for that type.	See Thyroid and Adrenal
Pancreatic	Usually obese; very large frame; large bust, belly, and butt	Gentian
Pineal	Small in stature with large head; usually not overweight; doesn't apply to weight loss, but may need weight-gaining therapies (see the section "Are You Underweight or Under Control?" in Chapter 22)	N/A

Always drink lots of extra water when you are losing weight, and keep the bowel clean. Toxins are stored in your fat cells, so expect to have some detoxing symptoms when losing your excess fat. Have fun in the process, and use herbs to support your efforts and to maintain your results. Happy new body to you!

Herbal Remedies for Common Ailments

Varicose Veins

Best Single Herb: Witch hazel (used externally)

Best Combinations: Butcher's broom and horse chestnut; capsicum; white oak bark; bilberry; rose hips; grape pine or pine bark extract; milk thistle (for liver if high cholesterol)

Other Helpful Supplements: Vitamin E; vitamin C with citrus bioflavonoids; B-complex vitamins

Possible Causes: High cholesterol, crossed legs; inadequate circulatory system; constipation

Complementary Help: Bowel cleansing; witch hazel compress or fomentation; exercise

Vertigo

Best Single Herb: Wood betony

Best Combinations: Gingko biloba, hawthorn; wood betony

Other Helpful Supplements: B-complex vitamins; lecithin; CoQ_{10}; vitamin E

Possible Causes: Inner ear problem; poor circulation; spinal misalignment; blood pressure too high or low; anemia

Complementary Help: Ear coning; chiropractic care; reflexology; bowel cleansing

Vomiting

Best Single Herb: Spearmint

Best Combinations: Ginger, capsicum, golden seal, licorice; spearmint; papaya

Other Helpful Supplements: Hydrated bentonite

Possible Causes: Food poisoning; virus/bacterial infection; emotional upsets

Complementary Help: Spearmint or peppermint tea (see treatments for nausea, in Chapter 18, "N: Now You Have a Remedy")

Warts

Best Single Herb: Reishi mushroom

Best Combinations: Reishi mushroom; pau d'arco

Other Helpful Supplements: Colloidal silver; vitamins A and D

Possible Causes: Virus; lowered immune system

Complementary Help: Externally use any of the following: tea tree oil, vitamin E oil, apple cider vinegar, castor oil (twice per day until gone)

Water Retention

Best Single Herb: Juniper berries

Best Combinations: Dong quai, golden seal, juniper berries, uva ursi, parsley, ginger, marshmallow; cornsilk

Other Helpful Supplements: B-complex vitamins; trace mineral supplement

Possible Causes: Constipation; kidney problems; heart problems

Complementary Help: Bowel cleansing; low-protein diet

Weight Loss

Best Single Herb: Chickweed

Best Combinations: Chickweed, cascara sagrada, licorice, safflower, parthenium, black walnut, gotu kola, hawthorn, papaya, fennel, dandelion; brindall berries, gymnema, marshmallow, psyllium; garcinia cambogia; Chinese ephedra (for some)

Other Helpful Supplements: Chromium; l-carnitine; balanced amino acid supplement; food enzymes with hydrochloric acid

Possible Causes: Improper food combining; eating late in evening; lack of exercise; thyroid problems; hormonal imbalance; improper digestion; constipation

Complementary Help: Cleanse the bowel; support digestion; balance glands; find out your glandular body type, and then use a program to support your type; exercise

---

The Least You Need to Know

➤ Witch hazel makes a great external remedy for varicose veins, hemorrhoids, and many other swellings.

➤ Small amounts of wood betony have been used as a brain tonic and may help with vertigo.

➤ Spearmint soothes the stomach and eases nerves, both of which make it a useful remedy for vomiting.

➤ Reishi mushroom has been used to boost the immune system and may be helpful in ridding the body of warts.

➤ Juniper berries serve as a strong diuretic and should not be taken for long periods of time.

➤ Chickweed is a favorite herb used in weight-loss remedies.

Part 5

Now That You're Well, Let's Work on Prevention

Congratulations! If you have read this book all the way through, you have successfully learned about 100 ailments and more than 100 herbal solutions. You can now refer to this book anytime as a quick reference guide for what ails you.

Now that you know how to use herbs as a quick fix for some of your ailments, and you understand how you got yourself in your situation in the first place, let's take a look at how you can keep well using herbs. When used properly as nutrition, herbs can be an important factor in maintaining health. How can you go about that? Find an herbalist you can trust, and let him or her guide you.

These next chapters will show you what to look for in an herbalist and will also give you some tips on growing your own herbs at home. You will even get a recipe for making an herbal soap, potpourri, and a first aid kit that you can take along on your travels with you. So now that we've walked the herbal path, let's roll around in it a bit!

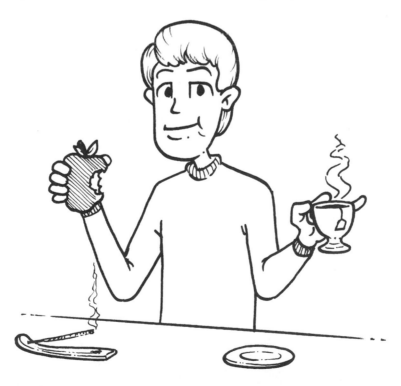

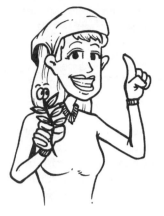

Chapter 24

Working with an Herbalist

In This Chapter

➤ What to look for in an herbalist

➤ Things you don't want in an herbalist

➤ Find an herbalist through two major organizations

➤ Discover a daily herbal program for health and longevity

➤ What herbalists can and can't tell you

So, now that you've tried some of the herbal remedies you found in this book and they've worked miraculously for you, you see the value of herbs. You are now ready to find your own special herbalist to cook you up an individualized herbal nutritional program for long life and great health, right? Good. This chapter will give you some tips on finding and working with one who suits you. I will give you some tips to help screen out some Johnny rotten apple seeds and find an herbalist that will grow on you. So put on your gloves and join me in the weeding process.

The Weeding Process

As I mentioned earlier in this book, many home-grown herbalists I have met didn't set out to become herbalists by trade; many began using herbs because of their illnesses. When they were offered no hope and were downtrodden, they were led to herbs, which turned out to be their cure and their answer. Some of them found a passion for helping others with the same illnesses, which led them to an in-depth study of herbs.

Others have had moms, dad's grandmothers, grandpas, and ancestors on up the line who harvested herbs and used them as medicines throughout their family history. Herbology is a second nature to some.

Sage Advice

Unfortunately, with the explosive popularity of herbs in our daily lives in recent years, there are plenty of bad apples out there in the herbal fields, just like there are good and bad medical doctors, teachers, dentists, and people of all fields. Licensing doesn't give one integrity. As with anything you do in a free country, *use your own best judgement* to rule out those herbalists whom you are uncomfortable with.

Finally, some practitioners set out to be herbalists, studying Chinese medicine and healing modalities, Ayurvedic practices from India, and Western herbology. Some are botanists or pharmacologists and even medical doctors who have found herbalism. Many herbalists own herb shops or natural health clinics, or own businesses or schools dedicated to the study and use of herbs. Most herbalists have a deep connection with nature and health and have a sincere desire to help others.

Here are some cautions to use when seeking an herbalist:

➤ Beware of people claiming to be able to help all your ailments who only offer a handful of products. Although the few products the person may carry might be wonderful, a handful of herbs comes nowhere near what is available. In addition, the herbalist probably won't be able to truly customize a program specifically for your needs. Individualized programs are important to get quality results.

➤ Similar to the herbalist with only a few products for sale is the herbalist that claims that a few miraculous combinations are sure to cure all that ails you. This is why many herbal remedies defy solid scientific research results. Each person varies in his or her biochemical makeup, lifestyle, eating habits, and genetic strengths and weaknesses. This makes the effects of a single herb differ for each person.

➤ Beware the herbalist who tells you how great a product is but cannot tell you what is in the products. If a so-called herbalist cannot tell you the ingredients in the mixture or can't explain the nature of the herb, be leery of what you are taking. If the products sold are bottled and properly labeled and the herbalist cannot answer questions or find out answers for you on the ingredients, consider working with someone who can.

➤ Anyone who pressures you to buy products just to make a sale cannot have your best interests at heart! Seek sincerity, and read a person for honesty.

➤ There are many, many herb manufacturers out there—more and more pop up every day. Some are exceptional and have spotless reputations; others are fly-by-night, and some are even negligent. A good herbalist will have done his or her homework for you and will choose a product or a source you should be able to trust. You can ask your herbalist about the manufacturer of the herbs suggested for you. Some of the top herbal companies have been around a very long time, for good reason. (See the checklist for a quality manufacturer in Chapter 1.)

On the other hand, you need to know where the herbalist's legal boundaries are. Professional herbalists do not practice medicine, and so they will not and cannot treat, diagnose, or prescribe. They cannot make claims for any herbs that they may suggest for you, without legal repercussion.

Herb Lore

If you ask an herbalist point-blank, "Will alfalfa cure arthritis in my joints?" he will have to tell you no. However, he may reword his answer to tell you that alfalfa is rich in minerals and that minerals support the structural system. Herbalists walk a fine line (as do other holistic health practitioners), and in most states they cannot even name an organ that they have seen healed with the use of herbs—unless there is scientific proof to back up the claim, of course. There are no magic bullets with herbs, and your herbalist should have a broad knowledge of different herbs and their combinations and uses.

What an herbalist *can* do for you is teach you about the herb(s), share information with you, and supply you with information that supports the use of herbs for specific purposes. Working with an herbalist should be an educational and empowering experience for you.

Witch One Is Best for Me?

Now that you know what things *not* to look for in an herbalist, how can you find the one that is right for you? Simply put, the one that works for you is really the person you feel most comfortable with and who has the knowledge to help you with herbs.

The following questions will help you determine which herbalist is right for you:

➤ Does this person engage you in your own healing process?

➤ Does this person ensure you that the body heals and that the herbs give it the opportunity to heal, or does he or she take the credit for your recovery?

➤ Does this person make you feel that you can trust him or her?

➤ Do you learn from this person?

➤ Does this person guide you or dictate to you?

➤ Can this person answer your questions to your satisfaction?

➤ Does this person teach you about herbs and about the nature of why you may be ill in the first place? Does he or she help you with a plan suitable for you?

➤ Do you get results working with this person?

➤ Does this person listen to you?

Poison Ivy

You will do yourself a disservice if you hop around from herbalist to herbalist seeking a quick cure or a miracle herb. True healing takes time and is a process. Once you find an herbalist you can trust, stick with that person, and give yourself several months to track your changes. Remember, the healing is yours to do, and the herbalist is only your guide—be patient.

And, of course, because you might be seeing your herbalist for occasional "check-ups," good chemistry helps!

Once you find a good herbalist and are on a good program for yourself, you will become familiar with the herbs you are taking and what effects they have on your body. If your herbalist is really good, you will need to be visiting him or her only occasionally to get feedback, and possibly to work with issues that come up from time to time.

Everyone is different, but I usually tell my clients upfront that it will take three months to see substantial changes; sometimes it is longer, and sometimes it is shorter. Then I set a game plan, based on what that person's health goals are. Eventually, we come to a point where my client is feeling good and healthy and is familiar with the herbs that work well for him or her. At that point, the client can maintain health nutritionally with herbs; hopefully their diet will have improved, and the need for an abundance of herbs is curbed.

Branching Out

You might find that it is difficult to locate an herbalist who specializes only in herbs. Herbs are holistic; to have an understanding of their use, a good herbalist will have knowledge of anatomy and physiology and the nature of certain illnesses in the body.

Herbalists are found amongst many practitioners in the healing arts including chiropractors, osteopaths, naturopathic physicians, traditional naturopaths, holistic nutritionists, clinical nutritionists, reflexologists, massage therapists, iridologists, kinesiologists, acupuncturists, and colonic therapists.

Licensing is not required for herbalists, so many herbalists seek out the highest levels of certifications attainable.

Two designations to look for after a professional herbalist's name, who is not already licensed in other areas, include M.H. and A.G.H.

The M.H., or Master Herbalist, designation means that the herbalist has been certified by an organization in the use of herbs. Master herbalists can receive their training through various schools and programs.

A.G.H., or American Herbalist Guild professional member, is a designation awarded to professional herbalists who have achieved a high level of training, who pass examinations to prove herbal competency, who have been in clinical practice for several years, and who agree to a high code of ethics in the field. The American Herbalist Guild is a non profit educational organization that claims to be the only peer-reviewed organization for professional herbalists specializing in the medicinal use of plants. The AGH can refer you to an herbalist in your area. To find out more, contact:

Sage Advice

Almost every holistic practitioner will use herbs in some capacity in their practices. Some specialize in herbs more than others. Many of these practitioners can and will help you with an herb or two here or there, but if you are looking for a game plan for incorporating herbs into your life, you may have to search.

> **American Herbalist Guild**
> P.O. Box 746555
> Arvada, CO 80006
> 303-423-8800
> Fax: 303-402-1564
> www.healthy.net/herbalists
> e-mail: ahgoffice@earthlink.net

Another organization of professionals is the American Botanical Council, another non-profit research and educational organization. They can be reached at:

> **American Botanic Council**
> P.O. Box 14435
> Austin, TX 78714-4345
> 512-926-4900
> Fax: 512-926-2345
> www.herbalgram.org

And no herb book would be complete without mentioning the Herb Research Foundation, which offers a massive amount of herbal information and resources. Contact:

> **Herb Research Foundation**
> 1007 Pearl Street, Suite 200
> Boulder, CO 80302
> 800-748-2617
> www.herbs.org

Herbs as a Lifestyle

The best use of herbal remedies comes when you take a holistic view at the nature of your overall health and illnesses and then take a look at the nature of the herbs you are using. It is really all about getting the right combination to achieve the effects you are aiming for. This is why it is almost essential to consult with a holistic health practitioner of some kind to find out what is right for you, especially if you intend to use herbs nutritionally on a daily basis.

You might want to look for someone who has a method of assessing what herb or combination of herbs is correct for you. As you have learned in this book, several different herbs are helpful for a certain ailment, but how do you know which one will be the best for *your* particular body?

Some methods that practitioners will use to assess what might be best for you include a mixture of the following:

➤ Body typing

➤ Muscle testing

➤ Iridology (analysis of the iris of the eyes)

➤ Tongue diagnosis

➤ Pulse diagnosis

➤ Blood tests

➤ Saliva testing

➤ Urine analysis

➤ Metabolic typing

➤ Hair analysis

➤ Live blood analysis

Sage Advice

General conditions of the nails, face, skin, hair, tongue, and eyes indicate a state of health or illness.

There are many other forms of assessing your constitution and chemistry, and these methods listed can be used in combination to gain information about your health.

A good herbalist will help you put together a combination that will bring you results. It is much nicer to have a game plan with someone schooled in herbology than to take guesses and choose things randomly off the shelves at your health food store (although many qualified herbalists are available in health food stores!).

The quality of the herbal products you take will also have a lot to do with the results you get using herbs.

The FDA does not regulate the herb industry, so it is best to get your products from a reputable company that runs their manufacturing plant to the same standards as the pharmaceutical companies. These are usually large manufacturers that have been in business for decades. See more on quality of herbs in Chapter 5, "A Is for Ailment."

A Daily Program

A good general maintenance program will differ slightly for each person because we all have special needs, but a general daily program that almost anyone can safely take to maintain health is included here. Any generally healthy adult who lives an average lifestyle can use these herbs. They won't be necessary for those living on a macrobiotic diet of all whole, raw, fresh, organic foods. Nor will it be necessary to help those who are perfect in every way, but for most of us, this general program is designed for the maintenance of health and can be used for a lifetime.

A Daily Program for Health and Longevity

Herb	Quantity	Supports
Liquid chlorophyll	Two to four tablespoons in water to taste, daily.	Digestive, intestinal, structural, and circulatory system support. Saves energy digestion; is safe and easily assimilated. Provides minerals; deodorizes, filters pollutants we come in contact with, builds red blood count.
Psyllium hulls	Four capsules twice daily.	Intestinal system. Gives the bowel something to resist against, sweeps excess waste from colon, and aids weight regulation, steadies blood sugar.
Papaya	Two chewable tablets before each meal, and after as needed.	Digestion. This fruit (comes in a chewable tablet form usually) supplies enzymes helpful in breaking down enzyme-less (cooked) foods. Saving digestive energy will help save life energy.
Gotu kola	Two capsules daily.	Gotu kola is my favorite anti-aging remedy; it feeds the nervous system and will help keep the mind sharp, aids vitality and longevity.

continues

A Daily Program for Health and Longevity   (continued)

Herb	Quantity	Supports
Garlic	Two cloves, or equivalent in capsules daily (if tolerated).	Garlic is sometimes not suitable for sensitive stomachs, but it is a wonderful all-around food beneficial for the immune system, circulatory system, and respiratory system. It can help protect you from catching illnesses of all sorts.
Bee pollen	Two capsules twice daily.	Bee pollen will round off your program, providing you every substance needed to survive. It contains many vitamins and amino acids. Only those with allergic reactions to bees or bee pollen should avoid its use. (Substitute barley grass herb if so.)

Along with your other good habits—such as daily water intake, exercise, good relationships, and a variety of wholesome foods—this program can help you maintain your health and help you live a long and nourished life!

The Least You Need to Know

➤ Use your best judgment when seeking an herbalist; seeing an herbalist should be a learning experience.

➤ Seek an herbalist who has a method of determining which herbs might be best suited to your particular body.

➤ Look for the M.H. or A.G.H. designations after an herbalist's name if you are seeking one with credentials specifically in herbology. Otherwise, many holistic-oriented practitioners may be knowledgeable about herbs.

➤ You can use herbs daily as your source for nutritional support to ensure that you receive minerals, vitamins, fiber, brain nourishment, and immune support.

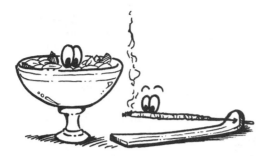

Chapter 25

Other Uses of Herbs

> ## In This Chapter
>
> ➤ How to use herbs to decorate your home
>
> ➤ Make your own potpourri from dried herbs
>
> ➤ Step-by-step instructions to make your own herb wreath
>
> ➤ Tips for growing your own herbs for spices
>
> ➤ Make your own herbal soap

Besides using herbs daily as nutritional supplements, we can use herbs in a variety of creative ways, from decorations to spices. In fact, many of us use herbs daily in our lives and are not even aware of the ways we surround ourselves with these multifarious plants.

In this chapter, we will take a look at how herbs surround you almost daily, and we'll see how you can use herbs in almost every aspect of your life.

Everyday Uses of Herbs

I recently returned from visiting some good friends who live in Montana. I specifically went to help one of them get on an herbal and nutritional game plan to boost her immune system. My friend is 37 years old and, by chance, went to her doctor for a regular check-up and was diagnosed with a cancerous tumor. Her surgery was completed almost immediately to remove the tumor. Fortunately, they did not find any more traces of cancer during her check-up, so she was not a candidate for chemotherapy treatment.

My friend realized that somehow she had created an internal environment in which cancer was given the opportunity to propagate. She realized that if she were to continue on her daily routine as she had previously, she wouldn't be doing anything to prevent the problem from happening again. Wisely, she decided to change her internal environment into one in which cancer and illness would be clearly uninvited. I was honored to have her choose me as her holistic guide.

My friend is now on a program to help ensure her a long and healthier life.

Herb Lore

Herbalists and many holistic practitioners believe that cancer feeds off the calcium in your body, which is why it usually ends up in the bones, a very serious stage of cancer. This belief makes it very important to get extra calcium when fighting cancer. Make sure that you also engage in therapies that enhance your immune system to fight and kill off free radicals.

The ironic thing about this story is that, although I went there to help my friend with herbs as nutritional supplements, I saw that she was surrounded by herbs! I first visited her sister and family, who had a basement with a room dedicated to growing herbs. Her sister had grown rows of tiny, live, green, and growing fresh herbs, including chives, marjoram, thyme, dill, rosemary, and many, many more. These herbs were growing for use as spices and to add to her canning, for homemade salsas (I should have asked for a jar!), and for general food flavoring.

Sage Advice

Herbs can and will change your internal environment, which will eventually be reflected on the outside as well. I have watched the phenomenon happen over and over again not only personally, but also with my clients, family, and friends.

Then we traveled to my friends' 40-acre piece of the mountains where she and her husband are building their house. (The view was breathtaking—her home overlooks a huge lake and the Canadian Rockies.) As we walked to feed her horses, I noticed echinacea flowers lining her fences (great for the immune and respiratory systems), yarrow (for fevers), and even uva ursi (for the urinary system) covering the ground. Almost everywhere I looked I saw herbs beautifying her lot. Then we entered their unfinished home, and I was stunned to see a massive and beautiful display of herbs hanging to dry over her dining room table! (See the photo I included here. The black-and-white print does it no justice, but the colors were fantastic.)

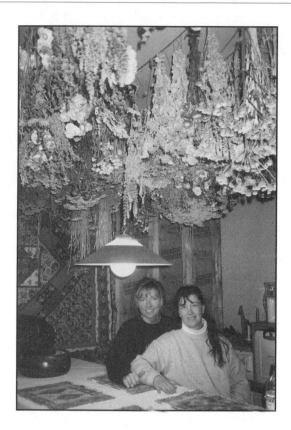

The author and her friend Marge sitting under Marge's Montana dried herb collection.

So what did this friend need me for?! She's a gardener and a wild herb harvester and has a sister who grows her own indoor herbs! Well, unlike me, my friends seem to have a knack for nature and a heavy dose of nurturing inherent in their blood, but had been harvesting herbs primarily for decoration and spice. Although I admire and am in awe of nature, I am a different type of herbalist. And I guess that's why my friend called me for help. When I think of herbs, I think tinctures, infusions, and pills. Ironically, when my friend received her box of herbs from the manufacturer, she thought she had never seen so many herbs in her life! You may be this way, too; you bought this book because you thought you were an "idiot" when it came to herbal knowledge, but when you look around you'll find that you might know a lot more about them than you thought!

So, you see, herbs can infiltrate our lives in many ways without us really noticing we are surrounded by them.

Here are just a few of the ways we can use herbs other than ingesting them for nourishment:

➤ Tie dried herbs together to make decorative wreaths

➤ Use dried herbs as bouquets for vases

➤ Add herbs to candle wax to make decorative candles

➤ Burn herbs as incense

➤ Fill bowls with herbal potpourri

➤ Add herbs to clear decorative bottles of bath oil to enhance the appearance and fragrance of oils

➤ Stuff small fabric bags with herbs to make eye pillows for relaxation

➤ Add herbs to canning for flavor and/or preservation

➤ Grow herbs for good luck, viewing pleasure, fragrance, or to repel insects

➤ Add herbs to soap for decorative soap-making, which also make great gifts

Now let's take a more detailed look at how you can fill up your life—instead of just your medicine cabinet—with herbs.

Decorations from Nature

It doesn't have to be Christmas to decorate your home with wreaths. Some like to make wreaths from herbs for other holiday times and celebrations, or to give as gifts.

Here's how to make a pretty wreath from herbs:

1. Purchase a straw or wooden wreath as a frame from your local craft store. The frame can be circular, but sometimes they come in half-circles.

2. Pick your favorite herbs (flowering herbs make nice decorations), and tie them in bunches with a light wire (also purchased at your craft shop). Make sure the stems are all going in the same direction.

3. Beginning on the inside of your frame, start inserting your herb bunches in a circular fashion, underneath the wires of the frame. You can also use florist pins, purchased at the same store, to ensure that the herbs stay in.

4. Continue this addition of dried herbs, working your way toward the outside of the wreath. It is better to start with the smaller leaves and flowers on the inside, and work your way outward with larger plants.

5. You can decorate with a bow, pinecones, dried berries, candles, ribbon, or any other decorations you can think of. You can either hang your wreath immediately, or you can first let the herbs dry for a week or so, and then decorate it with accessories and hang it. If you let it dry first, you might see some gaps open up that you can fill in before hanging.

Sage Advice

You can use pretty dried flowering herbs to decorate a glycerin-based bar of soap, fragrance it with some essential oil, and wrap it in a clear cellophane. Tie it with a ribbon, and add a bar to gift baskets or hand them out just as they are!

A variation of this is to purchase a foam wreath as a frame, and stick the stemmed end of your dried herbs and flowers into the wreath itself until the entire foam frame is covered. Be creative and have fun!

How about making your own herbal soap? Not only are these very decorative in a soap dish or a bathroom basket, but they also make very nice gifts. Here's a transparent soap recipe generously donated to me for this book. You can try it if you get the urge.

Ingredients:

1 cup tallow (various fats, can be animal- or plant-based)

³/₁ cup water

²/₃ cup glycerin (can be purchased from a drug store)

¹/₂ cup olive oil

1 cup isopropyl alcohol (purchased at a drug store)

4 tablespoons lye flakes (purchased at a drug store)

A dish or container to use as a mold, greased with Vaseline®

A double boiler

Step 1: Melt fat (tallow) in olive oil in a medium pan (or in a coffee can)—make sure to use pot holders to avoid getting burned by the can!

Fill your large sink or bathtub with lukewarm or cool water, and gently set the pot or can into the water to cool the mixture. Do not submerge it! Just float the container in the water to cool it. Be careful to not let it spill.

Stir in lye into the water, and then pour into the fat mixture and stir. When it becomes a creamy mixture, add your liquefied glycerin.

Pour into the mold, and let it sit for three days

Step 2: The soap will now be hard. Grate the soap with a cheese grater into the top of a double boiler. Gently boil water to a warm mixture. Add the alcohol, and stir consistently. This process will make your soap transparent. You will know when it is done by lifting the spoon from the mixture and looking for a ropy, thread-type consistency. Remove the mixture from the heat, and a skim should form almost instantly. You can then either mix in tiny pieces of dried herbs and immediately pour the whole thing into molds, or you can pour the mixture into your molds first and add your herb pieces more deliberately directly into the mixture before it cools.

Let the soap sit for two to three days, and then remove it from mold and place in open air to cure for two weeks.

Spicy Ways to Sprinkle Herbal Knowledge

Spice up your life with parsley, sage, rosemary, and thyme—wait a minute, didn't I hear that somewhere before? Anyway, these herbs in addition to basil, marjoram, chives, and dill are some of the most popular herbs to grow for spices. You can use any of these fresh and add them to your cooking and canning, or you can chop them and add them directly to your foods.

Garlic is another wonderful herb to have around, and the bulb keeps for a long time in your refrigerator crisper.

Botanical Bit

Potpourri is a mixture of dried flower petals, herbs, flower tops, bark, leaves, nuts, fruit skins, and seeds of plants, tossed together in a mix and left out to scent a room.

Sage Advice

For those of you who are green thumbs and who have patience, growing your own herbs at home is a rewarding hobby, and many good books on the subject are available. Call the American Botanical Counsel for a suggestion, and see Appendix B, "Bibliography," for some suggested reading.

You can also grow your own cayenne peppers. This plant loves the heat and direct sunlight; grow it in a large pot, and wait until the peppers grow and ripen. You can then pick the peppers, if you are Peter Piper (just kidding). Pick the peppers and set them out to dry, or use a dehydrator, if you wish. These peppers make great decorations hanging in bunches for a southwestern effect in the kitchen, or you can grind them up with a mortar and pestle and encapsulate them to rev up your circulatory system. Put the crushed mixture, along with the seeds, into a container with holes in the top. You can shake the hot mix onto any food that needs some spice. (My husband likes to add this to his pizza.)

Potpourri, Fragrance from Nature

Potpourri (pronounced *poe-poor-ree*) is a French word that translated literally means "rotten pot"! In English, however, potpourri is used to describe a usually decorative mixture of dried sweet- or flowery-smelling herbs, flower tops, bark, leaves, nuts, fruit skins, and seeds of plants, tossed together in a mix and left out to fragrant a room. Potpourri is also a pretty addition to an empty bowl, basket, or jar.

Potpourri can be left dried in a bowel—in the bathroom, for instance—or it can be added to a simmering pot of water for a more strong and immediate aroma. But beware—if you leave the potpourri in water and let all the water evaporate, the mixture will mold quite rapidly. Maybe this is where the French translation of "rotten pot" comes in!

Here's a recipe for a favorite mild-smelling and nerve-relaxing potpourri mixture:

Ingredients:

> 1–2 cups of dried lavender flowers
>
> $^3/_4$ cup tangerine peels
>
> $^1/_2$ cup chamomile
>
> $^1/_4$ cup dried blueberries
>
> $^1/_4$ cup powdered orris root
>
> 5–10 drops of lavender or chamomile (your preference) essential oil

Place all ingredients in a bowl, and mix so that the oil is absorbed into the dried mix. Place the entire mixture into a paper bag, and shake wildly. Once you are done shaking, grasp the bag and shake the mixture to toss all ingredients. You can then place this mixture in a bowl, basket, or jar and leave out for a sweet, relaxing aroma for any room.

You can pulverize extra leftovers of this mixture with a mortar and pestle and then use them to stuff herb pillows or sachets, or make a bath bag (use a small muslin or cotton sack, tie securely at one end, and place in bath tub water). You can also use the potpourri mixture and add the petals and tiny flower tops to decorate candles when making your own. This works best with larger candles.

Growing Your Own

To bypass the dangers of incorrectly identifying herbs in the wild, and to get started using fresh herbs without a botany lesson, you always have the option to grow your own. You can start by visiting a nursery that grows herbs and purchasing your own seeds (rather than collecting seeds from the wild, which will again involve the problems with misidentifying).

The biggest benefit of growing your own herbs is that because you have purchased your seeds, you will be able to correctly identify the herb that grows. Most plants you grow at home will be mild because of the pampering you give them and will be safe to use for occasional medicinal purposes—they'll be especially useful for spices and cooking.

Botanical Bit

Perennials are plants that have a life span of more than two years—if you are lucky, these plants come back over and over again for years. **Annuals** are plants that live and grow for only one year or season and then die. **Biennials** are plants that usually require two years to reach maturity; these bloom in the second year before dying.

If you look at your thumb and see that it is more orange, purple, blue, or anything but green, but you still desire to grow a few of your own herbs, then we should cover a couple of the basics here first. First of all, you might want to consider planting *perennials* instead of *annuals*; or, if you are patient, try *biennials*, which take two years to bear fruit or flowers.

You don't need to be a country boy or girl to grow your own herbs; even city-dwellers can grow herbs in a windowsill flower box, or in small pots set by a window. Whether growing indoors or outdoors, take a look at the following table for 10 popular herbs to grow, with their category and some uses. This chart will help you if you are feeling stood up because you have been waiting patiently for your basil (an annual) to re-grow again, but it never shows! (Don't take it personally—this is basil's nature.)

Popular Herbs and Their Uses

Herb	Latin Name	Type	Uses
Anise	*Pimpinella anisum*	Annual	Taken by nursing mothers to produce lactation; seeds sooth stomach. Used as a spice (licorice-type flavor) and to flavor liquors. Leaves are used in salads.
Basil	*Ocimum basilicum*	Annual	Used as a spice mainly to flavor tomato-based dishes, spaghetti sauces, and Italian dishes. The fresh plant is said to repel mosquitoes and flies.
Chamomile	*Matricaria recutita*	Annual	Tea or capsules are used to calm nerves and settle the stomach. Used in shampoos for blond highlights. Great ingredient in eye pillows. Fresh plant is an insect repellent. Use in potpourri.
Catnip	*Nepeta Cataria*	Perennial	Soothes stomach; moms find it helpful for colicky babies. Cat's love to eat it, so keep it away from them when trying to grow it; the dried herb stuffed into a cat's toys will serve as entertainment for you and your cat (it makes cats act intoxicated and silly!).

Herb	Latin Name	Type	Uses
Chives	*Allium Schoenoprasum*	Perennial	This herb from the onion family is popular as a topping on baked potatoes or any foods you would add onions to for flavoring. Folklore used hanging chives to chase away evil spirits.
Parsley	*Petroselinum crispum*	Biennial	Aids digestion and urinary tract. Decorates food plates. Attracts a caterpillar that will turn into a black swallowtail butterfly—an endangered species!
Sage	*Salvia officinalis*	Perennial	Used as a seasoning for meats. Used medicinally for sinuses, nerves, bowels, and the bladder.
Clary sage	*Salvia viridis*	Biennial	Decorative with blue and white flowers. Attracts hummingbirds. Oil is used to balance hormones in women, and some use it as a perfume.
Thyme	*Thymus vulgaris*	Perennial	Used as a spice. Medicinally has been used to boost the immune system. Many different types of thyme are available, some very decorative for growing; ask your nursery specialist.
Valerian	*Valeriana officinalis*	Perennial	Used as a sedative. Grown for sweet fragrance, but the root (the medicinal part of the herb), is repulsive to humans, yet irresistible to cats! (Then again, most of us are not fond of mice either!)

Harvesting is tricky business because it will vary depending on where you live and what your climate is like. It will also depend on what use you will have for the herb you harvest and which herbs you are harvesting. For instance, the medicinal value of ginseng root is not effective until it is at least five years old. Some manufacturers will sell ginseng that is immature and therefore not very potent. Again, be sure you know or trust your source, especially when purchasing ginseng because this is one of the more expensive herbs.

As a general rule, my herb-growing friends tell me that you should harvest your flowering culinary herbs (herbs you are using for spice and food additions) just before they flower to preserve the essential oils (which give them their strong flavor and smell)—unless, of course, you are growing the herbs for the use of their seeds, such as with fennel, anise, or dill.

After you learn when to harvest your herbs for your purposes, you will need to learn how to dry them. Again, this will vary depending on what type of herb you are harvesting and what you are going to use it for.

In general, you can bunch most of your herbs and place them in paper sacks. You should mark on the outside of the bag what the herb is so you don't get them mixed up. Some herbs should be bunched and then hung upside down from a string, and still other herbs can be placed directly into vases as decorations and left to dry as a dried flower decoration.

The Need for Weeds

You might consider having a couple other indoor or outdoor plants just for emergency or culinary use. You can purchase these as mature plants and begin using them as needed.

The aloe vera plant is a wonderful healing, medicinal plant that is easy to find, purchase, and keep alive. You won't need to water this plant very often, either. If you live in a warm climate, this plant can be an outdoor plant; otherwise, bring it in during the winter. Think of the aloe plant as a living first aid kit. If someone gets a cut, scrape, or burn, you can snip a piece off one of the leaves and apply the gel-like sap directly to the cut. Aloe sap can also be used as a beautifying ointment to soften skin and wrinkles, and it can be applied to sun burn and insect bites and stings to ease pain.

An old wives' tale says that if you are having bad luck, plant a garlic bulb in your window closest to your front door. This will ensure that no evil enters your home. I have a friend who began planting garlic in her windowsills without knowing a thing about this old wives' tale. She called me recently and told me about the weird way she just decided to plant garlic around her windows, and how well the plant grew. She also told me that since then, her typical bad luck was changed and that only good things were happening to her! Coincidence or synchronicity? Will we ever know? Film at eleven.

We have known for a long time that garlic serves as a valuable herb for our bodies. In the olden days, people used to wear garlic around their necks or hang it from their doorways and bedposts because they believed it to keep away evil spirits, vampires, werewolves, and plagues.

I've included this table just for fun, to take a look at some superstitious or earned reputations linked to some herbs, spices, and flowers.

Sage Advice

Branches of juniper are used by Native Americans to add to the sweat lodge fire and produce a cleansing, sweet-smelling smoke. You can dry some juniper branches and sprinkle some of the leaves onto a piece of lit charcoal to burn as incense. And, of course, if you are lucky enough to have your own sweat lodge, you can use it there also!

Herbal Reputations

Plant	Meanings
Roses	Love
Garlic	Protection from evil
Chives	Protection from evil and plagues
Marigolds	Joyful memories
Bachelor buttons	Happy independence
Basil	Good wishes
Marjoram	Joy
Rosemary	Memories
Sage	Long life
Thyme	Courage
Carnations	Friendship

Overall, the use of herbs in our lives is absolutely endless! Herbs are becoming popular as nutritional supplements, health-boosters, and body rejuvenators, but, as you can see, herbs can be a part of almost every aspect of our lives.

The Least You Need to Know

➤ Herbs can be used for much more than medicinal purposes: They make great decorations as wreaths, decorative soaps, candles, and pleasing-looking and fragrant potpourri.

➤ Growing your own herbs is a nice way to have a living spice cabinet, and herbs can be grown indoors or out.

➤ An aloe vera plant is a nice addition to any home; a piece can be cut off anytime and applied to cuts, scrapes, sunburn, and rashes.

➤ Sagebrush and juniper branches both make a nice-smelling and refreshing incense.

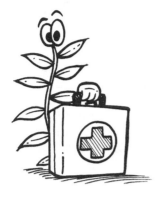

Chapter 26

An Herbal First Aid Kit

In This Chapter

➤ Make your own herbal first aid kit for travel or camping

➤ Herbs to help stop bleeding and help counteract poisonings

➤ Herbs for an asthma attack and to stop bruising

➤ An herb oil to help with toothache pain

➤ Use herbs to keep the bugs away

Are you a traveler? Do you like to go camping, hiking, backpacking, or any of the other fun outdoor sports that lead you away from your medicine cabinet or a family physician? Great! This chapter is for you.

In this chapter, you will learn how to make your own herbal first aid kit, and you'll learn the multi-faceted uses of six popular herbs or herbal oils. You can take this kit along with you in a backpack or a suitcase when traveling. It will come in handy if you get yourself into trouble, and it can help tide you over in case you can't reach a medical doctor right away. In fact, this kit can sometimes even negate the need for a doctor visit! Now, come along as we continue on the long path through herbalism.

Capsicum, Not Too Dumb to Keep on Hand

Encapsulated, dried herbs are especially useful to take as a first aid kit for hikers and backpackers because of their light weight. When stored in a compartmentalized container, herbs can be taken along just about anywhere.

At the end of this chapter, I'll give you some suggestions about how and what to store all these different herbs in, but for now, let's talk about how you can use each one in a pinch. Don't hesitate to make up this kit to store in your medicine cabinet at home, either—it can come in handy almost anytime, anywhere. I am a traveler, and it has come in handy for my family, my friends, and me in many countries, hotel rooms, and backpacking trips.

Sage Advice

You might want to make several small herbal first aid kits and store them in different places. For instance, make one for your boat, one for your home, one to keep with the camp gear, one for each vehicle, and one with your traveling bags.

Poison Ivy

The only caution with using capsicum in a lotion or gel is to watch out that you don't touch your eyes or any other sensitive parts after using the formula. If you do, flush out the area with cool water immediately. If you are sensitive to hot foods, try capsicum in very small doses.

Capsicum (*Capsicum minimum, C. frutescens*), also referred to as cayenne pepper or red pepper, is one of those herbal cure-all herbs and makes an excellent addition to any first aid kit. The fruit (pepper) of this plant is used for medicinal purposes, food, and spice. This herb is very hot, and if you buy it in encapsulated form, you will notice that it is red in color.

I would add a bottle of capsicum capsules to your first aid kit instead of a bulk powder. This herb is useful in winter if you are venturing on a snowmobile or a cross-country skiing trip. The pepper powder is stimulating and brings blood supply to the area to which it is applied. In other words, if you are on a winter outing, take capsicum with you to keep you warm. Simply open a capsule and sprinkle some in your socks and mittens to help prevent frostbite and keep your extremities warm. In addition, you can swallow a couple of capsules internally, and you will be able to feel the inner fire that it ignites.

Capsicum is also useful in your first aid kit as an emergency fix to stop bleeding. Capsicum is so "hot" that it has an ability to actually cauterize a wound in some cases. If you cut yourself and wish to stop the bleeding, empty a capsicum capsule onto your cut. The application will sting, but it should stop your bleeding right away.

Capsicum seems to have an ability to deaden the nerve endings temporarily, which is why it has been used as a pain-relieving remedy. While it may deaden pain, it also brings blood to the area to which it is applied and therefore can enhance your healing. Blood circulation brings nutrients and oxygen and is imperative to the process of tissue healing; capsicum can aid this process.

For a sore throat, gargle with capsicum added to water or juice. Although it may burn at first, the pain should subside within a short time, and your throat will feel better. You can even make capsicum into a spray for sore throats. (See the section "Tonsillitis: Tea Tree for Two, and Two for Tea Tree," in Chapter 21, "T: Terrific Solutions," for an herbal throat spray containing capsicum.)

When camping, you can sprinkle capsicum on foods—especially bland-tasting backpacking foods (although some companies are offering much better tasting foods these days). When taken internally, capsicum can increase the production of digestive acid and also may help expel gas from the intestines, relieving gas pains.

Herb Lore

If you are a comic fan, check out the back to see ads offering all types of gag gifts. You might see an ad for a type of gum that, as a trick, you offer to your enemies. When I was a young teen, I remember the ad showing a cartoon face of a man who had obviously chewed the gum and whose face was red as a beet. The drawing shows him perspiring heavily with his tongue sticking out and his hand grasped around his neck in choking agony! Guess what the main ingredient added to the gum was to cause this effect? You guessed it: good old capsicum!

The herb powder can be added to lotion or gel and can be applied to areas that need pain relief or circulation. The active ingredient capsiacin is a popular extract added to many pain-reliving formulas.

Capsicum is so stimulating, in fact, that it can be used in cases of severe shock, fainting, or even heart attack to bring someone back to consciousness. Add a small amount of powder to the tip of the tongue in these cases to try to stimulate blood flow back to the head and help the person recover from shock.

Giving aspirin to a heart attack victim has been publicized lately, probably due to the fact that aspirin thins the blood. Heart attacks that involve a blockage of blood flow to the heart can be helped by thinning the blood to allow at least some passage of blood to the heart. But don't forget about white willow bark, which is where the active ingredients in aspirin originally came from. White willow can be just as effective. Capsicum also is a circulatory stimulant, and both of these can work together to save a life in an emergency situation.

To sum up, here are some of the ways capsicum has been used and why it can be an integral part of any first aid kit.

Capsicum has been used to:

➤ Stop bleeding

➤ Relieve pain

➤ Warm extremities

➤ Increase internal heat

➤ Add flavor to foods

341

➤ Increase circulation

➤ Aid digestion and expel gas from intestines

➤ Stop heart attacks

➤ Bring people out of shock or keep them from going into shock after trauma

Take some along in capsules instead of the bulk form in case you need to swallow some.

Activated Charcoal, for De-Activating Poisons

Although charcoal is not an herb, It should be added to a first aid kit as a potent remedy to counteract the affects of poisoning.

When camping, traveling, or otherwise eating things that may not be clean, there is always the threat of food poisoning. Read up on food poisoning and more on the effects of charcoal in Chapter 11, "F: Fantastic Healing Flora."

However, you are more vulnerable to poisoning from snake bites, spider bites, and insect bites and stings when you are camping or out in the wild. This is where charcoal could serve to save your life.

Sage Advice

Another good remedy that you might want to take with you is blackberry tea. If you pack tea bags, make sure you put them in a sealed plastic bag or wax paper to preserve freshness. This tea makes a strong astringent herbal remedy, and I have seen it stop chronic cases of unexplained diarrhea right away.

Activated charcoal has properties that can attract (like a magnet) poisonous substances from your body, making them unable to be absorbed or can at least render them less harmful to the body. If a snake, scorpion, tick, spider, or any other animal or insect bites you—or even if you think you were bitten—you can begin taking a few capsules of charcoal to counteract any possible toxic side effects.

You can also make a poultice out of charcoal and apply it directly to a bite to draw out the poisons through the skin.

If you suddenly have an attack of diarrhea, you might want to consider taking a few capsules of charcoal as well. Diarrhea usually indicates that the intestines are reacting to some type of poison that the body is trying to rid itself of rapidly. Activated charcoal will assist the body in getting rid of the toxin and will help you to recover while you are seeking the medical attention you may need.

Clove Oil, Not a Snake Oil Remedy

We talked a lot about cloves and its properties back in the section "A Toothful Solution," in Chapter 21. Unexpected toothaches are one of the reasons you may benefit from having a small bottle of clove oil in your herbal kit.

Clove oil has an analgesic (pain-relieving) effect on tissues, and a small amount applied topically on or around sore gums or to an aching tooth can relive pain until you can get to see your dentist. Clove oil may also be used to apply topically if you have broken a tooth, to help numb the pain of an exposed nerve.

I can't vouch for this, but it is said that chewing on two raw cloves without swallowing also will curb someone of an alcohol craving. The strong taste of cloves left in your mouth will probably curb your appetite for almost anything, at least temporarily.

Besides its topical pain-relieving virtues, clove oil is a bug repellent, which is especially appealing to campers and hikers. A small amount can be applied to your hat or garments where bugs are bugging you!

Cloves can be used to kill bacteria, and therefore are used as an antiseptic for washing hands before preparing food when camping. This herb also has been used to ease indigestion, laryngitis, nausea, toothaches, vomiting, flatulence, abdominal pain, and asthma.

Cloves are a powerful remedy against parasites and can help you expel worms if you suspect you have picked up a parasite. You can add a tiny drop of clove oil to a liquid and then drink it; this is usually more than enough to expel a parasite. In general though, cloves are not recommended for internal use at all because of their strong and sometimes irritating effect on the body.

Children should not use the herb, although you can wet your finger and then add a drop of clove oil to apply to babies' gums when they are teething to ease their pain.

Sage Advice

If you make a mixture of clove oil and peanut oil or another type of non-essential oil that doesn't evaporate so easily, like olive oil, it will help keep the essential oil from quickly evaporating when you apply it to cloth for repelling insects.

Arnica You Glad You Use Herbs?

The yellow flowering herb arnica (*Arnica montana*) can be purchased as a topical application or for internal use as a *homeopathic* remedy. Arnica can be poisonous, so take internally only in a homeopathic solution as directed on the label. Never ingest arnica from the wild.

A homeopathic rule of thumb is that less is best. In other words, taking larger quantities is less effective than taking smaller amounts more often. I always have some arnica on hand to use for any type of trauma, stress, shock, bumps, bruises, emotional distress, and muscle soreness. Arnica is a wonder remedy, as far as I'm concerned, and should be a

Botanical Bit

A **homeopathic** is a highly diluted solution made from plant, animal, or mineral extracts. The dilution renders the solution non-toxic to humans, and the dilution also makes it more effective as a medicine.

part of everyone's first aid kit. My first introduction to the herb came when a family member, Sherry, came to my rescue at night, after I was accidentally smashed in the nose with great force. I heard the crunch of my cartilage and feared to look at my reflection, thinking I had been disfigured for life! Sherry was a self-taught natural herbalist and healer. I think her Cherokee blood and her close involvement in her tribe's traditional ceremonies gave her a special talent for knowing exactly what remedy to use for what ailments. She helped me learn a lot about plants, but I had no idea about arnica until that night.

By the time she could get to me, my crying from the initial pain and shock had begun to subside, and I dared to look in the mirror. I thought my nose was broken, and two dark blue half-circles had begun to appear under my eyes. When Sherry arrived, she had me hold out my hand, and she rolled six tiny white pills into my hand. She told me to put them under my tongue and let them dissolve. I did, and I immediately felt calmer, although I wasn't sure if it was Sherry's presence or the arnica that made me feel better. My prescription from Sherry was to take six of these little pills every two hours for the rest of the night, and then four pills every four to six hours for the next day. I followed her suggestions faithfully.

When I woke up the next morning, I was stunned to see that the dark purple coloring that was beginning to form under my eyes had faded into a pale blue. In two days, the discoloring was completely gone! I then understood the value of arnica: It not only can help calm you down from emotional or physical trauma or shock, but it also had an almost miraculous ability to heal and prevent bruising.

Another story about arnica stems from a time when another family member of mine had to undergo some serious facial surgery. She had to be bandaged for weeks afterward, and the bandages were to be changed weekly. I was just beginning to become more learned in the use of herbal remedies, and I suggested that she take arnica.

She took the arnica several times a day, three days before her surgery, and then continued on more frequent but smaller doses after her surgery. The first week after surgery, she went in for her check-up. After her bandages were removed, she reported that her surgeon was in absolute amazement at how well she had healed! The surgeon questioned her about what she had done specifically so that he could recommend this miracle-healing agent to his future patients.

For your herbal first aid kit, I suggest that you purchase arnica homeopathic in a pill form because pills are easier to pack than a liquid. You can also obtain a jar of cream to apply to sore areas after hiking, or to put on bumps and bruises of any kind. If you can get arnica in a liquid homeopathic with a glass dropper, this is also a sufficient way to take the remedy, but it might not be as convenient for packing.

Poison Ivy

Arnica also works well when applied as an ointment or cream. However, the cream should never be applied to any open wounds or cuts because it may cause a bacterial infection. Only apply to areas that are bruised or sore.

Ephedra, Help from China

Chinese ephedra, also commonly called ma huang, is a heart stimulant that increases circulation and opens bronchial passages. This makes it an excellent emergency remedy for anyone who is prone to asthma. Before I was on my daily herbal routine, I suffered from asthma and allergies (among many other ailments). For me, taking one or two capsules of herbs containing ephedra was equivalent to taking a shot off my bronchial inhaler. Ephedra stops bronchial constriction and eased my breathing and chest tightness within 15 minutes. If someone begins to get short of breath and has a tendency toward asthma, this remedy can be taken in small doses as a preventative remedy. It can be used in slightly larger doses if asthma strikes.

Read up on ephedra in the section "Asthma: It's So Wheezy to Fix," in Chapter 6, "Give Me Another A!" You will see that it is banned in some states and is not suitable for everyone, but this herb has been a godsend for many who used to suffer from asthma.

Ephedra can also be used as part of a weight-loss program because it curbs the craving for sweets, gives energy, and lessens appetite. Taking a capsule or two can ease a craving for camping junk food, too! What? No s'mores?

Ephedra also helps many with allergies, which could come in handy when hiking and camping. Plane travel, where you have the pleasure of breathing circulated air used by all passengers, seems to create more sniffles and sneezes as well, and ephedra can prove beneficial here, too. Just be sure to take it in small quantities, such as one capsule at a time, and see how you feel. You will usually find ephedra mixed in with other herbs to lessen the impact of the speedy feeling you can get from it.

Poison Ivy

Because ephedra is a heart stimulant, those with high blood pressure or other heart problems should avoid using it. This herb is also not recommended to be used daily for more than two weeks in a row, nor should it be used by pregnant or nursing moms.

If you live in a state or country where ephedra is not allowed, you can substitute lobelia in your herbal first aid kit in its place. Lobelia can also be used for allergies, asthma, and coughs. In higher doses, you can use lobelia as an emetic (induces vomiting), which can come in handy in case of poisonings. See more on lobelia in the section "Asthma: It's So Wheezy to Fix," in Chapter 6.

Peppermint for an Uplifting Time

One of my favorite herbs and essential oils of all time is peppermint (*Mentha piperita*). This cooling, minty, refreshing essential oil can make a nice addition to your first aid kit for many types of uses.

First of all, peppermint is stimulating, so it can be used as a pick-me-up by rubbing a little dab onto the temples. Just be careful not to touch your eyes after touching peppermint oil. You can put a dab on the middle of your tongue, close your mouth, and inhale. The "fumes" go directly to your brain area and help keep you alert and "mintally" stimulated.

Here's a list of the variety of ways peppermint can come in handy:

➤ Peppermint has been used topically to alleviate migraines and headaches.

➤ It can be rubbed onto a sore gum to ease toothache pain.

➤ Peppermint is great for camping breath, because a little dab can refresh your entire mouth.

➤ Some say that peppermint oil works great as a mosquito repellent, too.

➤ On a hot day, a few drops can be added to a tiny spray bottle filled with water and sprayed onto the skin for a stimulating cooling effect.

➤ For stomach aches, heartburn, and indigestion symptoms, a dab of the oil on the tongue can make you feel better.

➤ For fevers, a few drops can be added to a wet washcloth and applied to the forehead.

Sage Advice

Peppermint oil is also a great remedy to have on hand to stimulate blood circulation to an area. Some folks add it to their shampoos to bring circulation to the head and believe it helps stimulate hair growth.

Sage Advice

Everyone should be certified in basic CPR training because it can save your life or others. CPR training is offered many places and is inexpensive and sometimes free if taken through your employer. Call your local hospital, community education center, or college, or ask your employer about getting trained in this life-saving method.

Now that you know what you want in your herbal first aid kit and understand the uses of each herb, you need to know where and how to conveniently put it together.

I have a couple of hints for you to make your own, although I am sure you can find some commercially packaged kits out there. If you do, you can replace whatever herbs you don't like with the ones listed here, or you can add your own favorites.

My favorite way to carry herbs for travel is in plastic Tupperware®-type containers with adjustable trays to hold loose capsules. These vitamin chests can be found in most health food stores and come with stickers so you can label your compartments accordingly. The containers also are sturdy and travel well.

You will need to purchase a container that has at least six compartments if you are going to take the six herbs we talked about in this chapter. Or, you can purchase one with more compartments, and add your other first aid supplies such as bandages, sterile gauze, a sewing kit, aspirin (or white willow bark capsules), and the like. I like the hard containers because they keep the herbs from getting crushed, but if you are careful, you might find that a material case (such as a jewelry or make-up-type case made from a lightweight material) might be an easier way to carry your kit for camping.

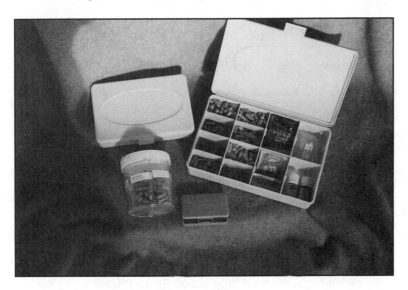

Herbal first aid kits in different sizes.

Your Herbal First Aid Kit

Herb	External Uses	Internal Uses
Capsicum	Sprinkled in socks or mittens will warm hands or feet; can help stop bleeding	Used to flavor bland tasting backpacking food
Activated charcoal	Poultice applied to bites or stings	Poisonings
Clove oil	Toothaches, insect repellent	Parasite expeller (minute doses only)
Arnica	Muscle soreness, bruises, blood blisters	Bruising, muscle soreness, pain, shock, emotional and/or physical trauma
Blackberry tea bags	Help shrink tissues (astringent)	Can help stop diarrhea
Ephedra (ma huang)	None	Aids asthma and allergy attacks
Peppermint oil	Mental pick-me-up; good for migraines, headaches, nausea, stomach ache; cooling	Numbs toothaches, alleviates canker sore pain and headaches; mental stimulant; freshens breath; helps get rid of fever

Time to sign off for now, but don't forget to check the appendixes in the back of the book for some more interesting reading on herbs and their uses. I encourage you to seek a competent herbalist to work with as you continue to learn about the safe and effective uses of plants. Until we meet again in the next book, I wish you the very best of natural health!

The Least You Need to Know

➤ Herbal first aid kits are a safe alternative for emergency use when traveling or camping.

➤ Capsicum applied to a wound may help stop bleeding immediately. This herb can also be used in the case of a heart attack to help the victim until you can get him emergency care.

➤ Activated charcoal taken internally may save you from toxic effects of poisonous bites, stings, or food poisoning.

➤ Clove oil should be used externally and can be an effective remedy for easing toothaches until you can see your dentist.

➤ A homeopathic remedy containing arnica montana can be an effective first aid for shock, trauma, emotional upsets, bruises, and pain.

➤ Ephedra can be used to alleviate or prevent an asthma attack or other allergic reactions or bronchial congestion.

➤ Peppermint oil is good to have in the first aid kit for any type of stomach discomfort or headaches.

Glossary

acne   A condition of the skin in which the sebaceous glands become inflamed and usually infected.

acupressure   An ancient Oriental art involving applied pressure to certain pressure points along the body to open energy flows, release tension, and promote balance.

adaptogenic herbs   Herbs that help the body adapt to stress. These include herbs such as ginseng, suma, astragalus, reishi mushroom, spikenard, and schizandra.

Alzheimer's disease   A progressive form of dementia occurring in middle age or later for which there is no medical treatment. It is associated with severe degeneration of the brain.

amenorrhea   Absence of menstruation (other than pregnancy) caused by a host of factors, including glandular abnormalities, diabetes, mental illness, anorexia, stress, and excessive exercise.

analgesic   Term used to describe an herb that has the ability to help relieve pain.

anemia   A reduction in the number of oxygen-carrying hemoglobin in the blood. This condition is characterized by fatigue, excess tiredness, pallor, low resistance to infection, and breathlessness. Some may show dark circles under the eyes and will bruise easily.

annuals   Plants that live and grow for only one year or season and then die.

antagonistic   Term meaning that some minerals are not compatible taken together, or that one mineral will suppress the absorption of the other.

anthelmintic   Term used for an herb that has properties that kill parasites. This term has been used interchangeably with *verimfuge, parasiticide,* and *anti-parasitic.*

antioxidants   Substances known to fight oxidation and therefore protect the body from free radical damage. Antioxidant vitamins include vitamins C, A, and E and help neutralize free radical scavenger cells.

anxiety attack   Pervasive fear dominating the feelings and characterized by a rapid heartbeat, shortness of breath, an out-of-control feeling, and uncontrollable shaking or crying. These attacks are more common in women than men and are usually related to some psychological factor. Also called *panic attack.*

arthritis   An inflammation of one or more joints characterized by swelling, redness, and warmth of the overlying skin; restriction of movement; and pain in affected areas.

asthma   A disease characterized by shortness of breath due to bronchial constriction. Most asthma is treated with *bronchodilators*, which are inhaled steroid substances that force the air passageways open to allow more air to pass through.

biennials   Plants that usually require two years to reach maturity; they bloom in the second year before dying.

bilirubin   A yellow or orange bile pigment. Bile pigments are colored compounds that are basically the waste components of blood that color feces.

bladder infection (cystitis)   A painful inflammation of the bladder usually caused by a bacterial infection such as E. coli. Symptoms include feeling the need for frequent urination, painful or burning urination, and may include blood in the urine.

bronchitis   Inflammation of the bronchi, which are the air sacks leading to the lungs. Symptoms include spastic, mucus-filled coughs. An airborne virus or bacteria is the usual cause of bronchitis.

carminative   An herbal property that, put simply, eliminates gas from the bowels.

chelated minerals   Minerals that are bound to proteins for better absorption in the body. A target-chelated mineral is one that is bound to a specific amino acid geared toward a particular body organ when it is ingested.

cleanse   Process occurring when the body dumps excess toxins through one or more elimination channels.

colonic   A water therapy used to cleanse the lower bowel that is administered by a trained colonic therapist. The therapist uses equipment to administer several gallons of water into the bowel. The irrigation is not retained, as in an enema, but it leaves the bowel through a tube and is sanitary and modest. Also called *colonic irrigation* or *colonic hydrotherapy*.

concentrated food   In holistic nutrition, a concentrated food is in contrast to a high-water-content food. In simple terms, you can think of a concentrated food as a food that when squeezed thoroughly, would produce little or no water. Foods such as cheese, meats, baked potatoes, and grains are considered concentrated foods.

conduction   The process in which heat is lost to a cooler environment from a warmer environment.

detoxing   Term used by herbalists for a process of internal cleansing. The body will eliminate waste materials or substances that are harmful to the body when it is strong enough to do so. Herbs help the body detoxify.

diabetes mellitus   A blood sugar disorder caused by the lack of or inability of the body to utilize a pancreatic hormone known as insulin. Symptoms of diabetes include excessive thirst and production of large volumes of urine. Diabetes is characterized into Type I and II.

diaphoretic   An herbal property that describes a certain herb's ability to increase elimination through the skin via perspiration.

dysmenorrhea   A painful menstrual period, which can lead to nausea, vomiting, and fainting.

eczema   A superficial inflammation of the skin. Eczema causes itching, with a red rash often accompanied by blisters that weep and become encrusted. Over time, the skin may thicken or discolor. The disorder has several forms with two basic divisions: outside causes and internal factors.

emetic   An herbal property used to describe an herb's ability to make you vomit.

emollient   Term used to describe an herb that has properties that soothe and soften tissue. Also called *demulcent*.

endometriosis   The presence of uterine-like tissue in abnormal places, usually in the pelvic cavity. Symptoms are usually painful menstruation and may exacerbate related menstrual symptoms.

enema   A therapy, usually self-administered at home, that cleanses the bowels with the use of an enema bag and water. The water is retained in the bowel and then ejected. The proper supplies can be purchased inexpensively at a pharmacy. Different herbs can be added to enema water for different effects.

enterically coated capsules   Capsules that are manufactured with a coating on them to protect them from being digested in the stomach so that they will be released in the intestinal tract. This is a more effective way of ensuring that the organisms such as intestinal flora (acidophilus) get replenished where you need them.

epimenorrhea   A menstrual period that comes in shorter than normal intervals.

ergonomically designed   A term used to describe furniture designed with correct posture and comfort in mind. This furniture is usually designed for the office worker.

expectorant   An herb that has properties that help the body expel phlegm or mucus from the lungs and sinuses.

glucose   The term used for blood sugar.

hemolysis   The rapid destruction of red blood cells caused by a mismatched blood transfusion, poisoning, infection, or the presence of certain antibodies. It usually leads to anemia.

herb   A plant with a fleshy stem that can be used as a food or spice, or that has some type of medicinal value. Think of herbs as wild vegetables.

Hering's Law of Cure   States that "All healing begins from the head down, the inside out, and in the reverse order as the symptoms have first been acquired."

homeopathic   A highly diluted solution made from plant, animal, or mineral extracts. The dilution renders the solution nontoxic to humans and also makes it more effective as a medicine.

insomnia   The inability to fall asleep or to stay asleep for an adequate amount of time. This causes almost chronic tiredness. Although some insomnia is linked to disease, much insomnia is caused by worry.

insulin   A hormone produced by the pancreas to regulate glucose in the blood.

menorrhagia   Abnormally heavy bleeding at menstruation.

nutritive   An herbal property that means that the plant has plenty of food value and may be used as a nourishing food.

perennials   Plants that have a life span of more than two years; if you are lucky, these plants come back over and over again for years.

peristaltic action   The wave-like muscular contractions that move contained matter along a tubular organ, such as the colon.

phytochemcials   Compounds found in plants that are captured by our body as nourishment when we eat the plant.

potpourri   A mixture of dried flower petals, herbs, flower tops, bark, leaves, nuts, fruit skins, and seeds of plants, tossed together in a mix and left out to fragrant a room.

radiation   General term meaning to radiate, which in physics is the term for the emission and movement of waves through space.

reflexology   The theory that all parts of your body can be positively affected by applying massage and acupressure-like techniques to the feet and hands. Reflexology has been used for pain reduction and promotes relaxation and euphoria.

reverse osmosis (R.O.)   A process of filtering water using a pressure vessel made up of layers of extremely fine membranes. As water is pushed through, viruses, heavy metals, bacteria, and other pollutants that are too large to pass through are left behind. The end result is pure H_2O. These filters can be found through catalogs, home stores, health food stores, and independent distributors.

Strontium-90   A radioactive substance harmful to the body. It can accumulate in food substances high in calcium; when you ingest the food, the calcium that is used by your bones will carry the pollutant to the bones, where it will damage bone marrow. The algin found in brown kelp will help block this absorption.

thermogenesis   Process of raising the body temperature to speed up the body's metabolism, which increases the burning of calories. Thermogenesis occurs naturally during periods of exercise.

tonsillitis   Inflammation of the tonsils usually due to infection.

toxins   Any substances that are harmful or poisonous, or that do not serve a positive function in the body

verimfuge   Term used for an herb that has properties that push parasites from the body. This term has been used interchangeably with *anthelmintic, parasiticide,* and *anti-parasitic.*

vitamins   Complex organic substances that occur naturally in plants (herbs) and animal tissue and that are essential for health and life. Vitamin pills differ from foods such as herbs and meat because they are usually a single, extracted vitamin from the plant (or animal) instead of the entire plant, which contains many phytochemicals and other vitamins and minerals intact.

weed   A plant thought of as undesirable, unattractive, and usually growing where it is not wanted. Some people consider certain herbs to be weeds. Once a person finds out the value of a "weed," however, he or she will usually refer to the plant as an herb.

Bibliography

Listed here are some books and other media that I referred to along the way to give you the information presented in this book. These titles are a small part of my holistic library, and you might find some of them very good reading, too. I broke them down into general categories. Happy reading!

Growing, Harvesting, and Decorating with Herbs

Shaudys, Phyllis. *The Pleasure of Herbs*. Pownal, VT: Storey Communications, 1992.

Medicine

Fries, James F., MD, and Donald M. Vickery, M.D. *Take Care of Yourself: The Healthtrac® Guide to Medical Care*. Reading, MA: Addison-Wesley Publishing, 1976.

Graedon, Joe, and Teresa Graedon, Ph.D. *The People's Pharmacy*. New York: St. Martin's Press, 1998.

Inlander, Charles B., Lowell S. Levin, and Ed Weiner. *Medicine on Trial: The Appalling Story of Medical Ineptitude and the Arrogance That Overlooks It*. New York: Prentice Hall Press, 1988.

Holistic Approaches

Airola, Paavo, N.D., Ph.D. *How To Get Well*. Sherwood, OR: Health Plus, 1974.

Balch, James F., M.D., and Phyllis A. Balch, C.N.C. *Prescription for Nutritional Healing*. Garden City Park, NY: Avery Publishing Group, 1990.

Bricklin, Mark. *The Practical Encyclopedia of Natural Healing*. New York: MJF Books, 1983.

Horne, Steven. *The Endocrine Symphony*. Provo, UT: Tree of Light Institute, 1996.

Time Life Books. *The Alternative Advisor: The Complete Guide to Natural Therapies and Alternative Treatments*. Richmond, VA: Time Life, 1997.

Wolfe, Frankie Avalon, Ph.D. *The Complete Idiot's Guide to Reflexology*. New York: Alpha Books, 1999.

Vitamin and Minerals

Clarke, Linda. *Know Your Nutrition.* New Canaan, CT: Keats Publishing, 1973.

Hausman, Patricia, M.S. *The Right Dose: How to Take Vitamins and Minerals Safely.* New York: Ballatine Books, 1987.

Pressman, Alan H., D.C., Ph.D., C.C.N., and Sheila Buff. *The Complete Idiot's Guide to Vitamins and Minerals.* New York: Alpha Books, 1997.

Medicinal Uses of Herbs

Carper, Jean. *Miracle Cures.* New York: HarperCollins, 1997.

Cox, Kathryn. *Pocket Guide to Wild, Edible and Medicinal Plants.* Laporte, CO: Motherlove Herbal Company, 1996.

Duke, James A., Ph.D. *The Green Pharmacy.* New York: St. Martin's Press, 1997.

Horne, Steven H., A.H.G. *The ABC Herbal.* Winona Lake, IN: Wendell Whitman Company, 1992.

Hutchens, Alma R. *Indian Herbology of North America: The Definitive Guide to Native Medicinal Plants and Their Uses.* Boston, MA: Shambhala Publications, 1973.

Krochmal, Arnold, and Connie Krochmal. *A Guide to the Medicinal Plants of the United States.* New York: Quadrangle/The New York Times Book Co., 1973.

Mowrey, Daniel B., Ph.D. *The Scientific Validation of Herbal Medicine.* New Canaan, CT: Keats Publishing, 1986.

Santillo, Humbart, B.S., M.H. *Natural Healing with Herbs.* Prescott, AZ: Hohm Press, 1989.

Shook, Edward E., Dr. *Advanced Treatise in Herbology.* Banning, CA: Enos Publishing, 1992.

Tenney, Louise, M.H. *Health Handbook.* Provo, UT: Woodland Books, 1987.

Wood, Matthew. *Seven Herbs: Plants as Teachers.* Berkeley, CA: North Atlantic Books, 1987.

Holistic Nutrition

Diamond, Harvey, and Marilyn Diamond. *Fit For Life.* New York: Warner Books, 1985.

Jensen, Bernard, Ph.D., N.D. *The Chemistry of Man.* Escondido, CA: Bernard Jensen International, 1983.

Jensen, Bernard, Ph.D. *Food Healing For Man: Volume I.* Escondido, CA: Bernard Jensen Enterprises, 1983.

Jensen, Bernard, D.C. *The Healing Power of Chlorophyll: From Plant Life*. Escondido, CA: Bernard Jensen Enterprises, 1984.

Jensen, Bernard. Ph.D. *Love, Sex & Nutrition*. Garden City Park, NY: Avery Publishing, 1988.

Pfeiffer, Carl C., Ph.D., M.D. *Nutrition and Mental Illness*. Rochester, VT: Healing Arts Press, 1987.

Food and Environmental Concerns

Green, Nancy Sokol. *Poisoning Our Children: Surviving in a Toxic World*. Chicago: The Noble Press, 1991.

Jensen, Bernard, and Mark Anderson. *Empty Harvest: Understanding the Link Between Our Food, Our Immunity, and Our Planet*. Garden City Park, NY: Avery Publishing, 1990.

Winter, Ruth, M.S. *Poisons in Your Food: The Dangers You Face and What You Can Do About Them*. New York: Crown Publishers, 1969.

Newsletters and Magazines

Better Nutrition. 5 Penn Plaza, 13th Floor, New York, NY 10001-1810; 212-613-9700.

Delicious. 1301 Spruce Street, Boulder, CO 80302; 303-939-8440; www.newhope.com/delicious.

Food & Water Journal. 389 Vermont Route 215, Walden, VT 05873.

Healing Feats News. (My personal newsletter to my clients.) 7 Whitehawk Circle, Boise, ID 83716; www.healingfeats.com.

HerbalGram: The Journal of the American Botanical Council and the Herb Research Foundation. P.O. Box 144345, Austin, TX 78714-4345; 512-926-4900; fax 512-926-2345; www.herbalgram.org.

The Integrative Medicine Consult. P.O. Box 1603, Newburg, NY 12551; 617-641-2300; www.onemedicine.com.

Townsend Letter for Doctors and Patients. 911 Tyler Street, Pt. Townsend, WA 98368-6541; www.tldp.com.

Herbal Cross Reference Chart

This alphabetical list of the herbs you learned about in this book serves as a helpful reference. The numbers in **bold** indicate the chapters where the herb is highlighted. See the index for more on the herb to make sure you find all references.

Herb	Chapter	Ailments Historically Used for...
Alfalfa	6	Arthritis, bursitis, rich in minerals; tooth decay, gout, ulcers, nutritional deficiencies (feeds), deodorizes, allergies, anemia, mild diuretic, kidney cleanser, radiation damage, fatigue
Algin	20	Radiation, heavy metal poisoning, detoxing
Aloe vera	4, 7	Burns (all types), digestive disorders, gastritis, ulcers, arthritis, laxative, scar tissue, deodorant, hemorrhoids, hiatal hernia, wrinkles, heartburn
Arnica	26	Bruises, pain, shock, trauma, distress, injuries
Bayberry	9	Diarrhea, indigestion, infections, jaundice, hemorrhage, goiter, prolapsed uterus
Bee pollen	5	Allergies, asthma, hayfever; immune system stimulant; provides nutrients for survival; nutritional deficiencies, anti-aging, hypertension, radiation sickness, anemia, increases fitness
Bilberry	10	Eyesight; improves night blindness; strengthens blood vessels; works as an antioxidant; varicose veins, kidney problems, light sensitivity
Black cohosh	7	Bites and stings, female disorders, menstrual pain, menopause, PMS, lungs (expels mucus), high blood pressure, relaxes nerves, eases hot flashes, stimulates estrogen production

continues

continued

Herb	Chapter	Ailments Historically Used for...
Black currant oil	17	Multiple sclerosis, immune system disorders, female disorders, eczema, mental disorders, obesity, provides essential fatty acids, alcoholism, cholesterol, high blood pressure, hair loss
Black walnut	11	Fungus, parasites, eczema, pimples, athlete's foot, psoriasis, jock itch, cold sores, constipation, worms, skin infections of all types; anti-bacterial; dries up breast milk; regulates blood sugar; removes plaque from teeth
Boneset	17	Measles, fever (induces sweating to break), colds, respiratory congestion, flu, arthritis, rheumatism, coughs, Rocky Mountain Spotted Fever, mumps
Buchu	7	Urinary tract problems, prostate trouble; works as a diuretic; strengthens the bladder; dropsy, yeast infections, bed wetting
Bugleweed	18	Nosebleeds, coughs, indigestion, pain, excess menstruation, irregular heart beat, overactive thyroid, multiple sclerosis, heart palpitations
Burdock root	5	Acne, fungus or bacterial infections, skin ailments, eczema, psoriasis, pimples, arthritis, gout, kidney problems, rheumatism, urinary tract; works as a blood cleanser, liver cleanser
Butcher's broom	13	Hemorrhoids, arteriolosclerosis, varicose veins, brain circulation, heavy feeling in legs
Calendula	20	Shingles, indigestion, cuts, wounds, chicken pox, rashes, burns, diaper rash; prevents pus/infections; beauty aid used topically
Capsicum	8, 26	Shock, trauma, stroke, heart and circulatory ailments; provides pain relief; stops bleeding when applied locally to cuts; increases circulation; improves digestion; helps with gas; increases vitality; reduces pain when applied to sore muscles or joints

Herb	Chapter	Ailments Historically Used for...
Cascara sagrada	8	Constipation, gallbladder problems, gallstones, hemorrhoids, liver, jaundice, spleen problems, worms, high blood pressure; tones bowel
Cedar berries	19	Pancreas trouble, incontinence, gout, dysentery, TB, diarrhea, diabetes, fungus, hemorrhoids, dandruff
Chamomile	20	Stress, nervousness, colic, stomach cramps, ulcers, drug withdrawal; improves appetite, insomnia, indigestion, nervousness; externally used for sunburn, cuts, scrapes, hemorrhoids, teething, blond hair highlights
Charcoal, activated	7, 11, 26	Poisoning; absorbs toxins; absorbs body odor; eliminates bowel toxins
Chickweed	4, 23	Weight loss, ulcers, obesity; works as an appetite suppressant; acts as a blood purifier; dissolves fatty tumors; cancer preventative, water retention, blood purifier
Chlorophyll, liquid	4, 7	Bad breath; purifies blood; deodorizes; builds blood count; rich in minerals, protects against pollution
Cloves	12, 21, 26	Teething, toothaches; works as a pain reliever; gets rid of parasites; repels bugs
Comfrey	15	Joint injuries, sprains, ulcers, wounds; heals bones; promotes new cell growth; arthritis, bruises, blood cleanser, burns; dislodges mucus
Cranberries	7	Bladder infection, kidney problems; works as a diuretic; prevents urinary system infections
Damiana	14	Frigidity, hormone balance, menopause, bronchitis, emphysema, exhaustion; works as an aphrodisiac for men and women
Dandelion	13	Hepatitis, jaundice, gallbladder problems, congestive heart failure, PMS, joint pain, blood pressure; cleanses the urinary tract; works as a diuretic; aids digestion
Devil's claw	15, 18	Neuritis, arthritis, swollen knees, diabetes, kidney problems, rheumatism; strengthens bladder; cholesterol (regulates)

continues

continued

Herb	Chapter	Ailments Historically Used for...
Dong quai	14	Infertility, female disorders, PMS, heart palpitations; improves poor circulation; eases tension, nourishes brain, reduces hot flashes, eases menopausal symptoms
Dulse	16	Thyroid problems, leg cramps, ulcers
Echinacea	8, 10	Colds, earaches, immune system problems, flu, infection, gingivitis, swollen glands, tonsillitis, laryngitis, diabetes, blood purifier
Elderberry	4, 11	Influenza, colds, flu, sinus congestion, allergies, asthma, mononucleosis, ear infections; boosts immune system
Elecampane	16	Lupus, parasites, bacterial and amoebic infections; works as a strong internal cleanser; supports the immune system
Ephedra, Chinese	6, 26	Asthma, allergies, all respiratory ailments, congestion; increases energy; increases blood pressure; activates heart; speeds metabolism
Evening primrose oil	8	Cold sores, PMS, multiple sclerosis, inflammatory diseases of the immune system, eczema
Eyebright	10	Eye problems, eye infections, pink eye, colds, nasal congestion; strengthens, soothes, and reduces redness and inflammation; improves eyesight
Fennel	12	Intestinal gas, indigestion, colic, bronchitis; works as an appetite suppressant
Fenugreek	7	Bronchitis, mucus problems, allergies, asthma, stomach problems, cholesterol (dissolves); reduces fever; eliminates water retention
Feverfew	17	Migraines, inflammation, arthritis, tinnitus; thins blood; reduces fevers
Garlic	4, 7, 8	Regulates blood pressure, respiratory congestion, immune system problems, asthma, ear infections infections (kills), parasites, fungus, high cholesterol; stimulates lymphatics; works as an antiviral agent, cancer preventative

Herb	Chapter	Ailments Historically Used for...
Gentian	15	Jaundice, hepatitis, STDs; strengthens and warms the body; promotes bile production; increases appetite; tonic; physical exhaustion (improves)
Ginger	17, 18	Nausea, car sickness, motion sickness, morning sickness, menstrual cramps, colds, flu, blood pressure, gas, stomach cramps; aids digestion
Ginkgo biloba	4, 5	Alzheimer's disease, vertigo, memory, tinnitus, atherosclerosis, headaches, depression, blood clots; improves memory; aids brain function; improves concentration
Ginseng	14	Infertility, depression, fatigue; boosts immune system and vitality; helps body adapt to stress; increases mental and physical efficiency
Golden seal	9	Diabetes, sinus congestion, infections, gum problems, mouth sores, allergies, liver problems, ulcers; works as an antibiotic
Gotu kola	21	Tinnitus, depression, fatigue, high blood pressure, memory loss, mental fatigue, physical fatigue, senility; increases circulation; promotes longevity; increases vitality
Guggal lipid	8	High cholesterol; strengthens the heart; supports lymph system and builds the immune system; stimulates gradual weight loss
Hawthorn	7	High blood pressure, angina, heart palpitations, inflammation of the heart, kidney problems; nourishes the heart and nerves
Hops	6	Anxiety, headaches, hyperactivity, pain, insomnia, nervousness; works as a diuretic; stimulates appetite
Horseradish	19	Pneumonia, asthma, bronchitis, catarrh, coughs, flu, hay fever, worms, sinus congestion, lymph congestion, colds
Horsetail	18	Nail biting, brittle hair, structural system weakness, bladder and kidney problems, joint pain, ulcers, immune and nervous system problems; improves condition of nails

continues

continued

Herb	Chapter	Ailments Historically Used for...
Hydrangea	15	Kidney problems, kidney stones, bladder stones, arthritis, gallstones, gout
Irish moss	22	Ulcers, thyroid problems, dry skin, itchy skin
Jojoba	9	Dandruff, flaky skin; softens skin
Juniper berries	23	Edema, bladder infections, cystitis, indigestion, menstrual irregularities, high blood pressure, PMS, dropsy, pancreas problems, water retention; works as an antiseptic
Kava kava	13	Hyperactivity, insomnia, tension, anxiety, stress
Kelp	7, 21	Thyroid problems, low blood pressure, goiters, radiation exposure, heavy metal poisoning or exposure, metabolism (helps body to regulate)
Lemongrass	21	Tendonitis, immune system problems, backaches, sprains
Licorice root	13	Hypoglycemia, coughs, Addison's disease, stomach ulcers, arthritis, congestion, female complaints, sore throat; nourishes adrenal glands; boosts energy and endurance
Lobelia	6, 11, 20	Food poisoning, coughs, pneumonia, fungus infections; helps in quitting smoking; relaxes nerves; clears lungs and mucus
Marshmallow	21, 22	Ulcers, tonsillitis, being underweight, sore throat, coughs, colds, sinus congestion, allergies, peptic ulcers, gastritis, colitis, bladder infections, kidney problems; soothes membranes, absorbs and draws out impurities from body
Milk thistle	5	Environmental allergies, jaundice, hepatitis, gallbladder, psoriasis; rebuilds liver; protects from alcohol damage
Motherwort	22	Uterine trouble, menstrual cramps, late periods, high blood pressure, epilepsy
Mullein	17	Mumps, hemorrhoids, all respiratory ailments, allergies, sinusitis, stomach cramps and diarrhea, whooping cough

Herb	Chapter	Ailments Historically Used for...
Myrrh	12	Gingivitis, sinusitis, asthma, coughs, colds, congestion; used as a mouthwash or gargle for gum problems, tooth pain, throat infection, and mouth ulcers
Nettle	19	Osteoporosis, hypoglycemia, rheumatism, rickets, TB, gout, infertility, urinary tract problems, food allergies, kidney inflammation, jaundice, hemorrhage, PMS, palsy, enriches breast milk
Olive Leaf	13	Anti-viral, antibacterial, AIDS, cancer, Epstein-Barr, candida, yeast infections, chronic fatigue syndrome, parasites, arthritis, colds, diabetes, fungal infections (including toe fungus), hepatitis, high blood pressure, infections, shingles, herpes (both types), and worms
Oregon grape	10	Eczema, acne, liver problems, psoriasis, skin diseases, chicken pox; cleanses blood
Papaya	5	Allergies, colon problems, gas trouble; supports digestion; supplies enzymes; juice lightens freckles
Parsley	15	Kidney problems, kidney infections, indigestion, PMS, bladder infections, dropsy, water retention; works as a diuretic
Pau d'arco	8, 10	Cysts, endometriosis, bacteria, fungus, parasite infection, viruses, worms, cancer preventative; combats infections; used in Parkinson's disease, psoriasis, spleen infections, eczema, diabetes, gastritis, leukemia, polyps, rheumatism, Epstein-Barr
Peach bark	15	Kidney problems, bladder problems, congestion, nausea, stomach problems, water retention, uterus prolapsus
Pennyroyal	17	Promotes menstruation; works as an insect repellent; works as a diuretic; breaks fevers, promotes abortion, use with caution
Peppermint	7, 26	Indigestion, stomach aches, gas problems, nausea, migraines, morning sickness, colds, flu; works as a mental stimulant
Plantain	15	Weak knees, water retention, eczema, burns, ulcers, skin ailments

continues

continued

Herb	Chapter	Ailments Historically Used for...
Psyllium	4, 8, 24	Constipation, hemorrhoids, cholesterol, diverticulitis; provides fiber; exercises and strengthens bowel for better overall function
Red clover	8	Cancer, bronchitis, whooping cough, pimples, acne, boils, cysts, skin diseases, psoriasis, immune system problems; cleanses the blood
Red raspberry	17	Morning sickness, mouth ulcers, bleeding gums; prevents miscarriage; tones uterus; stops diarrhea in children
Reishi mushroom	23	Warts, immune system (strengthens), cancer, bacterial infection, high cholesterol, ulcers, longevity
Rosemary	9	Dandruff, indigestion, tension, muscle pain; works as a decongestant
Safflower	12	Gout, arthritis, rheumatism, indigestion; works as a diuretic; eliminates excess uric acid from the system
Sage	16	Laryngitis, indigestion, mucus (breaks up), colds, coughs, sore throats; stops lactation
Sarsaparilla	4, 14	Hormone balancer, menopause, impotence; purifies blood; supports circulation; fights venereal diseases; stimulates immune system, rich in iron; used for joint aches, gas, rheumatism
Saw palmetto	19	Prostate trouble, nasal congestion, bronchitis, sore throats, reproductive organ trouble; works as a sexual stimulant; helps the underweight gain weight
Scullcap	14	Insomnia, tension, irritability, headaches, epileptic seizures, muscle aches, PMS
Slippery elm	2, 8, 14	Irritable bowel syndrome, colitis, coughs, sore throats, indigestion, ulcers; soothes irritated tissues; diarrhea, digestion, bronchitis, appendicitis, burns, lung problems
Spearmint	23	Vomiting, nausea, indigestion, upset stomach, flatulence, heartburn, morning sickness, colds, headaches

Herb	Chapter	Ailments Historically Used for...
Spirulina	4, 22	Underweight problems, toxic metal poisoning, diabetes; feeds the thyroid; promotes feeling of well-being; balances the body; provides nourishment; rich in protein; increases stamina
Squawvine	22	Supports the uterus during childbirth
St. John's wort	9	Depression, scar tissue; heals wounds
Suma	16	Lyme disease, immune system problems; tonifies glands; helps the body adapt to stress
Tea tree	5, 21, 26	Tonsillitis, fungal infections, cuts, insect bites, acne, skin ailments; used as a vaginal douche for candida or other yeast or bacterial infections, gargle for throat or mouth infections
Thyme	20, 25	Sinusitis, colds, chest congestion, nerve pain, hysteria, colic, fever; feeds the thymus to boost the immune system
Uña de gato (cat's claw)	11	Fibromyalgia, inflammations, joint pain, muscle pain; boosts the immune system, supports digestion
Uva ursi	22	Urinary trouble, kidney or bladder infections, menstrual bloating, bed-wetting; works as a diuretic; tones the uterus
Valerian	6	Anxiety, insomnia, nervousness, headaches, menstrual cramps, convulsions, hysteria, shock, spasms, tension
White oak bark	8, 12	Swollen glands, hemorrhoids, cold sores, inflamed tissues, varicose veins, gingivitis
White willow bark	13, 26	Headaches, pain, gout, muscle strain, menstrual cramps, fever, inflammations
Wild lettuce	6	Anxiety, trauma, stress, nervous disorders
Wild yam	19	PMS, menstrual cramps, nausea, menopause, infertility, ovary pain, painful periods, lungs, urinary tract problems, rheumatism, muscle relaxer
Witch hazel	23	Varicose veins, hemorrhoids, wrinkles, inflammations, bruises, bumps, insect bites
Wood betony	23	Vertigo, spleen problems, immune system trouble, hysteria, nervousness, migraines; works as a mild sedative to the central nervous system

continues

continued

Herb	Chapter	Ailments Historically Used for...
Wormwood	19	Parasites, scabies, gallstones, bloating, arthritis, lead poisoning, fever, gas; works as an insect repellent
Yarrow	11	Fevers (promotes sweating to break), digestive disorders, menstrual cramps, anxiety, insomnia
Yohimbe	14	Impotence, frigidity; works as a sexual stimulant

Index

Symbols

5-hydroxy-tryptophan, 291

A

acetylsalicylic acid, *see* aspirin
Achillea millefolium, L., see yarrow
acid-forming foods, 202
acidity, pain, 200
acidophilus, 114, 129
acne, 63-65
  adolescent, 64
    burdock root, 64-65
    junk food, 65-66
    tea tree oil, 65
  adult, 65-67
    burdock root, 66
    red clover, 66
actions of herbs, 25
activating herbs, 34
  capsicum, 34
  horseradish, 34
  peppermint, 34
acupressure points, headaches, 170
adaptogenic herb, 216
ADHD (Attention Deficit Hyperactive Disorder), *see* hyperactivity
adolescent acne, 64
  burdock root, 64-65
  junk food, 65-66
  tea tree oil, 65
adrenal glandular body type, 313
adult acne, 65-67
  burdock root, 66
  red clover, 66
aggravations
  joint injuries, 199-202
  ulcers, 289
AHG (American Herbalist Guild), 323
alfalfa, 34, 47-49, 86-87
  pets, gas, 56
algin, radiation poisoning, 264-265
Alium sativum, see garlic
alkaline-forming foods, 202
alkaloid yohimbine (yohimbe), 184

allergies, 67-70
  bee pollen, 68-69
  eliminating airborne allergens, 70-71
  environmental, 74-76
    milk thistle, 74
    supplements, 74-77
    ephedra, 345
  food, 71-73
    digestion, 72-74
  horseradish, 69-72
  pantothenic acid (B vitamin), 70
  symptoms, 67
  vitamin C, 70
aloe vera, 40, 58
  burns, 101
  laxative agent for hemorrhoids, 176-177
  plant, 336
Alzheimer's disease, 76-77
  causes, 76-77
  gingko biloba, 77
  gotu kola, 77-80
amenorrhea (lack of menstruation), 222
American Botanical Council, 323
American Herbalist Guild, *see* AHG
Anas barbariae, see oscillococcinum
ancient Egyptians, history of herbs, 22
anemia, 46
Angelica sinensis, see dong quai
anise, 334
annuals, 334-335
anthelmintics (parasite expellers), 255
anticoagulant drugs, 29
antihistamines, 31
antioxidants, 57, 110
  radiation poisoning, 265-266
anxiety, 81-89
  hops, 83
  lettuce, 83-84
  symptoms, 82
  valerian root, 82-84
apple pectin, 112
applications of herbs, 5-8
  capsule/tablet herbs, 7-8
  chewable, 8
  compressed and fomented, 7

  decoctions, 6
  infusions, 6
  internal versus external, 5-8
  liquid/tinctures, 8
  poultices, 7
Arctium lappa, see burdock root
Arctostaphylos uva-ursi, see uva ursi
arnica, 343-344
Artemisia absinthium, see wormwood
Artemisia frigida, see wormwood
Artemisia tilesii, see wormwood
Artemisia tridentata, see sagebrush
Artemisia vulgaris, see mugwort
arthritis, 86-89
  alfalfa, 86-87
  herbal combinations, 87-89
aspartame, 230
aspirin, 22
asthma, 84-86
  ephedra, 84-85
  herbal combinations, 85-86
  lobelia, 85
  preventing/stopping attacks with ephedra, 345
astragalus, 53
athlete's foot, 152
attention deficit hyperactive disorder (ADHD), *see* hyperactivity
autoimmune diseases, lupus, 213
avoiding junk food, adolescent acne, 65-66

B

bachelor buttons, superstitions, 337
bacteria, killing with clove oil, 343
bad breath, *see* halitosis
blackberry tea, 342
Barosma betulina, see buchu root
basil, 334
  superstitions, 337
baths, fever, 145-146
bayberry, diarrhea, 128-129
bearberry, *see* uva ursi
bee pollen, 326
  allergies, 68-69

373

temperature descriptions (herbs), 39-40
tendonitis, 277-279
    lemongrass, 278-279
    reducing inflammation, 279-280
tepid sponge baths, 145
thermogenesis, 50
Thomson, Samuel (father of herbology), 23
throat spray recipe, tea tree oil, 283
thyme, 53, 335
    sinusitis, 267-268
    superstitions, 337
thymus gland, 110
thymus glandular body type, 313
Thymus vulgaris, see thyme
thyroid glandular body type, 313
thyroid problems, 281-282
    kelp, 281-282
    prevention, 282
tinctured herbs, 8
tinnitus, 279-281
    causes, 279-280
    gotu kola, 280-281
    herbal combinations, 281
tipped uterus, 295
Tissue Cleansing Through Bowel Management, 76
tonsillitis, 282-285
    symptoms, 283-284
    tea tree oil, 283-284
toxins, 35
transfer methods of parasites, 253
traumatic shock, *see* shock
traveling, herbal first aid kits
    arnica, 343-344
    capsicum, 339-342
    charcoal, 342
    clove oil, 342-343
    ephedra, 345
    peppermint, 345-348
Trifolium pratense, see red clover
Trigonella foenum-graecum, see fenugreek
Turnera aphrodisiaca, see damiana
twitching (muscle), *see* leg cramps
Type I diabetes, 125
Type II diabetes, 126

U

ulcers, 287-290
    aggravations, 289
    golden seal, 288

herbal combinations, 288-291
Irish moss, 288
Ulmus fulva, see slippery elm
uña de gato, fibromyalgia, 148
under-eating, 15-16
underweight, 290-293
    recipe for weight gain, 292-293
    spirulina, 291-292
    what herbs can and cannot do, 290
uric acid, 163
urinary problems, 293-294
    herbal combinations, 294
    uva ursi, 293-294
Urtica dioica, see nettle
uterine problems, 295-298
    motherwort, 295-298
    squawvine, 296-298
uva ursi, urinary problems, 293-294

V

vaccination, measles, 220
Vaccinium myrtillus, see bilberry fruit
valerian, 335
valerian root, anxiety, 82-84
Valeriana officinalis, see valerian root
varicose veins, 299-302
    herbal combinations, 301-302
    witch hazel, 300-301
Verbascum thapsus, see mullein
verimfuges (parasite killers), 255
vertigo, 302-303
    causes, 302
    wood betony, 302-303
vitamins, 14
    A, 101
    C, 101
        allergies, 70
    E, 101
voice box, 209
vomiting, 304-305
    herbal combinations, 305
    as herbal side effect, 30
    spearmint, 304-305

W

warts, 305
    folk remedies, 306-308
    Reishi mushroom, 306-307
water, 16-17

formula for body's need, 16
    retention, 293, 307-310
        causes, 307-308
        juniper, 308-310
weeds, considered herbs, 4
weight loss, *see* weight management
weight management, 290-293, 310-315
    chickweed, 312
    Garcinia cambogia, 312-313
    glandular body types, 313-315
    l-carnitine, 312-313
    pineapple, 312-313
    reasons for excess weight, 311-313
    recipe for weight gain, 292-293
    spirulina, 291-292
    what herbs can and cannot do, 290
"wet" herbs, 39
Western herbalists, history of herbs, 23-24
wheat grass juice, 46
white oak bark, 39, 114
    gingivitis, 161-162
    swollen glands, 162
white willow bark, 32, 50, 53
    headaches, 171-174
    shingles, 266-267
Wild American Panax quinquefolium, see ginseng
wild bergamot (*Monarda fistulosa*), 277
wild yam, PMS, 258-259
witch hazel, varicose veins, 300-301
wives' tales, *see* superstitions
wood betony, vertigo, 302-303
wormwood, parasites, 254-256
wounds, healing with arnica, 344
wreaths, creating with herbs, 330-331

Y–Z

yarrow, 31
    fever, 144
yeast infections, 152
yellow dock, 46
yohimbe, impotence, 184-185

zinc, 101
Zingiber officinale, see ginger root